NUCLEAR MEDICINE
A Clinical Introduction

NUCLEAR MEDICINE
A Clinical Introduction

Michael Maisey
B.SC, MD, FRCP

Consultant Physician and Director
of the Department of Nuclear Medicine,
Guy's Hospital, London

1980
UPDATE BOOKS
LONDON • DORDRECHT • BOSTON

Available in the United Kingdom and Eire from

Update Books Ltd
33/34 Alfred Place
London WC1E 7DP
England

Available in the USA and Canada from

Kluwer Boston Inc.
Lincoln Building
160 Old Derby Street
Hingham, Mass. 02043,
USA

Available in the rest of the world from

Kluwer Academic Publishers Group Distribution Centre
PO Box 322
3300 AH Dordrecht,
The Netherlands

First Published 1980

© Update Books Ltd, 1980

Softcover reprint of the hardcover 1st edition 1980

British Library Cataloguing in Publication Data
Maisey, Michael Nuclear medicine. 1. Nuclear medicine I. Title 616.07′575   R895

ISBN-13:978-94-011-6394-1   e-ISBN-13:978-94-011-6392-7
DOI: 10.1007/978-94-011-6392-7

Contents

Preface

The emphasis throughout this book is on solving clinical problems, for nuclear medicine is a clinical discipline and in order to gain maximum benefit from the investigations described it is essential that the staff performing them and reporting the results should understand completely the question that is being asked. In turn, the right question can only be asked when the clinician caring for the patient understands the basis and limitation of any individual technique. Both individuals must in addition be familiar with alternative modalities of diagnosis so that problems can be solved in the most economical way, both from the point of view of the patient and the system, by intelligent 'channelling' of the problem through the various possible diagnostic routes.

The book also shows that nuclear medicine is mainly, and increasingly, about function—that is to say about how things work rather than how they look. It is important to note that the development of new radiological tools, e.g. computer tomography and ultrasound, which display anatomical features with such dramatic spatial resolution, has enabled us to stop performing those investigations to which nuclear medicine was inherently ill-suited and which depended upon demonstration of anatomical abnormalities via changes in function. The best examples include investigations on space-occupying cerebral lesions, renal tumours and cysts, and pancreatic lesions, which were previously visualized by nuclear medicine techniques because no better non-invasive modality was available and these are therefore not covered in this text.

The future for nuclear medicine is exciting and, later in the book, the way is pointed towards future developments. These will undoubtedly be in the direction of increasingly specific functional investigations to demonstrate abnormalities of pathophysiology, together with increasingly specific labelled tracers to localize sites of disease with a high degree of accuracy.

Nuclear Medicine—A Clinical Introduction started off as a series of articles published by Update. The articles attracted so much interest that it was decided to use them as the basis for a book. Whilst new chapters have been added and existing articles revised, the book does not set out to be an exhaustive treatise on nuclear medicine. Rather it will provide, for any clinician without previous experience of nuclear medicine procedures, a practical guide to their place in solving clinical problems. For those to whom these procedures are not yet available, and for those who are still being trained to use them, it will enable an essential grasp of fundamentals to be made, for it is anticipated that the majority should not in the future have to practise modern medicine without the advantages of non-invasive investigative techniques.

Michael Maisey
Guy's Hospital, London
January 1980

Preface

Foreword

It has been said that perhaps the greatest contribution of the space age is the picture of the earth obtained from the surface of the moon, a picture that reveals the beauty but also the fragility of spaceship earth. A picture of comparable significance, it seems to me, is the picture of the brain obtained by new techniques of nuclear medicine—a picture that shows the increased metabolic activity in the region of the brain concerned with hearing, evoked by the subject's listening to the story of Davy Crockett. For the first time, we can examine the chemical events associated with thoughts in the living human being. It is easy to imagine the potential extensions of analogous studies of regional brain chemistry in patients with neurological and psychiatric disorders, such as Parkinson's disease, Huntington's disease, schizophrenia, chronic pain states and other conditions.

More and more we are learning what nuclear medicine is really about, that it is concerned with the study of the motion and change of body structures and functions, with regional biochemistry and physiology.

Advances over the past two decades have presented practising physicians with the problem of keeping up to date. More than ever before the clinician must struggle to become acquainted with advances in all fields of medicine if he is to care properly for his patients. The specialist has similar difficulty in maintaining adequate familiarity with other areas of medicine. The major role of the clinician, then, is to provide a holistic approach to the patient and his problems. This book will help.

Dr Maisey explains what nuclear medicine can do for patients, how the procedures are performed, and how they are interpreted. Physicians, radiologists, nurses, technologists and other persons can use this book to keep up with the enormous advances that continue to be made. It is a useful and important contribution to modern medical practice.

Henry Wagner
Professor of Medicine and Radiology
and Director of the Division of
Nuclear Medicine
Johns Hopkins University
Baltimore, Maryland, USA
January 1980

Acknowledgements

The production of a book is as multidisciplinary as Nuclear Medicine itself and it is impossible to acknowledge the contributions from everyone who made this book possible. I would, however, like particularly to acknowledge the contributions made by my coauthors in the original articles upon which the book is based: R. J. Wainwright (Nuclear Cardiology), S. Ng Tang Fui (Thyroid Disease), T. Higgenbottam (Lung Scanning), A. J. W. Hilson (Renal Scanning) and J. G. Ayres (Scanning Techniques). I would like to thank Helen Upperton for patiently typing all the manuscripts, the Medical Photography Department at Guy's Hospital for taking such care over reproducing the original material, and the staff of the Nuclear Medicine Department without whose consistent high standard of work none of this would have been possible; finally the publishers with whom it has always been a great pleasure to work.

1. Introduction

Nuclear medicine has been defined as the 'application of radioactive materials to the diagnosis and treatment of patients and the study of human disease' (Wagner 1968). The purpose of this new account of nuclear medicine is to outline the present 'state of the art', paying particular attention to the routine clinical application of the techniques described, with emphasis on two major aspects:

1. The clinical aspects of investigations which are well established and have well proven clinical values. These are facilities which should be available to any doctor practising where more than rudimentary diagnostic facilities are available.

2. Sufficient practical detail of these investigations to enable the clinician to make the best use of facilities available to him.

Some of the more exciting developments of the future, such as radionuclide emission CT scanning (ECT), in which fundamental physiological functions incorporating radionuclides of carbon, nitrogen and oxygen are being used to produce functional images of biochemical processes, will be mentioned to put the present investigations into perspective. No attempt will be made to cover the field completely; only the investigations which are currently the most important and most widely used will be covered in detail.

Nuclear medicine is probably the best clinical example of the integration of medical and scientific disciplines (Physics, Chemistry, Radiopharmacy, Computer Science) used routinely on a daily basis for the care of individual patients and for progress of the discipline. Clinical nuclear medicine, like radiology and ultrasound, should be problem orientated and problem solving, and is most effective when there is an understanding of the clinical problem in addition to the appreciation of the most effective pathways of diagnosis using alternative methodology. All techniques are relatively ineffective, expensive and unrewarding when organized to provide a purely technical service.

The strength of nuclear medicine lies in the use of radioactive tracers to study function rather than structure, and is well encapsulated by three often quoted aphorisms:

a. 'Nuclear Medicine is to Radiology what Physiology is to Anatomy'.

b. 'Biochemical and functional changes occur in disease before structural changes can be identified'.

c. 'How things function is more important to the patient than how they look'.

The important features of radionuclide studies are as follows:

1. The radioactive tracers are handled physiologically and biochemically in the same way as the stable element.

2. Radioactive tracers are given in such small quantities that they do not alter the physiological process and consequently allow observation of the function under investigation without alteration of that function.

3. They are non-invasive, requiring in most instances no more than an intravenous injection.

4. There is a negligible morbidity and virtually non-existent mortality.

5. The radiation dose is similar to that given in an equivalent radiological investigation and often far less, in spite of the general misconception that if radioisotopes are introduced into the body compartments they must result in increased radiation doses as compared to the radiation when it is transmitted through the body. A big advantage, however, is that when the radionuclide has been administered the radiation dose (rads received by the patient) remains constant irrespective of the number of images or observations which are made. This is in contrast to radiographic techniques where the radiation dose to the patient is directly related to the number of observations or images that are made.

Cost Effectiveness

The cost effectiveness of all investigations must be considered in terms of improvement of the diagnostic probability, and nuclear medicine is no exception. In every clinical situation it is necessary to weigh the advantages of increasing the diagnostic probability in solving the patient's problem in terms of the improvement of management against the cost. Cost can be considered both in economic terms and in cost to the patient, as all studies, although they are relatively noninvasive, do require an intravenous injection and a small but measurable radiation dose. The economic cost effectiveness of most of the investigations is high, in

Table 1.1 Major uses of radionuclides in medicine.

	Diagnostic
'In vitro'	— Radioimmunoassay and other techniques
'In vivo'	— Non-imaging. e.g. thyroid uptakes, blood volume, glomerular filtration rate, etc.
	— Imaging, e.g. liver scanning, renal scanning, etc.
	Therapeutic
Sealed sources	— Internal, e.g. yttrium-90 for acromegaly
	— External, e.g. cobalt-90 source in radiotherapy
Unsealed sources	— Systemic, e.g. phosphorus-32 for polycythaemia rubra vera, iodine-131 for thyrotoxicosis and thyroid cancer
	— Localized, e.g. yttrium-90 in rheumatoid arthritis

that they are relatively cheap and can usually be performed on an out-patient basis, thus frequently reducing the high cost of in-patient investigation and management.

Radioisotopes are very widely used in medicine and their major applications are summarized in Table 1.1. The areas that come most clearly within the scope of nuclear medicine are those in which radioisotopes are administered to patients for diagnostic purposes, both the imaging and non-imaging procedures. The in vitro use of radioisotopes may or may not occur solely in a nuclear medicine department and this will depend on the main interest and the development of, for example, radioimmunoassays in the biochemistry department. However, it is convenient for in vitro investigation of thyroid function to be situated within a nuclear medicine department, in view of the extensive investigation of thyroid disease and the frequent involvement of radioiodine in the management and treatment of this disease.

Whether or not the therapeutic use of radioiodine is undertaken in nuclear medicine departments will depend on the interests of the nuclear medicine physician and the facilities which are available for radioiodine therapy within the endocrine unit and radiotherapy unit. As a general rule, radioiodine administration for thyrotoxicosis is usually performed now in a nuclear medicine department, whereas treatment for thyroid cancer may or may not be.

Radionuclides and Instrumentation

Some practical aspects of both the choice of radiopharmaceutical and the fundamentals of the instrumentation will be discussed, so that it is possible to

appreciate the scope, and also the limitations, of any of the individual investigations which will be considered in later chapters. Rather than cataloguing the radioisotopes and instruments which are used, the steps from the preparation of the radiopharmaceutical to the analysis of the final study for a typical investigation will be outlined.

The single most important radionuclide at the present is technetium-99m ($^{99}Tc^m$). (In less well developed countries where access to radioisotopes is more difficult, indium-113m is more likely to be the basis of most investigations.) It was the discovery and exploitation of technetium-99m which led to the rapid expansion of nuclear medicine imaging techniques during the last 10 years. The advantages of $^{99}Tc^m$ are:

1. It decays with a short half-life (approximately six hours).

2. During this decay it emits only gamma photons and not beta particles (which are responsible for the larger radiation dose incurred by other radionuclides such as I-131).

3. The gamma photons have an energy of 140 KeV which is particularly well suited to the characteristics of the main imaging instrument—the gamma camera.

4. The relative ease with which it can be attached to many and varied chemical compounds, although the chemistry of technetium is extremely complex and poorly understood.

Other commonly used radionuclides in nuclear medicine are shown in Table 1.2, with their principal physical characteristics and most common uses.

The Generator System

Technetium-99m would not be nearly so useful (in view of its short half-life, and therefore delivery) were it not for the generator system. This is a system whereby longer-lived 'parent' radionuclides (in this case molybdenum-99) decay to the shorter-lived 'daughter' radionuclide (in this case $^{99}Tc^m$). The generator or 'cow', which is an alumina column with molybdenum-99 absorbed on to it, is kept in the laboratory with the parent continually decaying to $^{99}Tc^m$. Thus, $^{99}Tc^m$ is available whenever required by eluting the column with a saline solution which does not wash out the parent, but washes out the daughter radionuclide in high concentration in the eluate. These generator systems are delivered weekly or twice weekly depending on the workload of the department. A typical generator system is shown in Figure 1.1. The eluate containing $^{99}Tc^m$ must be checked for:

1. An excess of the long-lived parent.

2. Aluminium from the column.

Table 1.2 Other commonly used radionuclides in medicine.

Radionuclide	Principal energy	Half-life	Common uses
[1]Iodine-131	364 KeV	8 days	Thyroid function and treatment of thyrotoxicosis and thyroid cancer
Gallium-67	91 KeV 185 KeV 300 KeV	78.1 hours	Localization of infection and tumours
Thallium-201	81 KeV	3.1 days	Myocardial visualization
Chromium-51	320 KeV	27.7 days	Labelled red cell studies, gastrointestinal blood and protein loss, glomerular filtration rate
Cobalt-57	122 KeV	270 days	Schilling tests
Iodine-125	35.5 KeV 27.0 KeV	60 days	Radioimmunoassay
[1]Tritium-3	5.7 KeV	12.3 years	Total body water
[1]Carbon-14	49.3 KeV	5,730 years	Gastrointestinal uptake, CO_2 breath tests
Xenon-133	80.9 KeV	5.3 days	Lung ventilation
Krypton-81m	191 KeV	13 secs	

[1] β emitters. (All the radionuclides are gamma emitters.)

3. Sterility.

4. Pyrogens.

The $^{99}Tc^m$, which is in the oxidized pertechnetate form, can then be used directly, for example in brain scanning or thyroid scanning, or attached to an appropriate chemical or biological material to be used to study a particular functional process or organ imaging for which it is required.

The labelling is usually a rapid and simple process due to the development of the 'kit concept' whereby all the reagents necessary for the labelling process have been pre-prepared, pre-sterilized and checked for pyrogens, thus saving valuable time and increasing simplicity,

reliability and quality of the preparation. It is performed under sterile conditions using a 'no-touch' technique, preferably in a laminar flow cabinet (as shown in Figure 1.2). Because of this batch kit method, quality control of each preparation is not necessary prior to the use in patients. However, the first of each batch should be checked for:

1. Labelling efficiency, i.e. whether all the technetium is attached to the chemical or biological material.

2. Sterility.

3. Pyrogenicity.

The preparation and quality control of radiopharmaceuticals is best organized by a radiopharmacist, with

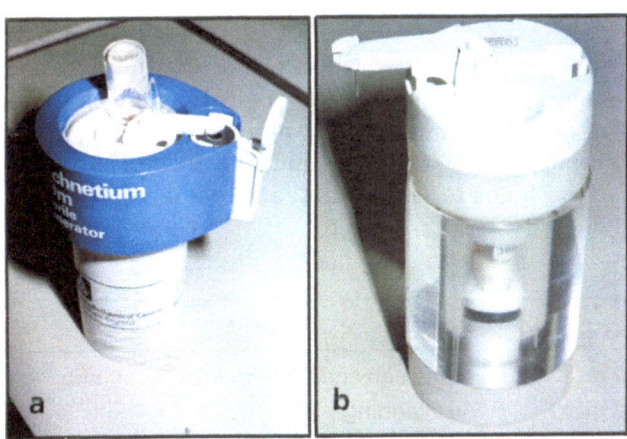

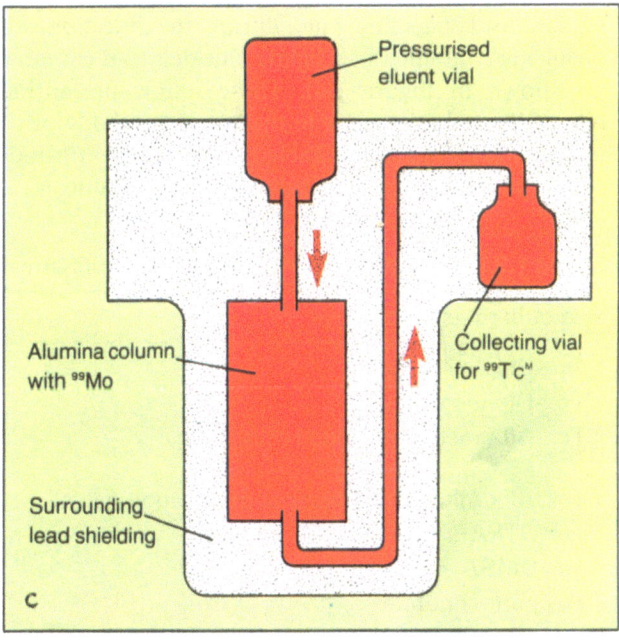

Figure 1.1 (a) *A typical molybdenum-99/technetium-99 generator system in routine use, together with* **(b)** *a plastic see-through model and* **(c)** *a schematic cutaway section showing how the introduction of saline into the top of the column washes out the daughter product* ($^{99}Tc^m$) *in the eluate.*

appropriate training, working in the nuclear medicine department.

After preparation, the individual doses for the patients are drawn up from the multi-dose vial in the same way as any other drug but, unlike any other drug,

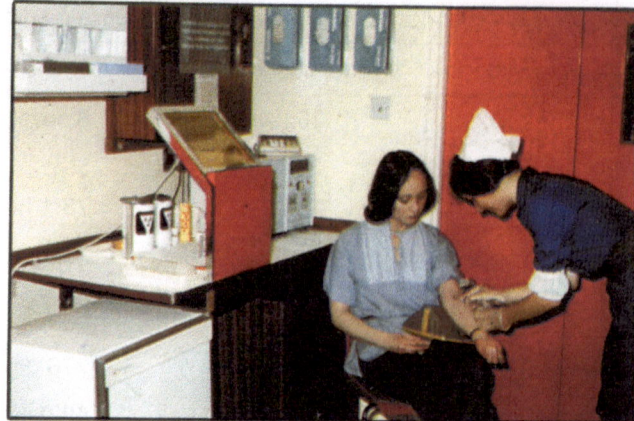

Figure 1.3 *A typical set for injection, including the radiopharmaceuticals, with a protective lead shield and the dose calibrator for measuring the amount of radioactivity to be injected.*

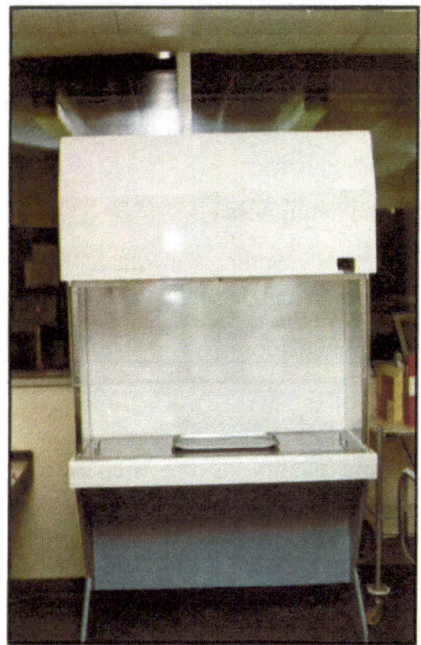

Figure 1.2 *A laminar flow cabinet for the sterile preparation of radiopharmaceuticals.*

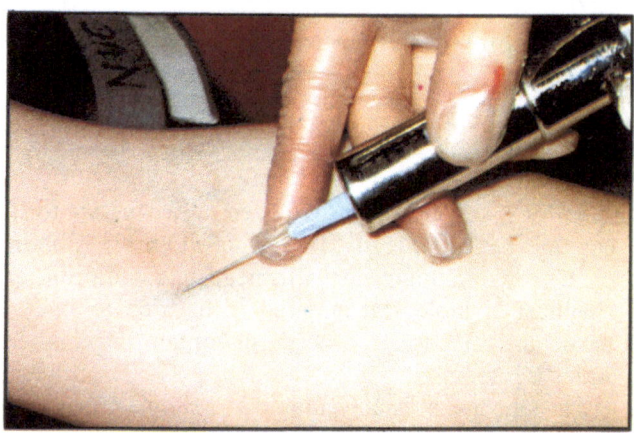

Figure 1.4 *The syringe should be surrounded by a special lead shield during i.v. injection to protect the operator from unnecessary radiation.*

reliance is not placed on the stated concentration: each dose for each patient is measured using a radiation dose calibrator (Figure 1.3). This is best performed by a nurse who has been trained in the safe administration of drugs—the only additional training necessary is that of basic radiation safety. The preparations are stored behind lead shielding and, during the injection, the syringe is contained in a lightly shielded lead container (as shown in Figure 1.4). These simple precautions reduce the radiation dose to the hands and body of the operator to trivial levels. Table 1.3 summarizes the most commonly used $^{99}Tc^m$ labelled radiopharmaceuticals.

Equipment

Following injection the investigation may be performed immediately, e.g. a lung scan, or after a variable period of time to allow for the appropriate uptake, or incorporation, by the organ under investigation, e.g. one to two hours for brain scans, and four or five hours for

Table 1.3 Commonly used $^{99}Tc^m$ labelled radiopharmaceuticals.

Radiopharmaceutical	Dose	Uses
$^{99}Tc^m$-Sulphur colloid	2-10 mCi	Liver, spleen and bone marrow scanning
$^{99}Tc^m$-Diphosphonate	10-20 mCi	Bone scanning
$^{99}Tc^m$-Albumen or red blood cells	10-20 mCi	Dynamic vascular imaging, cardiac ventricular function
$^{99}Tc^m$-Albumin microspheres or macroaggregates	2-4 mCi	Perfusion lung scanning
$^{99}Tc^m$ DTPA	10-20 mCi	Dynamic renal imaging
$^{99}Tc^m$ DMSA	2-5 mCi	Static renal imaging
$^{99}Tc^m$ pertechnetate	2-15 mCi	Thyroid and brain imaging

a bone scan. The instrument which is most commonly used now is the gamma camera (Figure 1.5c). The principle of this instrument lies in the ability of a large

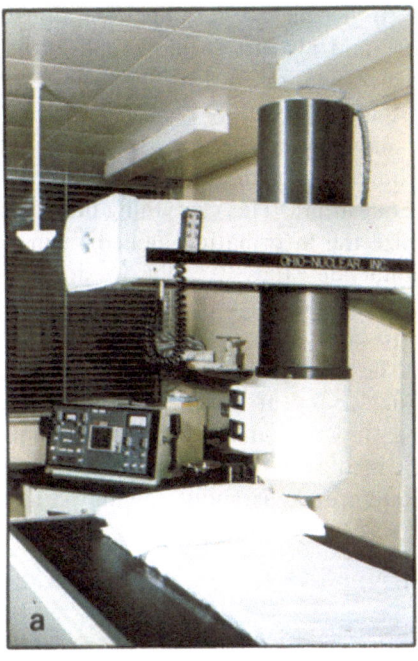

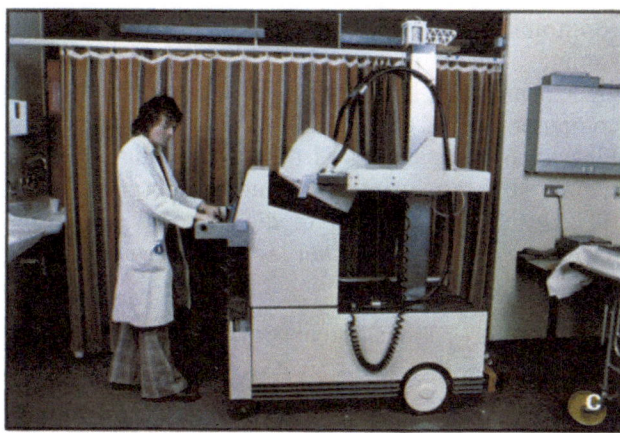

Figure 1.5 (a) *A typical rectilinear scanner (top left) consisting of a moveable detector head over the patient, and a console for operation and recording the image on to film. The schematic diagram* **(b)** *shows the principle of detection and spatial localization by the gamma camera detector (bottom left).* **(c)** *A mobile gamma camera (above) can be used at the bedside or in the intensive care unit.*

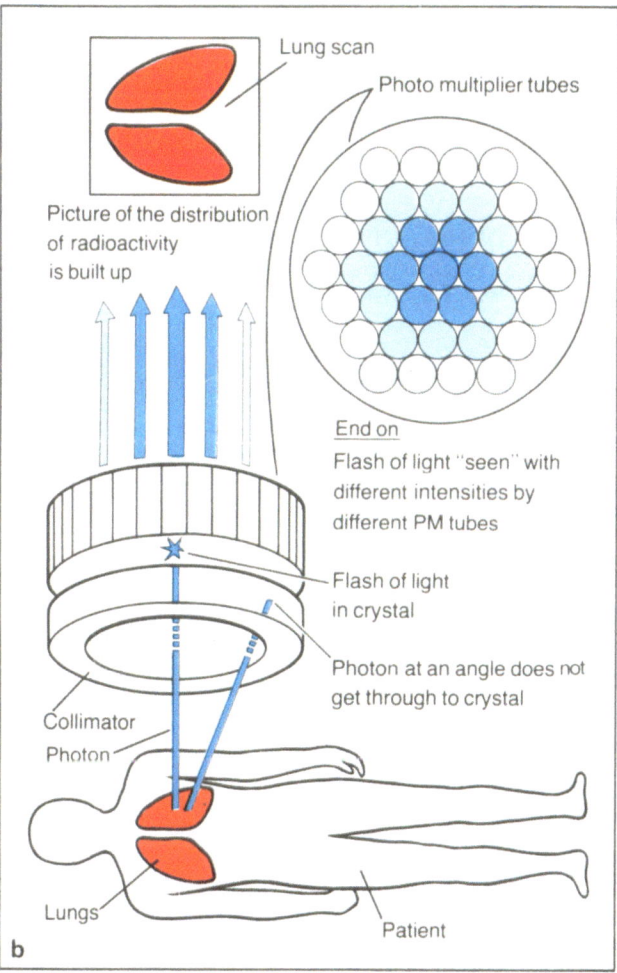

sodium iodide crystal (approximately 12 inches x 0.5 inch), contained within the detector head, to respond to gamma rays emitted from the radioisotope by the emission of tiny scintillations of light. These scintillations are magnified and altered electronically into electrical signals. From the positions of the scintillations which occur within the crystal, the picture of the isotope distribution in the organ is built up. A diagram to illustrate this is shown in Figure 1.5b.

The other instrument which is used is the rectilinear scanner, which usually has two sodium crystals, one above the patient and one below, and the whole head moves backwards and forwards in a rectilinear fashion, recording the radioactivity and building up an image of the distribution of radioactivity within the organ. This is illustrated in Figure 1.5a. Most of the routine investigations can be performed with either instrument equally well, although the advantages of the gamma camera are:

1. The ease with which it can be interfaced with the computer, making comparable measurement possible.

2. The speed with which investigations can be performed.

3. The ability to do dynamic studies when rapid time sequence images are required.

4. The relative ease of positioning the patient.

It is possible to use both the rectilinear scanner and the gamma camera for investigations such as bone scans, gallium scans and iodine scans for metastases from thyroid cancers, as they are both capable of recording total body scans. Some form of data processing, either as a small dedicated programmable computer[1] (see footnote) or a hard wired system integral with the gamma camera, is becoming a routine part of most nuclear medicine investigations. An example of a mini computer interfaced to a gamma camera is shown in Figure 1.6. Data are recorded by the gamma camera as signals of a certain intensity, and certain positions on the crystal, and changed to digital form and stored within the computer's memory for subsequent analysis.

The Clinical Problem

In discussing the sequence of events during a routine investigation, one must not lose sight of the patient and the clinical problem. For the most effective use of nuclear medicine, as well as any other diagnostic techniques, the clinical problem to be solved must be clearly understood by the nuclear medicine physician and an adequate history and clinical examination should be performed.

It is essential for a clinician experienced in nuclear medicine to decide on the justification for the investigation, and also to decide which is the most appropriate investigation to solve the problem. He should also monitor the procedure as it is being done so as to alter it or add to it at the time, depending on the results and the clinical problem, and before the patient leaves to ask the question: "Has everything possible been done to maximize the information gained from performing this radionuclide study?" Not to do this and, for example, to fail to mark a thyroid nodule on the scan, a mass in the abdomen, or demonstrate that a space-occupying lesion is a rib impression on a liver scan, necessitating a repeat study for this purpose, is to practise a low standard of clinical patient care. Diagnostic medicine is not about pattern recognition in a pile of pictures; it is about solving patient's clinical problems.

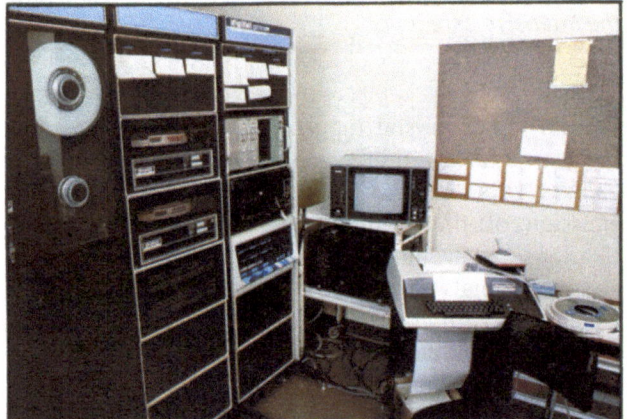

Figure 1.6 *A small dedicated minicomputer interfaced to a gamma camera for quantitative analysis and image processing for increased diagnostic information.*

Footnote

[1] A dedicated computer is a microprocessor which is programmable. It records the data from the gamma camera in digital form—so that images can be reprocessed, and quantitative data can be recorded in the form of uptake of radiopharmaceuticals and time activity curves.

Reference

Wagner, H., *Principles of Nuclear Medicine*, W. B. Saunders, Philadelphia, 1968.

Further Reading

Gottschalk, A. and Potchen, E. J. (Eds.), *Diagnostic Nuclear Medicine*, Williams and Wilkins, USA, 1976.

2. Liver and Spleen Scanning

Liver and spleen scanning, using $^{99}Tc^m$ labelled sulphur colloid, should have become a routine investigation now in any hospital providing anything more than a rudimentary diagnostic service. It is easy to forget what a profound difference liver scanning has made to the investigation of liver diseases, unless one recalls the diagnostic tests which were available before the introduction of radionuclide liver scanning. Serum function tests have always been the primary tool in the investigation of liver disease, from the early measurement of serum bilirubin to the present complex series of enzyme level measurements. However, serum liver function tests, although moderately sensitive to disorders of liver function, have a relatively low specificity and no spatial resolution for the site of disorders within the liver. Prior to liver scanning the investigation with spatial resolution was the hepatic arteriogram which is invasive, associated with a significant morbidity, insensitive and relatively non-specific. It could never have been used for extensive routine screening of patients with neoplasms, prior to their treatment, in the same way that radionuclide liver scanning is now used. More recently, the use of ultrasound, in combination with the radionuclide liver scan, has further refined the investigation of spatial lesions within the liver. The radionuclide liver scan is the first investigation, with ultrasound frequently providing further information when necessary, e.g. the differentiation of a solid from a cystic lesion, or the identification of dilated bile ducts which may occasionally simulate multiple focal lesions on a liver scan. However, ultrasound remains highly operator-dependent, is not cost-effective in terms of skilled physician manpower and, in general, has a limited ability to detect functional or parenchymal liver disease as opposed to space-occupying lesions.

Principles

The routine radionuclide liver scan depends on the demonstration of the integrity of the reticuloendothelial system (RES) within the liver and spleen. Colloid particles, usually sulphur colloid, labelled with a radionuclide, normally $^{99}Tc^m$, are taken up by the reticuloendothelial (RE) cells because of their particle size, which is approximately 0.01μ. The uptake of these particles by the liver depends basically on two factors:

1. The extraction efficiency.
2. The hepatic blood flow.

The extraction efficiency for a normal liver approaches 100 per cent, i.e. almost 100 per cent of colloid particles in the blood passing through the liver will be removed. Therefore, the actual amount that appears in the liver will depend both on the extraction efficiency and the blood supply to the liver. Diseases of the liver, which almost always affect both the function of the RE cells *and* the blood flow, will be reflected in the change in distribution of radioactive colloid particles. In the case of a diffuse process, such as cirrhosis, less radioactive colloid will be taken up generally by the liver. Therefore, more is available for other RES sites in the body, such as the spleen and bone marrow. Space-occupying lesions in the liver completely replace the RES cells and therefore appear as areas devoid of radioactive material ('cold spots') on the scan.

Other radiopharmaceuticals are used for liver scanning to solve particular problems, and these are shown in Table 2.1. However, in most instances the $^{99}Tc^m$ sulphur colloid liver scan is performed first with one of the secondary agents used to solve particular problems in the interpretation of the colloid scan and to increase the specificity of the investigation.

Technique

No preparation of the patient is required. Between 2 and 5 mCi of $^{99}Tc^m$ sulphur colloid should be injected

Table 2.1 Radiopharmaceuticals for liver scanning.

Radiopharmaceutical	Use
$^{99}Tc^m$ sulphur colloid	Routine liver and spleen scanning
Gallium-67 Selenomethionine	Localization of abscesses and diagnosis of hepatomas
$^{99}Tc^m$ HIDA I^{131} Rose Bengal	Hepatobiliary scanning for biliary obstruction and gallbladder function
$^{99}Tc^m$ labelled red blood cells or albumin	Estimation of the blood volume of a lesion
$^{99}Tc^m$ labelled heat-denatured red blood cells	Spleen visualization without visualization of overlapping liver

intravenously, and there are no known contraindications or side-effects from this investigation. After a waiting period of approximately 15 minutes (to allow for adequate uptake into the RES and clearance from the blood) a four-view scan of the liver and spleen is performed, using a gamma camera with the patient standing in front of the camera.

The costal margin is usually marked by using a lead strip or two radioactive sources 10 cm apart so that the final image can be displayed life-size and absolute measurements made. It may be necessary to mark any abdominal masses, e.g. the edge of an enlarged mass in the epigastrium, to differentiate them from functioning liver tissue of the left lobe. Other manoeuvres which are used frequently and are very helpful include a picture in full inspiration with breath-holding, and a picture in full expiration with breath-holding, to establish whether a lesion 'moves' with or independently of the liver.

Oblique views may differentiate the spleen from an enlarged left lobe and define its size more accurately. A space-occupying lesion in the upper part of the right lobe may be simulated, or masked, by overlying breast tissue absorbing the emitted photons and masking the underlying liver lesion. Marking a lesion for subsequent liver biopsy is a useful part of the investigation but, because of the mobility of the liver, this should be done very carefully in the position in which the subsequent biopsy will be performed.

It is often helpful to proceed directly to an ultrasound examination to evaluate a problem. The most efficient use of ultrasound is the direct referral of the patient to the ultrasonographer with, for example, a skin marking, and with the questions clearly defined: 'Is this a solid lesion or is it a dilated bile duct; is it a cystic lesion or is it a tumour?', thus making the most effective use of both techniques.

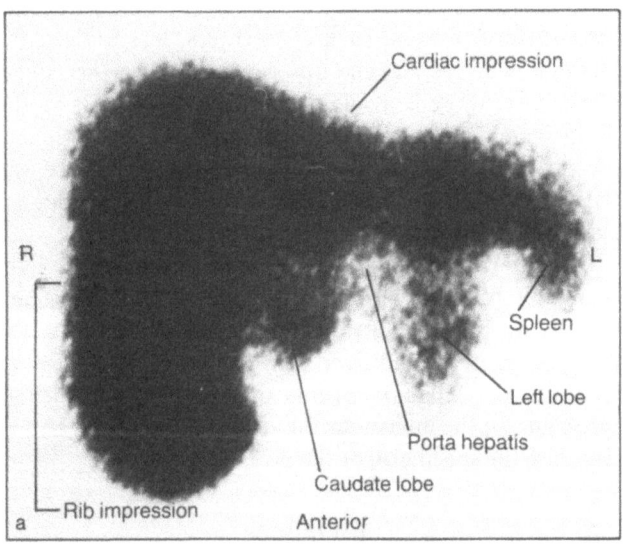
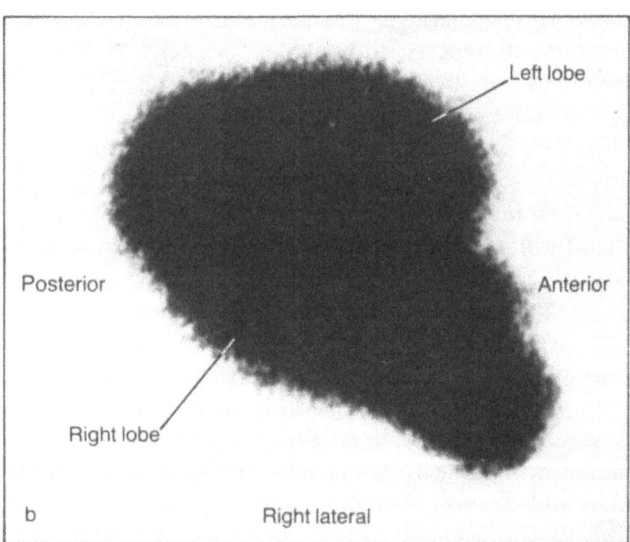
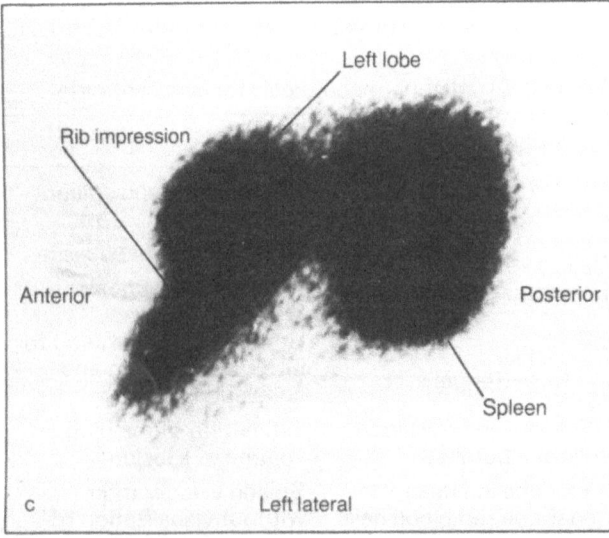
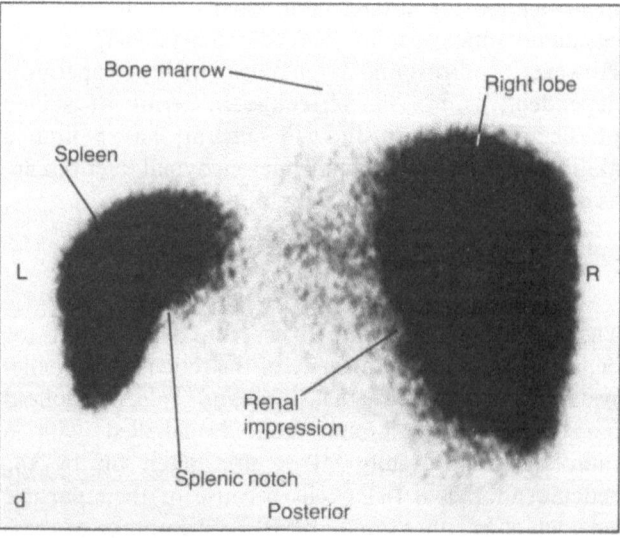

Figure 2.1 *Normal liver/spleen scan showing the site of common normal anatomical features.*

Other radionuclide studies which may be performed with the colloid routine scan include:

1. A simultaneous lung scan to define the extent of a subphrenic abscess (but this is not routinely necessary as a careful palpation and chest radiograph are usually adequate).

2. The use of a hepatobiliary agent to define the position of the gallbladder and differentiate it from a possible space-occupying lesion.

3. The use of $^{99}Tc^m$ labelled denatured red blood cells which are sequestered in the spleen to define the spleen more clearly when it is totally obscured by the left lobe of the liver.

4. The use of $^{99}Tc^m$ labelled red blood cells (undamaged) to establish the relative vascularity of a lesion, and consequently avoid the potential disaster of biopsying a haemangioma of the liver.

The addition of a gallium-67 or selenomethionine scan is one of the most effective methods for differentiating a tract of fibrous tissue in a cirrhotic liver from a superimposed hepatoma. (These radioactive tracers are highly specific agents for the diagnosis of a hepatoma in a clinical situation.) A typical example of a normal liver scan with normal variants is shown in Figure 2.1.

Clinical Indications

The clinical indications for liver and spleen scanning are shown in Table 2.2.

Staging of Malignant Disease

The extent of malignant disease is frequently the major factor in determining management, and liver scanning forms an important part of this owing to the high frequency of malignant disease involving the liver. A liver scan is an essential preoperative investigation of

Table 2.2 Indications for liver/spleen scanning.

Staging of malignant disease.
Investigation of jaundice.
Investigation of hepatomegaly and intra-abdominal masses of unknown aetiology.
Investigation of abnormal liver function tests of unknown aetiology.
Prior to liver biopsy to locate abnormal sites.
Investigation of subphrenic, parahepatic and intrahepatic abscesses.
Investigation of the possibility of a superimposed hepatoma in portal cirrhosis.
Splenic disease such as trauma, lymphoma, hyposplenism and splenomegaly of unknown cause.

the common neoplasms of the gastrointestinal tract, bronchus and breast, and of the other less common neoplasms which metastasize to the liver. Palpation, liver function tests and even direct palpation at laparotomy are not sensitive enough to assess the presence or absence of secondary deposits. Gastrointestinal deposits are often large, solitary and very clearly defined, as shown in Figure 2.2. The metastases from carcinoma of the bronchus and breast are frequently much smaller and more diffuse than gastrointestinal secondaries. Very rarely, diffuse nonfocal involvement with metastases may occur with carcinoma of the breast, and in the absence of another cause for diffuse liver disease then liver biopsy may be necessary to confirm this. Lymphomas, relatively

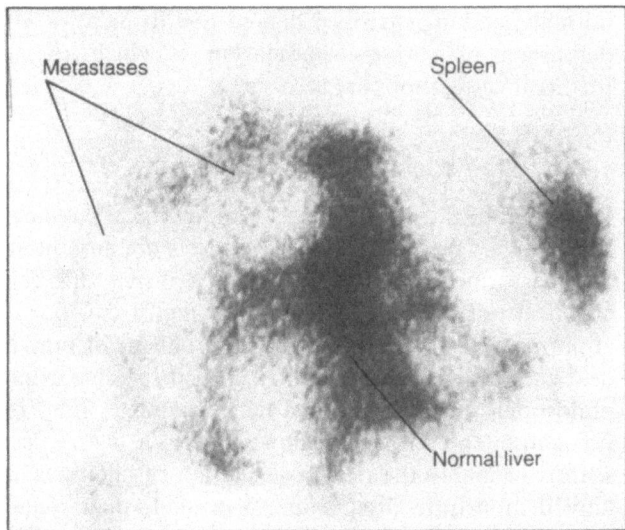

Figure 2.2 *An example of multiple metastases from a colonic neoplasm showing the absent radioactivity ('cold spots') in metastases.*

rarely, cause focal defects in the liver. However, they frequently cause enlargement of the spleen with or without focal defects, and without the overall increased uptake which is seen in the spleen area and is associated with parenchymal liver diseases and splenomegaly. It has been noted that some tumours (melanomas are the most frequent) cause increased uptake of colloid in the spleen relative to the liver without necessarily indicating any direct tumour involvement of either organ.

The Investigation of Jaundice

When the cause of jaundice is doubtful, both clinically and biochemically, or is associated with a known underlying malignancy, a liver scan is a useful screening test. Multiple secondary deposits will be easily identifiable, and further investigation, which might be invasive, will not be necessary. Dilated bile ducts may be identified and then confirmed by ultrasound examination; ultrasound, in fact, is the next investigation whether dilated bile ducts are seen on the liver scan or not. Occasionally, a radiopharmaceutical excreted in the bile ducts may be helpful in the investigation of jaundice but the place of this test in routine investigation has not been fully established.

Hepatomegaly

After clinical examination, the simplest and cheapest investigation for hepatomegaly of unknown aetiology is a liver/spleen scan. In a large proportion of cases, this investigation identifies either the disease process (diffuse parenchymal liver disease or focal disease such as metastases) or, more commonly, the liver which is of normal size but is easily palpated due to either a low diaphragm or a wide costal margin, in which case no further investigations are necessary.

Abnormal Liver Function Tests

One result of the increased use of biochemical screening procedures, whereby liver function tests are automatically performed when any one of a dozen different chemical tests is requested, is a very high frequency of abnormal liver function tests. The problems of how to deal with this situation are difficult and to some extent philosophical. However, after repeating the investigation to confirm the abnormality, a liver/spleen scan is probably the next investigation of choice. This may demonstrate disease or, if normal, may render further investigation unnecessary because, by definition, 2.5 per cent of the population will have biochemical tests outside the normal range (above two standard deviations from the mean).

Liver Biopsy

Where possible, the liver/spleen scan should be performed before a liver biopsy for several reasons:

1. If there is a focal lesion, this can be clearly marked in the biopsy position on the skin. This will significantly decrease the problem (which is sometimes found on liver biopsy of random sampling).

2. Even when diffuse liver disease is suspected this may not be uniform, and areas of more marked abnormality on the liver/spleen scan may indicate the most appropriate site for biopsy.

3. The use of the routine technetium sulphur scan, in combination with the labelled red blood cell scan to show blood volume (Figure 2.3), may prevent the occasional catastrophe following biopsy of a haemangioma.

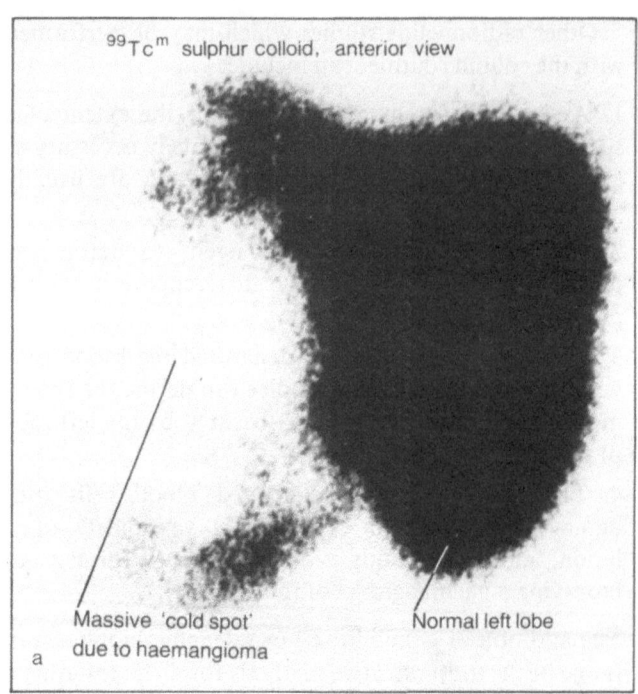

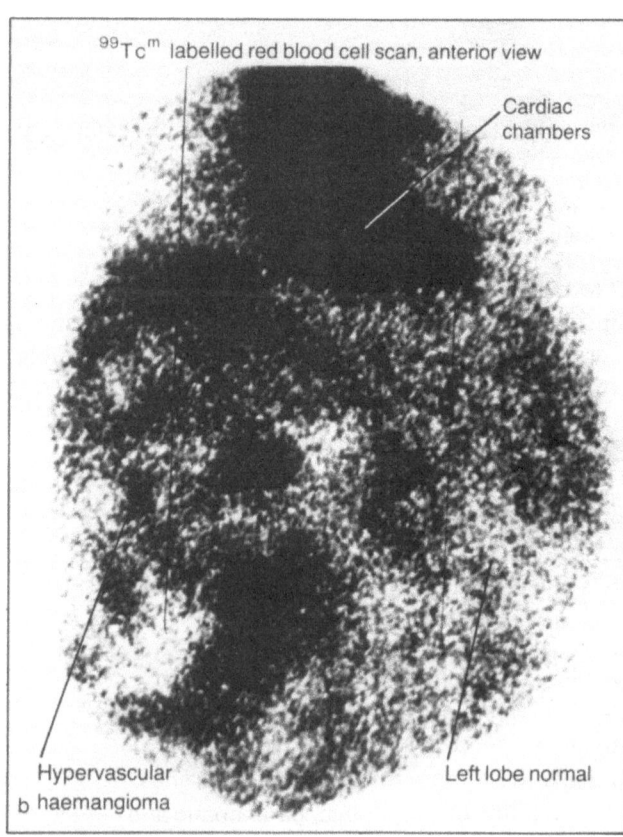

Figure 2.3 (a) *$^{99}Tc^m$ sulphur colloid scan, anterior view, showing massive replacement of functioning Kupffer cells,* **(b)** *anterior view of the liver after injection of labelled autologous red blood cells, demonstrating the high blood volume of the massive haemangioma.*

The Investigation of Subphrenic Abscess

A right-sided subphrenic abscess will cause distortion and compression of the upper margin of the right lobe of the liver (Figure 2.4). This must always be interpreted in conjunction with the chest radiograph to avoid misdiagnosis of lesions which may simulate a subphrenic abscess, such as a pleural effusion compressing the upper portion of the liver or large bowel interposed between the diaphragm and the liver. Without the chest radiograph, these scans could be misinterpreted as confirming a clinically suspected subphrenic abscess. It is rare for the combined liver/lung scan to be of help if the clinical examination, liver scan and chest radiograph

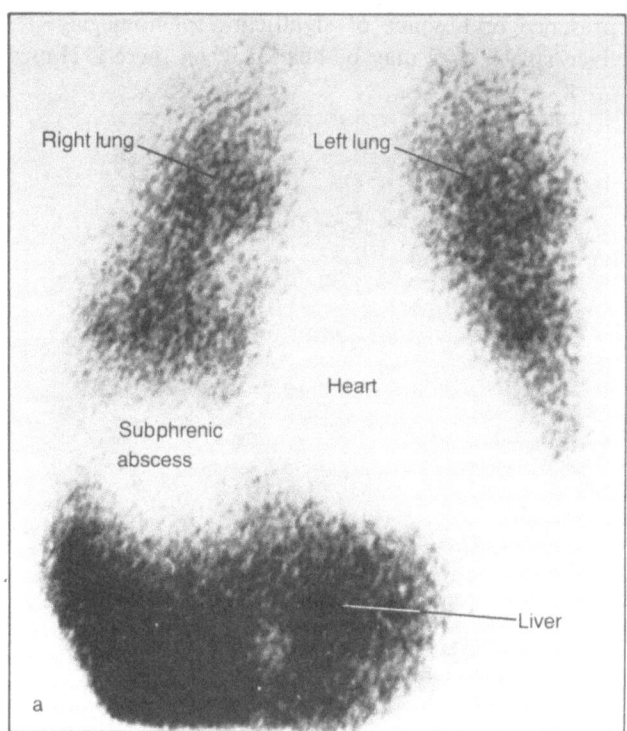

Figure 2.5a *Combined liver/lung scan to demonstrate the extent of the subphrenic abscess (Figure 2.4) on the right. (Anterior view.)*

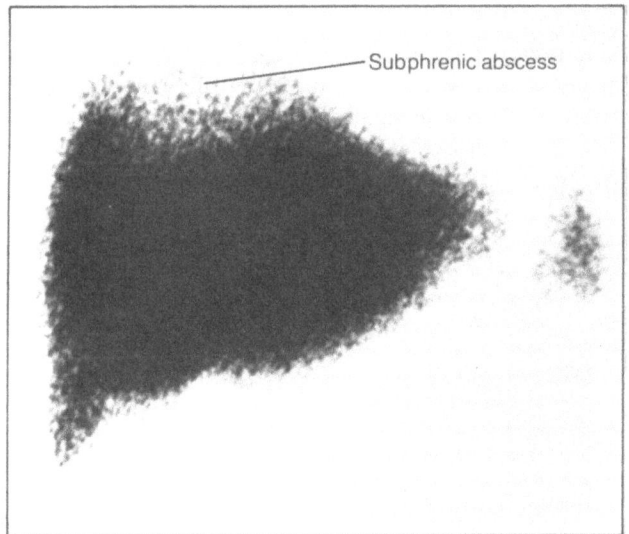

Figure 2.4 *The impression of a subphrenic abscess (which may even appear to be intrahepatic) distorts the upper margin of the right lobe of the liver. (Anterior view.)*

are all carefully performed. However, when it is performed it may outline dramatically the extent of the abscess, as shown in Figure 2.5. Liver/spleen scans are not a great deal of help in the investigation of left-sided subphrenic abscesses, except as an adjunct to the gallium-67 scan. In the latter case they are used to identify the spleen as lying separate from the abnormal accumulation of gallium-67 in the subphrenic abscess.

Diffuse Liver Disease

The liver/spleen scan has a characteristic appearance in diffuse liver disease which results from the impaired extraction efficiency combined with the impaired blood flow into the liver. This results in increased uptake of radioactive tracer by the spleen and by the bone marrow. In addition, in chronic liver disease the spleen is frequently enlarged and there is increased uptake of

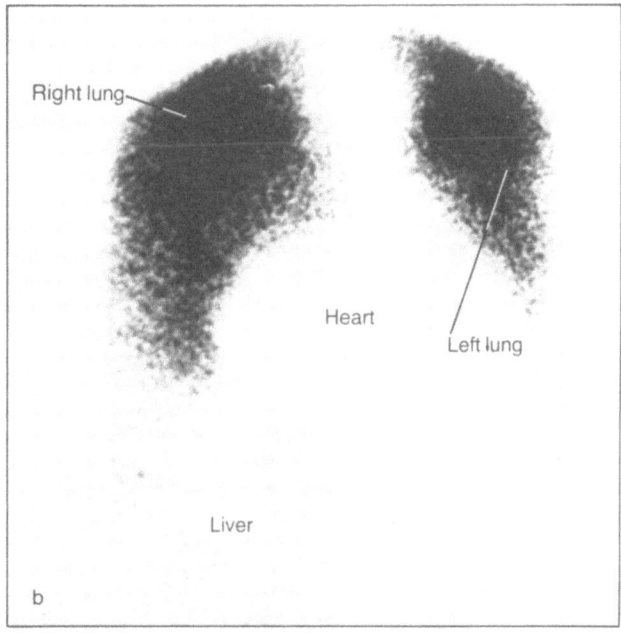

Figure 2.5b *A normal liver/lung scan in a patient suspected of a subphrenic abscess with associated cardiomegaly. (Anterior view.)*

colloid. However, apart from establishing diffuse parenchymal liver disease such as cirrhosis, progressive active hepatitis, alcoholic liver disease, etc., and the

11

presence or absence of significant splenomegaly, the liver/spleen scan may be helpful when there is clinical

deterioration of unknown cause. In the latter case, this may be associated with a generalized rapid progression of the disease (Figure 2.6a and b) or, in the case of cirrhosis, the superimposition of a malignant hepatoma.

Hepatic Abscess

Acute pyogenic abscesses, chronic abscesses (e.g. those due to hydatid disease) and amoebic abscesses are clearly defined on a liver scan. Therefore, this is of value both for diagnosis and, more importantly, for following the progress during treatment. Cysts are also usually well defined on the liver/spleen scan; suspicion of a cyst can be confirmed by ultrasound examination.

Splenic Disease

The presence or absence of a spleen can be identified easily where there is doubt, e.g. following a gastrectomy. For the investigation of splenomegaly and splenic trauma, a liver/spleen scan is probably the investigation of choice (Figure 2.7a and b). Functional hyposplenism,

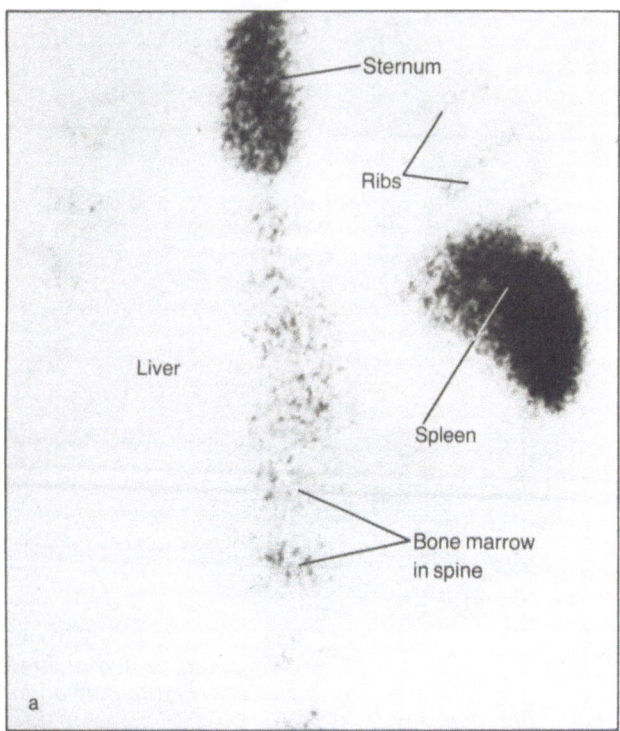

Figure 2.6a *Severe diffuse liver disease showing almost complete absence of liver uptake. (Anterior view.)*

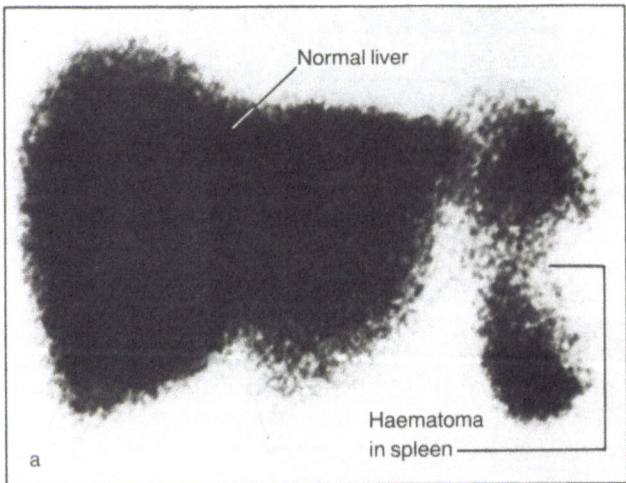

Figure 2.7a *A focal defect in the spleen due to a splenic rupture following trauma. (Anterior view.)*

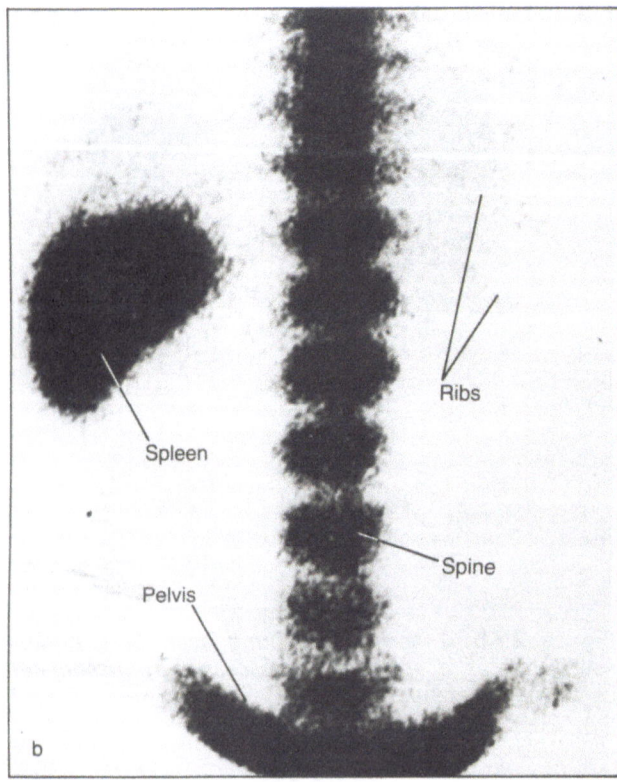

Figure 2.6b *Severe diffuse liver disease showing almost complete absence of liver uptake. (Posterior view.)*

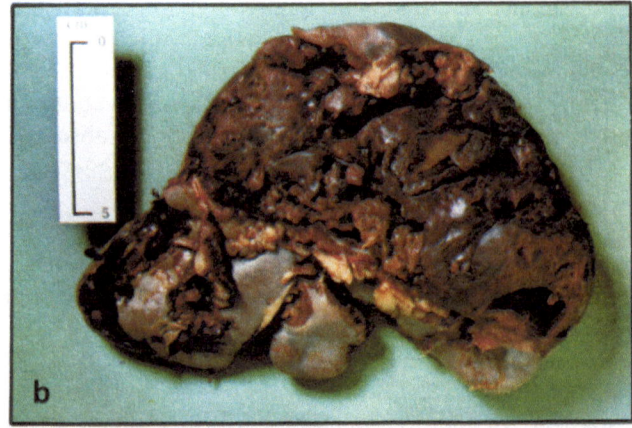

Figure 2.7b *The ruptured spleen after surgical removal.*

which may be associated with coeliac disease or, less commonly, with ulcerative colitis, can be demonstrated, although usually a scan is not necessary as Howell-Jolly bodies can be identified in the blood film. Focal defects of the spleen are relatively uncommon but may occasionally be seen with gastrointestinal neoplasms or lymphomas.

Artefacts of Liver/Spleen Scanning

Whilst there are many artefacts of liver/spleen scanning which may cause difficulties with interpretation, these usually present no problem to technicians or radiographers who are experienced in this field. An example of an artefact is shown in Figure 2.8, which is the well-known 'coin sign', due to the habit of hospital patients keeping their loose change in the breast pocket of their pyjamas. The artefact caused by absorption from a large pendulous breast has been mentioned. The

costal impression (Figure 2.9), particularly in old people with flabby abdominal muscles, and in patients with a scoliosis, may be extremely prominent. This impression, combined with that of the xyphoid, may result in the so-called 'hot cross bun' which, if one is not familiar with this, may be misinterpreted as focal deposits. An impression from an extrahepatic lesion may also simulate an intrahepatic lesion (Figure 2.10).

As mentioned earlier, high uptake in the spleen or bone marrow almost invariably means impairment of liver function. However, in anaemic patients there may be high uptake in the bone marrow, and the bone marrow may be clearly visualized but in these cases the spleen usually shows the normal relationship between splenic and liver tissue. The only exception is long-standing haemolytic anaemia in which the splenic uptake may be higher than that in the liver without any impairment of liver function.

Conclusion

Liver and spleen scanning has immense diagnostic value and is a relatively simple, quick and cheap investigation. The future lies, almost certainly, in more refined radiopharmaceuticals to image more specific functional changes occurring in liver diseases and in more detailed assessment of functional abnormalities of the gall-bladder and biliary system with, for example, sensitive quantitation of rates of contraction and filling of the gallbladder (Figure 2.11a, b and c).   ▷

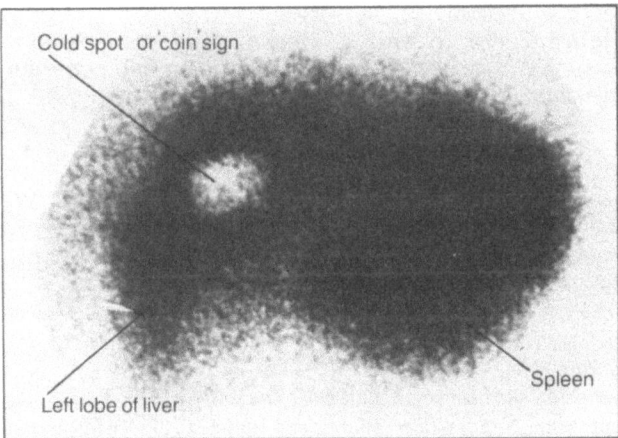

Figure 2.8 *The cold spot or 'coin' sign.*

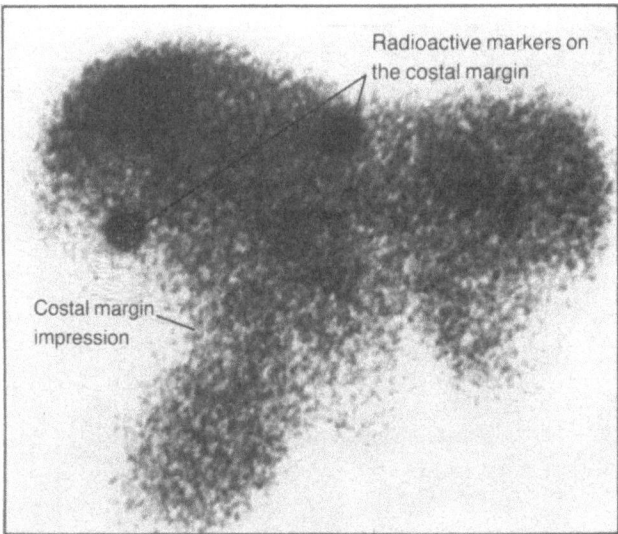

Figure 2.9 *Costal impression exaggerated due to scoliosis.*

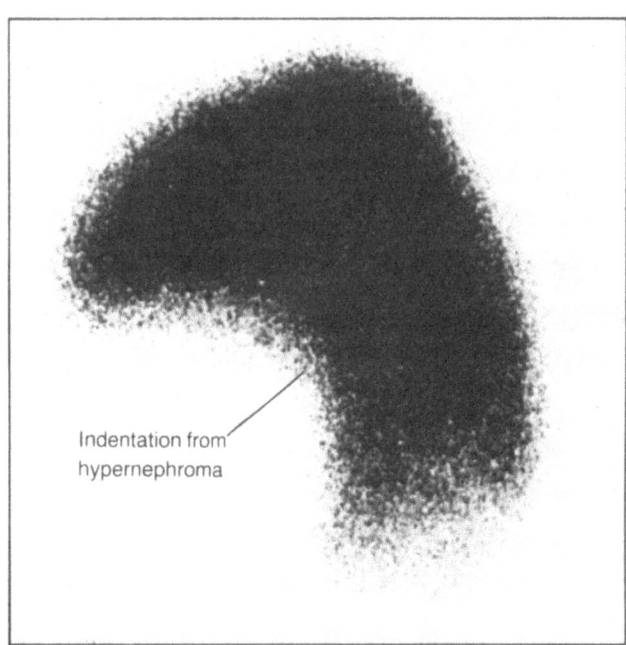

Figure 2.10 *Extrahepatic impression simulating an intrahepatic lesion due to a hypernephroma which was not invading the liver.*

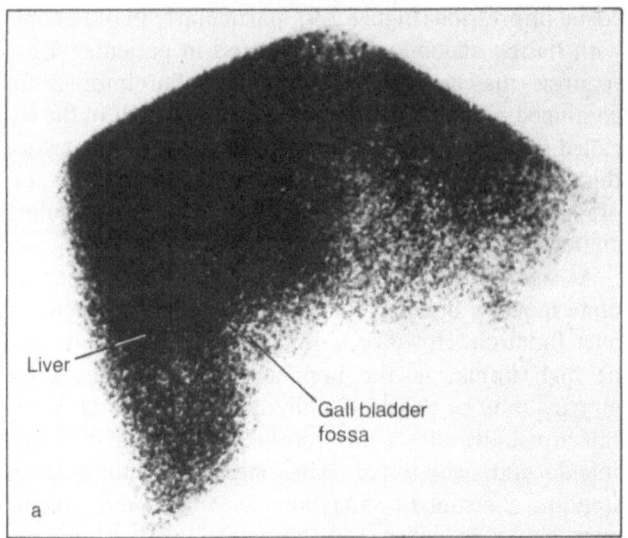

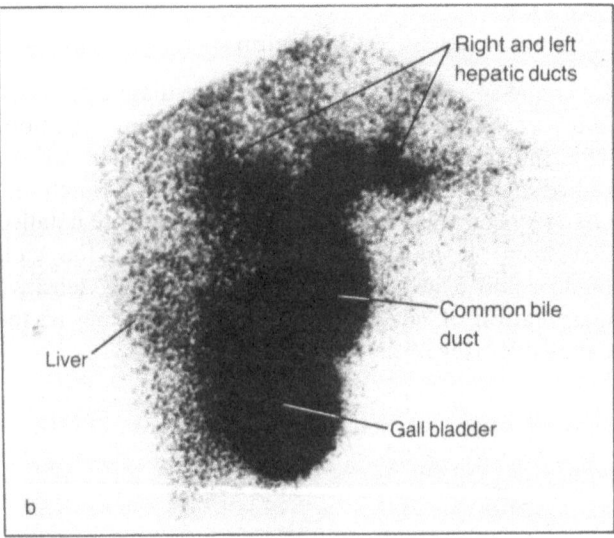

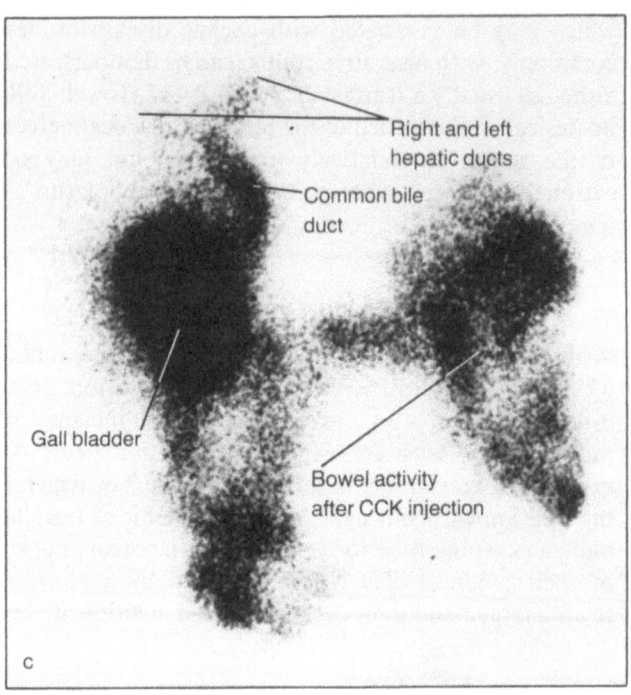

Figure 2.11a, b and c. *Hepatobiliary scan demonstrating the rapid filling of the gallbladder and common bile duct.*

Further Reading

Bryan, P. J., Dinn, W. M., Grossman, Z. D., Wistow, B. W. McAfee, J. G. and Kieffer, S. A., *Radiol.,* 1977, **124(2)**, 387.

Freeman, L. M. and Blautox, M. D., *Semin. Nucl. Med.,* 1972, **2**, 2.

Gold, R. P. and Johnson, P. M., *Radiol.,* 1975, **117**, 105.

Lomas, F. and Wagner, H. N., *N. Engl. J. Med.,* 1972, **286**, 1323.

Shantilal Lunia, Parthasarathy, K. L., Bakshi, S. and Bender, M. A., *J. Nucl. Med.,* 1975, **16**, 62.

Treves, S. and Spencer, R. P., *Semin. Nucl. Med.,* 1973, **3**, 55.

Openheim, B. S., Gottschalk, A. and Hoffer, P. B., in *Diagnostic Nuclear Medicine,* Gottschalk, A. and Potchen, E. J. (Eds), pp. 399-452, Williams and Wilkins, Baltimore, 1976.

3. Brain Scanning

The introduction of brain scanning using radionuclides was an important step in bridging the large gap which lay between the clinical examination of a patient, which may have raised the possibility of an intracranial space-occupying lesion, and definitive methods to demonstrate the lesion, which included carotid angiography and pneumo-encephalography. Both of these investigations are expensive, invasive and unpleasant, with a significant morbidity and some mortality. The EEG and skull radiograph have been used routinely for investigating patients with suspected intracranial pathology but, in general, the results have been unrewarding. Thus, the introduction of the radionuclide brain scan, which remains a simple, cheap, non-invasive method for investigating intracranial pathology on an out-patient basis with no mortality or morbidity, was an important advance. It enabled the clinician to investigate with a lower index of suspicion using a simple investigation which has an accuracy of 85 to 90 per cent. With the introduction of the high structural resolution CT brain scan the place of radionuclide brain scanning has altered somewhat, although the exact relationship of the two investigations has still to be fully evaluated. Leaving aside the areas in which the radionuclide scan is better than the CT scan and vice versa, at the present the radionuclide brain scan is probably the primary definitive investigation for an intracranial space-occupying lesion, with an approximate accuracy of 85 per cent and, used effectively, will answer a large proportion of the clinical questions. This way, the CT scanners, which are not so generally available, will be used more effectively in solving the problems for which they are more suitable, e.g. indicating ventricular size and cerebral atrophy. Also, they can be used for a more detailed evaluation of patients where the radionuclide scan has either not resulted in a definitive answer, or where more detailed information about a lesion detected on the radionuclide brain scan is required for effective management.

There are a few areas where the radionuclide investigation is probably superior and these include the mobility of gamma cameras (which, because of this, can be taken to the bedside in the intensive care ward) and the measurement of blood flow in cerebrovascular disease. It is probably easier to obtain a diagnostic quality brain scan, with disturbed patients, by this method rather than by using a CT scan when it may be necessary to anaesthetize the patient. However, in the next few years one anticipates a relationship between radionuclide brain scanning and CT scanning similar to that which exists between other radionuclide and radiological studies, in which there is an effective coordination between the high structural resolution of the CT scan and the functional information available from the radionuclide scan. This will probably be particularly true when using Positron gamma cameras and when utilizing radionuclides of carbon, oxygen and hydrogen, both of which will undoubtedly become more widely used in the investigation of functional disturbances of brain metabolism.

Principles of the Brain Scan

The possibility of detecting an intracranial space-occupying lesion with the radionuclide brain scan depends on the administered radiopharmaceuticals localizing in the lesion, with the highest possible ratio between the lesion and the surrounding brain. Initially, radiopharmaceuticals, such as mercury-199-chlormerodrin, arsenic-74 and I-131 labelled albumin were used. However, the most commonly used radionuclide now is technetium-99m ($^{99}Tc^m$) in its oxidized pertechnetate form (TcO^4), or less commonly other radiopharmaceuticals labelled with $^{99}Tc^m$, such as DTPA and glucoheptonate. It has ideal imaging characteristics for the gamma camera and the clear resolution of normal structures, such as venous sinuses, scalp and skull, make it superior. Also, even though the lesion to brain ratio is lower, and therefore theoretically less good than, for example, with mercury, its other characteristics, such as the very low radiation dose (and therefore the opportunity to administer much larger quantities), also make it superior. $^{99}Tc^m$ pertechnetate is distributed in the extracellular fluid, including the plasma, and there is a relatively low concentration within the brain tissue.

When there is an intracranial lesion present, such as a tumour, abscess or infarct, there is a larger extracellular fluid space in the lesion and surrounding brain. In addition, the blood volume of the lesion is usually greater per gram than that of the surrounding brain, both features resulting in a high uptake of isotope relative to the surrounding brain and hence in a positive brain scan. In addition to the static brain scan based on these factors, the dynamic brain scan takes advantage of the fact that images of the brain, recorded with a gamma camera during the first passage of a rapidly injected bolus of a diffusible tracer, give an estimate of the regional blood flow through the brain. Thus, with the static brain scan we are obtaining a functional image of the distribution of extracellular fluid within the brain, and with the dynamic brain scan we are obtaining a functional image of the regional distribution of blood flow.

Technique

No preparation of the patient is necessary. Approximately half an hour before the injection of $^{99}Tc^m$ pertechnetate, approximately 400 mg of sodium perchlorate is given orally to block the uptake of technetium-99m into the choroid plexus and, incidentally, into the thyroid gland (because $^{99}Tc^m$ is taken up into the same physiological sites as iodine, and choroid plexus may be confused with a tumour). The dose of pertechnetate is 15 mCi, given intravenously (ideally, it is given intravenously, but may be given orally or intramuscularly if necessary, although the rate of absorption in this case is somewhat variable). It is, of course, essential to inject it intravenously if a dynamic study is performed, and ideally this should be carried out in every patient.

For the dynamic blood flow study the patient is positioned so that the gamma camera takes a sequence of views from the appropriate position, depending on the clinical findings, e.g. posteriorly in a patient with a homonymous hemianopia, and anteriorly in a patient with signs of a frontal lobe tumour. The injection is given as rapidly as possible, either with a flushing dose of saline to keep the bolus compact, or alternatively using the 'Oldendorf technique' whereby the injection is given into the vein with a sphygmomanometer cuff blown up above the systolic BP. The cuff is then released rapidly to allow the compact bolus to reach the carotid arteries with as little spread as possible.

Repeated images are taken at approximately one to three second intervals after the arrival of the bolus in the carotid artery. Ideally, some form of data processing should be used to obtain maximum information but this is not essential. After the first passage of the bolus through the brain, the dynamic series is discontinued and after one to two minutes an equilibrium image is obtained without moving the patient. This represents largely the intracranial distribution of blood volume. The static brain scan is performed usually between one and two hours after the injection; the longer the period the greater the tumour to blood ratio, but with a short-lived radionuclide, such as $^{99}Tc^m$, the longer the interval the more decay occurs and therefore the longer each view will take. One to two hours is the compromise

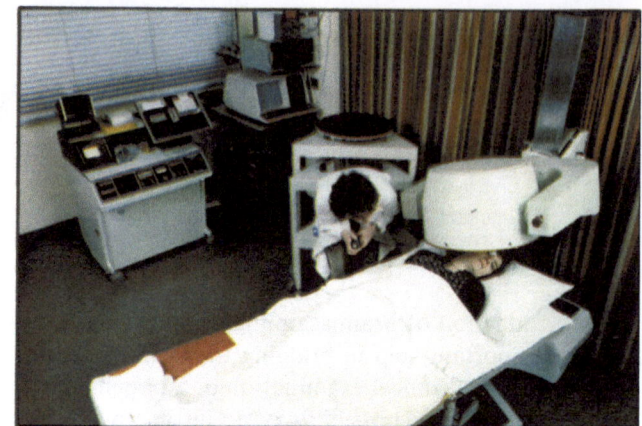

Figure 3.1 *A brain scan being obtained (lateral view) with a gamma camera.*

usually accepted. Five views are obtained with a gamma camera (Figure 3.1)—anterior, posterior, both laterals and the vertex (Figure 3.2 a, b, c and d). Occasionally, if the result is doubtful, repeating one or two views after four hours will demonstrate an equivocal lesion as a clearly abnormal one, or vice versa (Figure 3.3). This is particularly true of a subdural haematoma when it is probably wise to delay the brain scan for at least two hours routinely. If some form of data processing is available, then the regional cerebral blood flow can be analysed by using the area of interest facility (the area which is marked out by hand and recorded by the computer for subsequent analysis) on the computer and generating curves as shown in Figure 3.4.

Finally, the result of the dynamic/static brain scan, with consideration of the clinical history and physical findings, is evaluated. The clinical assessment should include palpation of the skull, where necessary, because superficial contusion will give rise to increased radionuclide accumulation and may mimic a tumour. For similar reasons, skull lesions and previous craniotomies or burr-holes must be accounted for in the clinical assessment. It is often helpful to have a skull radiograph or previous bone scan available as many of these patients will have primary tumours in other parts of the body with skull metastases which may mimic a brain tumour (Figure 3.5). It is important also, when interpreting the scan findings, to remember that $^{99}Tc^m$ is excreted by the salivary glands.

Clinical Indications

The clinical indications for referring a patient for radionuclide brain scan will vary according to the availability of other diagnostic facilities, particularly the CT scanner. However, in this particular discussion the assumption is being made that we are dealing with a smaller hospital, which will have a nuclear medicine facility together with a standard radiological facility,

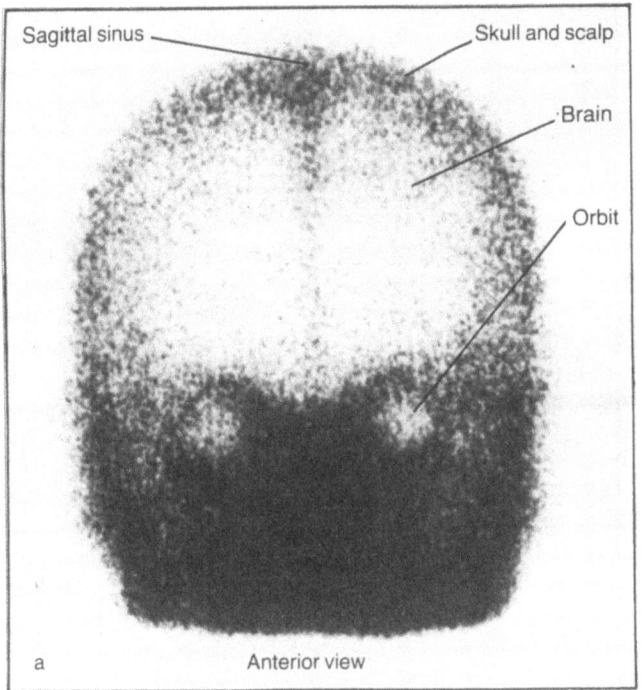

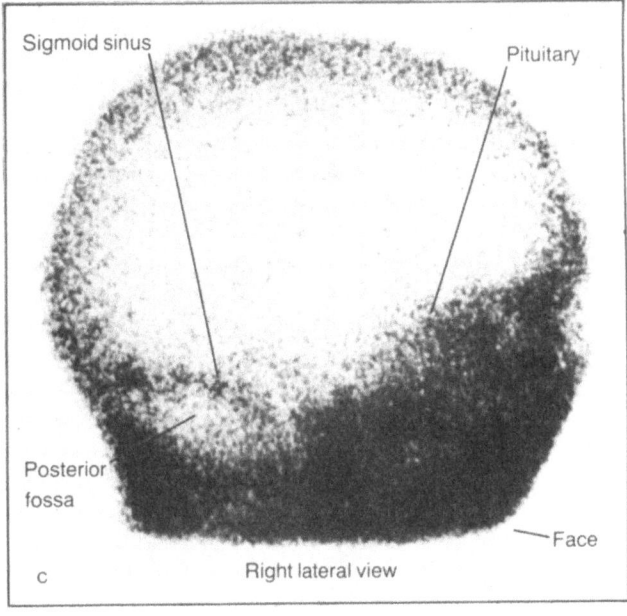

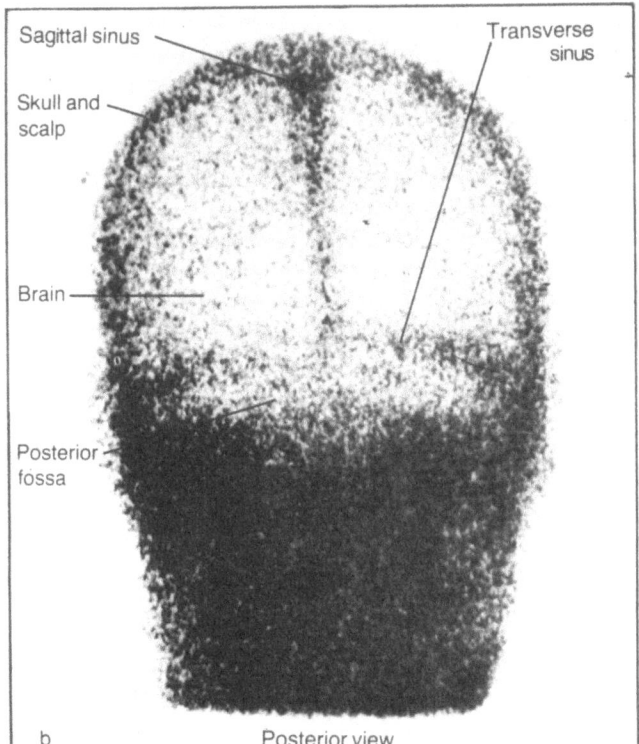

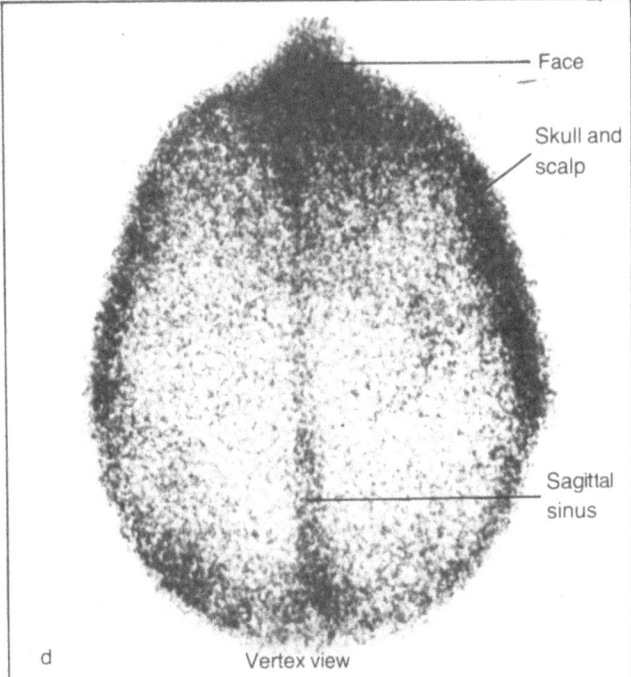

Figure 3.2 a, b, c and d *Normal brain scans showing normal anatomical features usually seen.*

but which does not possess, at the present, a CT brain scanner.

What are the indications for referring a patient for radionuclide brain scan?

Suspected Intracranial Neoplasm

Undoubtedly, this is the commonest indication for referring a patient for radionuclide brain scan. It is not possible to make definite rules about what constitutes a good indication for investigating a patient for a possible intracranial tumour but a few general points should be made. First, it is rare for headache to be the only feature of an intracranial tumour, with no physical signs or other history; also, in young people presenting with generalized epilepsy an intracranial neoplasm is an

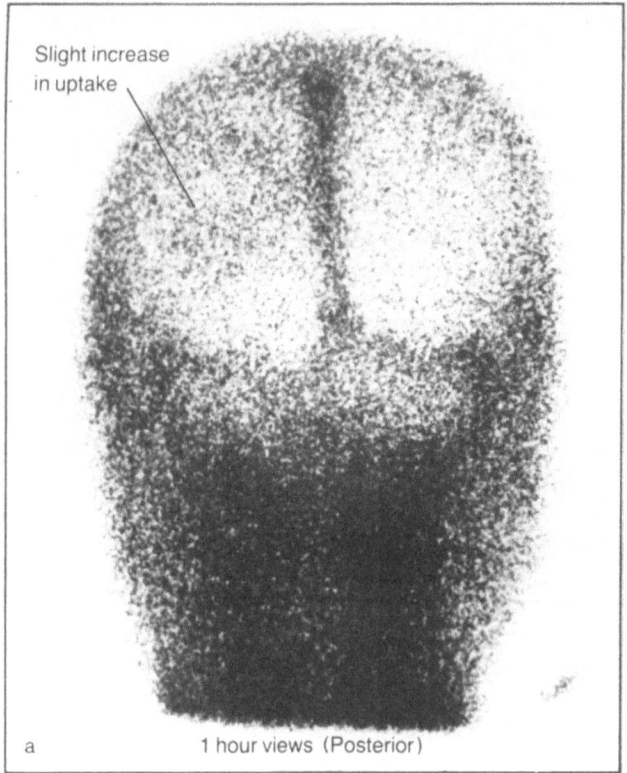

Slight increase in uptake

a   1 hour views (Posterior)

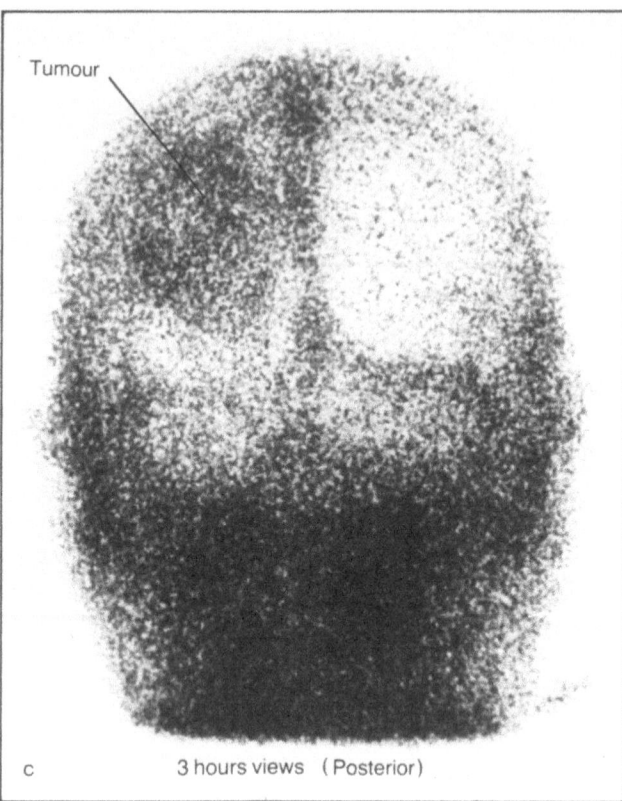

Tumour

c   3 hours views (Posterior)

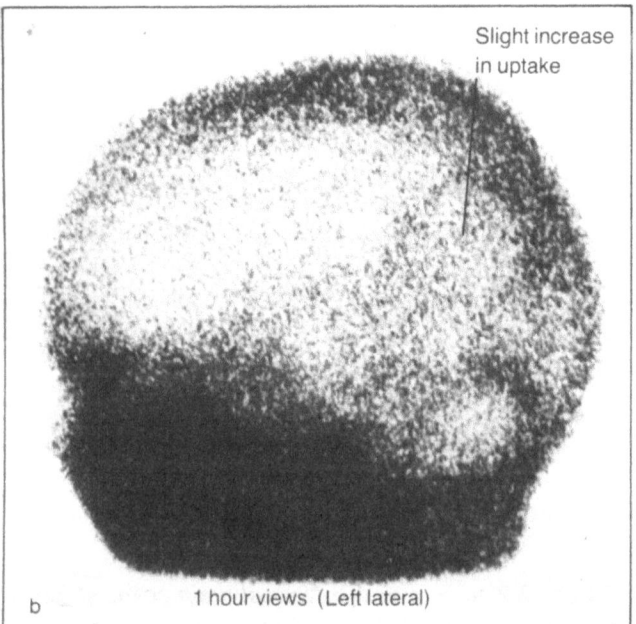

Slight increase in uptake

b   1 hour views (Left lateral)

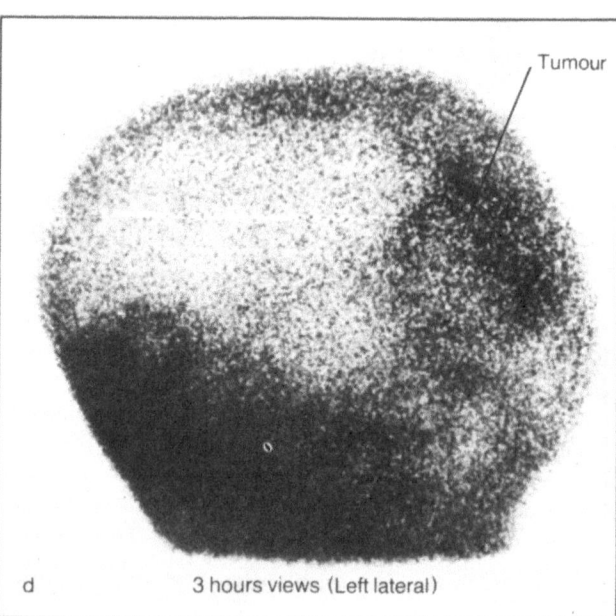

Tumour

d   3 hours views (Left lateral)

Figure 3.3 a, b, c and d *Early and delayed views of a patient with a posterior parietal/occipital brain tumour showing how an equivocal scan may become clearly positive as the tracer progressively accumulates in the tumour.*

unusual cause. Similarly, confusion in the elderly, mental retardation in the young and frank psychiatric syndromes with no physical signs and no underlying malignancy are rarely caused by an intracranial tumour. The typical appearance of a primary tumour is shown in

Figure 3.6. The presence of multiple lesions in the absence of clinical features suggesting multiple abscesses makes a diagnosis of metastases the most probable, as shown in Figure 3.7. It used to be thought that posterior fossa lesions, both in children and adults,

18

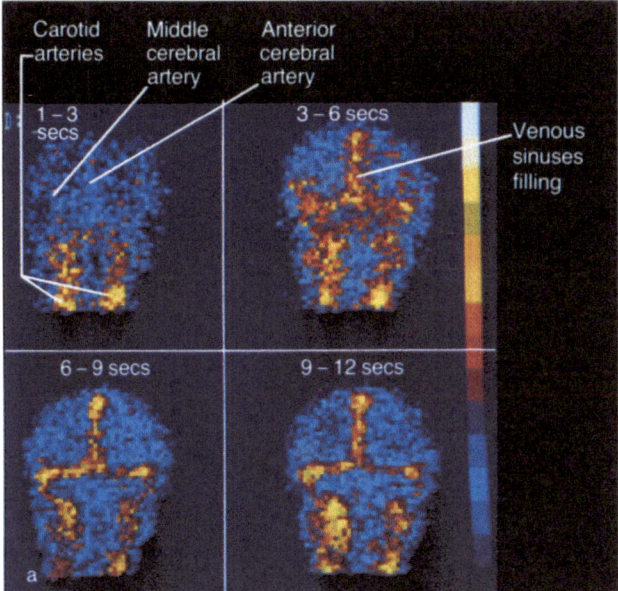

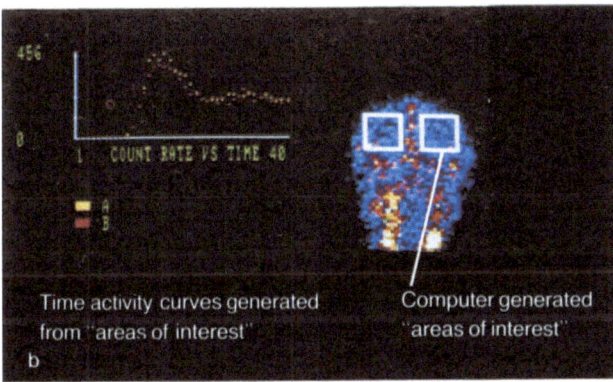

Figure 3.4 a and b (left) *Computer processed image of a normal posterior dynamic blood flow study with curves generated for comparison of the regional cerebral blood flow.*

were lesions with a relatively low yield on the radionuclide brain scan. However, with modern techniques and good attention to detailed positioning

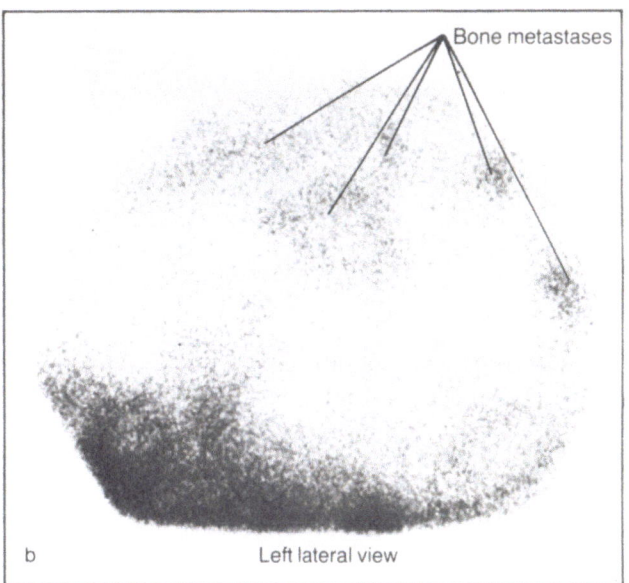

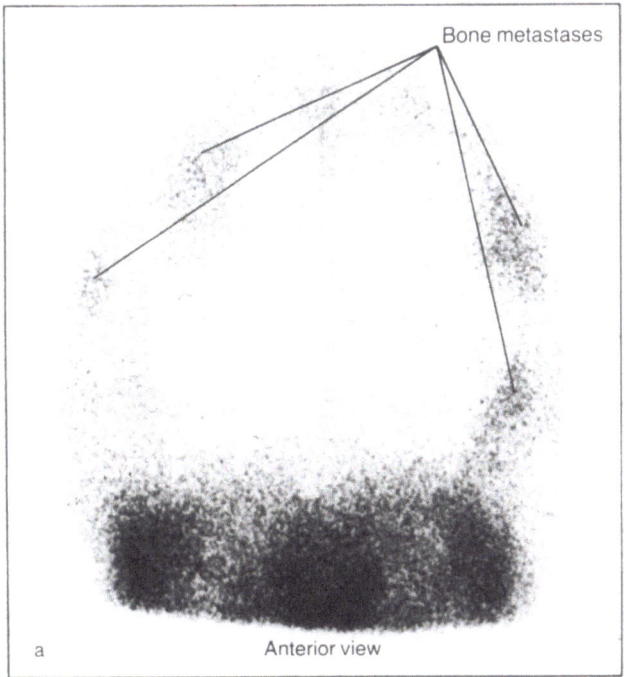

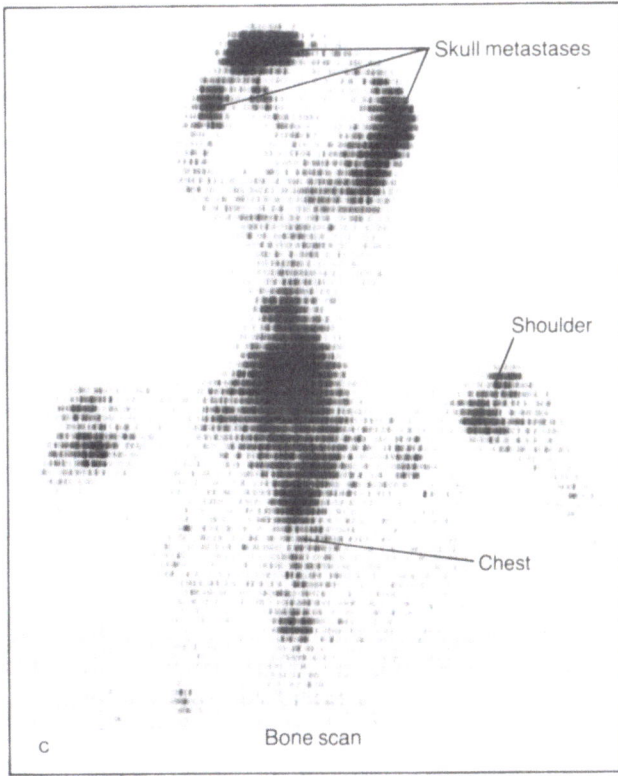

Figure 3.5 a, b and c (left and above) *Bone metastases in the skull mimicking cerebral tumours.*

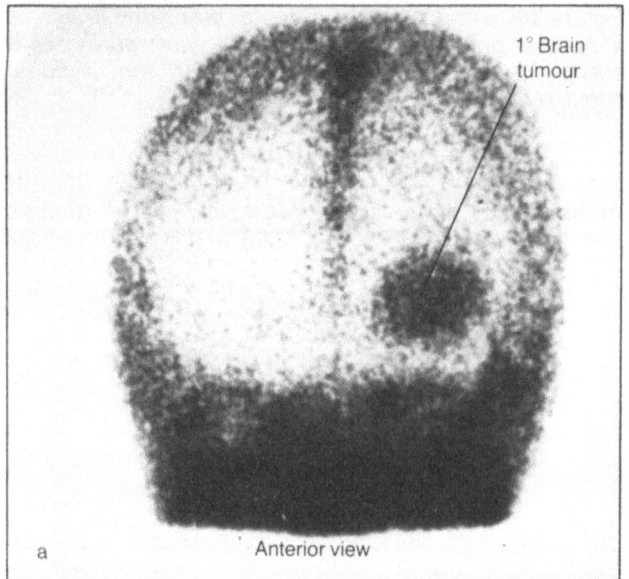

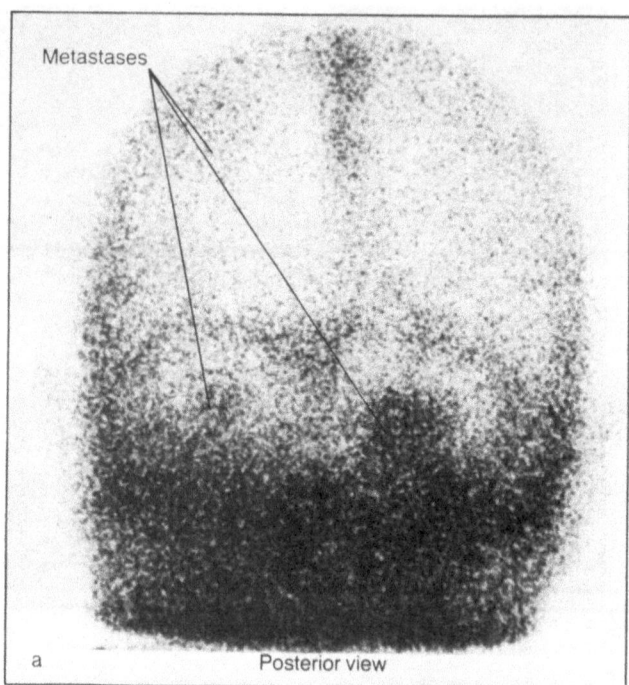

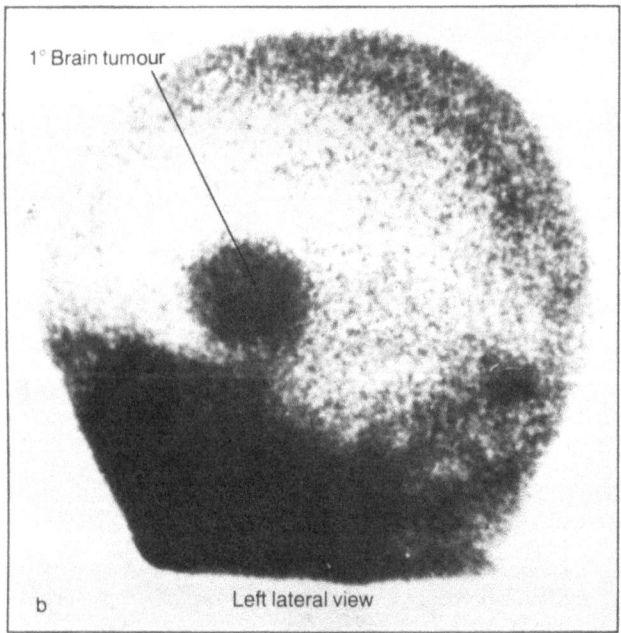

Figure 3.6 a and b *A typical example of a primary brain tumour (glioma) lying in the left fronto-temporal region.*

Figure 3.7 a and b *Multiple intracranial metastases in cerebral hemispheres and posterior fossa from carcinoma of the bronchus.*

the accuracy is approximately as high as with supratentorial lesions and not very different from that of CT scanning (Figure 3.8). Where possible, when investigating patients with clinically probable metastatic brain lesions, the brain scan should be performed before treatment with corticosteroids begins as these may decrease significantly the uptake of radionuclide into the tumours.

Trauma

The radionuclide brain scan, when performed carefully and with dynamic studies, is a good technique for the diagnosis of subdural haematomas, with a diagnostic accuracy of >90 per cent. There will be decreased blood

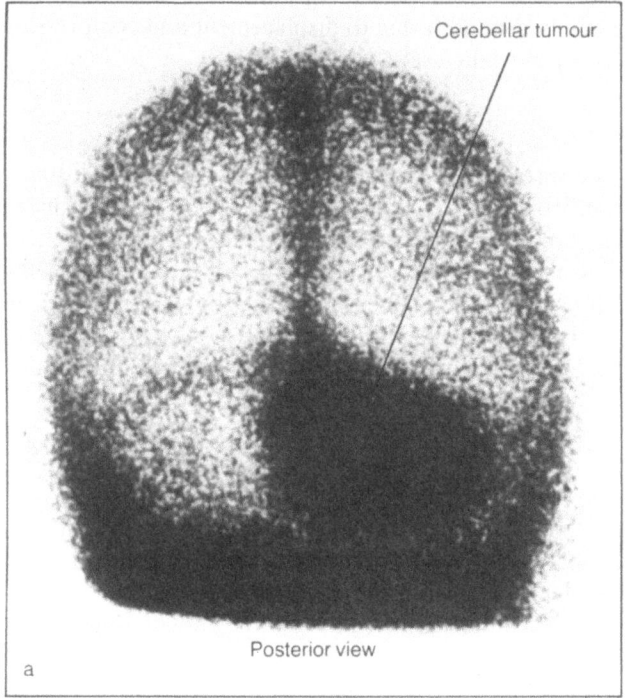

Cerebellar tumour

Posterior view

a

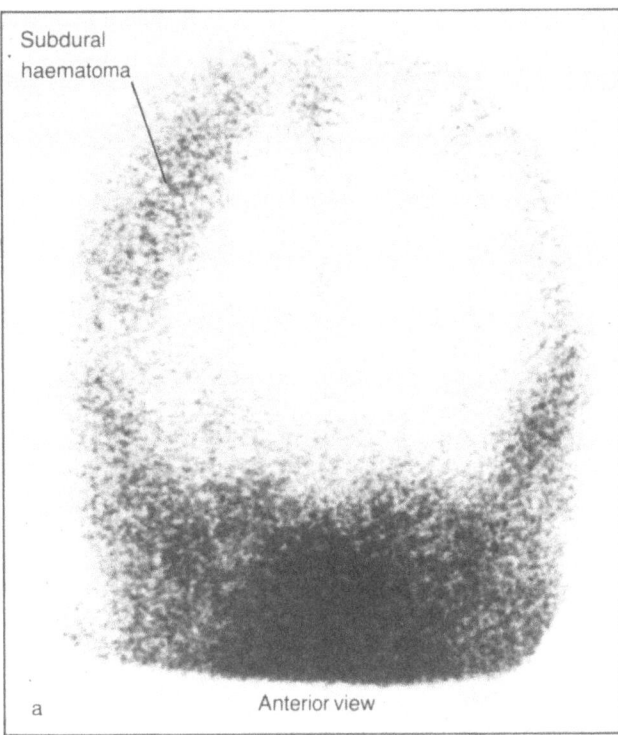

Subdural haematoma

Anterior view

a

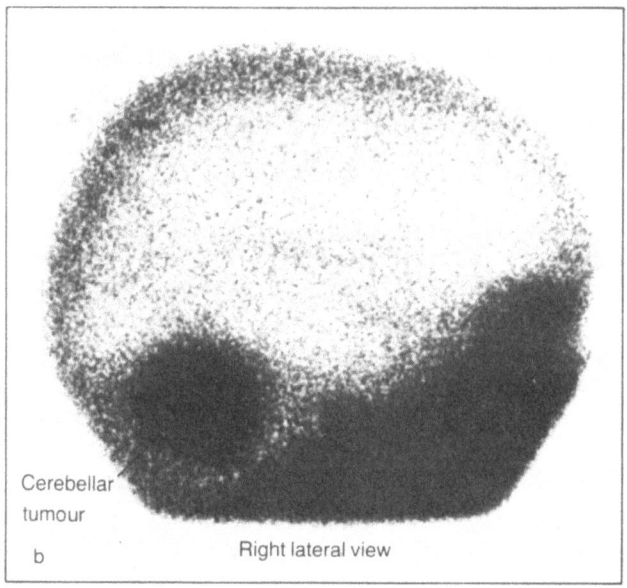

Cerebellar tumour

Right lateral view

b

Figure 3.8 a and b *A posterior fossa tumour—a typical example of a right-sided cerebellar tumour.*

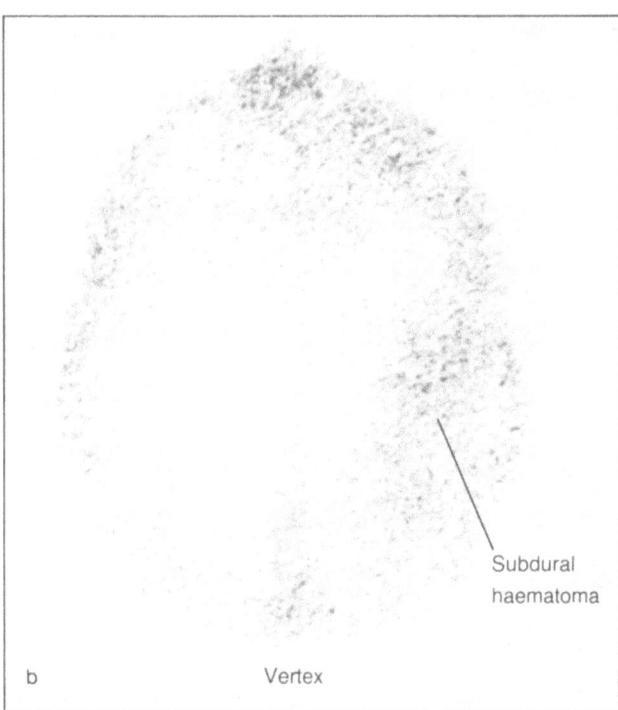

Subdural haematoma

Vertex

b

Figure 3.9 a and b *A subdural haematoma showing the typical lens-shaped uptake over the cortex.*

flow on the side of the subdural haematoma, which on the static brain scan is usually lens-shaped, as shown in Figure 3.9. There may be associated soft tissue trauma, which must be carefully differentiated from a subdural haematoma, and the brain scan is more likely to be positive if delayed views are taken as there is a significant time delay in the entry of the tracer into the subdural lesion. Again, the scan is more likely to

become positive a week or more after the onset of the trauma, probably because it requires the development of the membrane to allow the tracer to enter the haematoma. An extradural haematoma is usually a

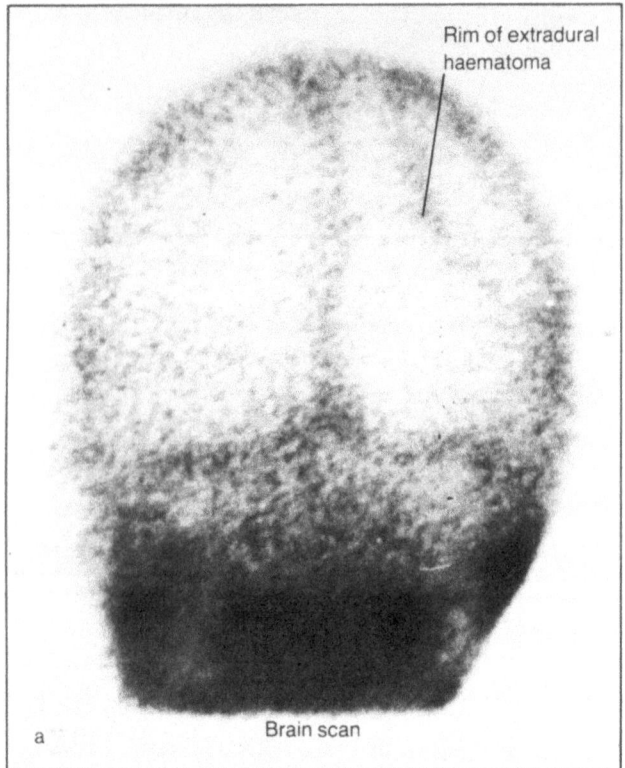

Rim of extradural
haematoma

a   Brain scan

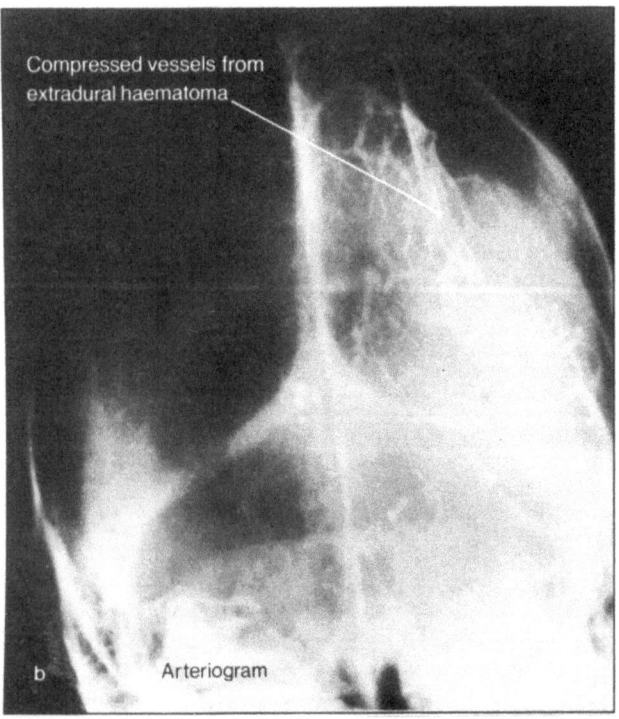

Compressed vessels from
extradural haematoma

b   Arteriogram

Figure 3.10 a and b *A right-sided extradural
haematoma showing the 'rim sign', which is due to
compression and shift of vascular meninges. (The same
patient is shown in a and b.)*

medical emergency and a brain scan is rarely used, but
the typical picture is shown in Figure 3.10, where the
lesion itself is negative but there is a rim of increased

22

activity around it due to displacement and compression
of superficial vessels.

Infection

The presence of an intracranial abscess is usually
confirmed with a high degree of accuracy when using
the brain scan, and an example is shown in Figure 3.11.
The characteristic appearance has been described as the
'donut' because of the ring of activity with no tracer in
the centre. This has since become recognized as a non-
specific sign which may occur in almost any intracranial
lesion where there is central necrosis.

Cerebrovascular Disease

Usually the clinical picture of an acute 'stroke' presents
no diagnostic problem and definitive investigation is not
normally required. However, there may be some doubt
as to whether it is a 'stroke' or, in the case of a patient
with a known carcinoma, an intracerebral metastasis
presenting as a 'stroke'. In the case of a cerebral infarction, the diagnosis can be made on the characteristic
vessel distribution together with decreased blood flow
on the dynamic study. Additional evidence is obtained if
sequential scans are performed because initially the
brain scan may be negative (although the dynamic brain
scan quite frequently shows decreased flow), becoming
most strongly positive in the second week after the onset
and then gradually resolving. Thus, a scan which may
be equivocal at one week, if repeated after a further
three or four weeks, normally shows disappearance of
uptake or less clear-cut uptake than was previously
shown. Figure 3.12 shows an example of a middle
cerebral infarct. Figure 3.13 shows the dynamic blood
flow study from the patient in Figure 3.12, demonstrating decreased flow due to the infarction.

Epilepsy

Generalized epilepsy of early onset is not normally
regarded as an indication for a brain scan, but focal
epilepsy in children or adults is an indication, as is late
onset epilepsy with no underlying metabolic or other
cause to account for it, such as alcoholic fits. Figure
3.14 shows the dynamic and static brain scan of a
patient with an AV malformation presenting with focal
epilepsy.

Apart from the positive indications for performing
radionuclide brain scans, it is probably as important to
know which lesions the radionuclide brain scan will not
detect:

1. For practical purposes, all causes of dementia apart
from frontal lobe tumours will not be diagnosed, and a

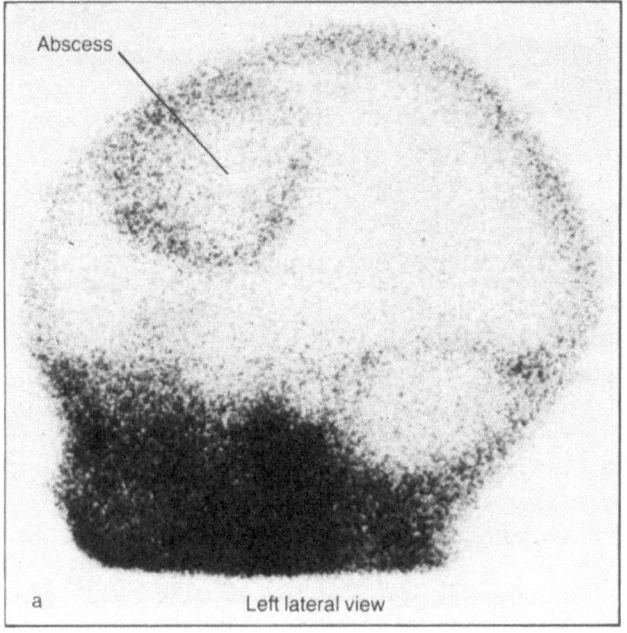

Abscess

a   Left lateral view

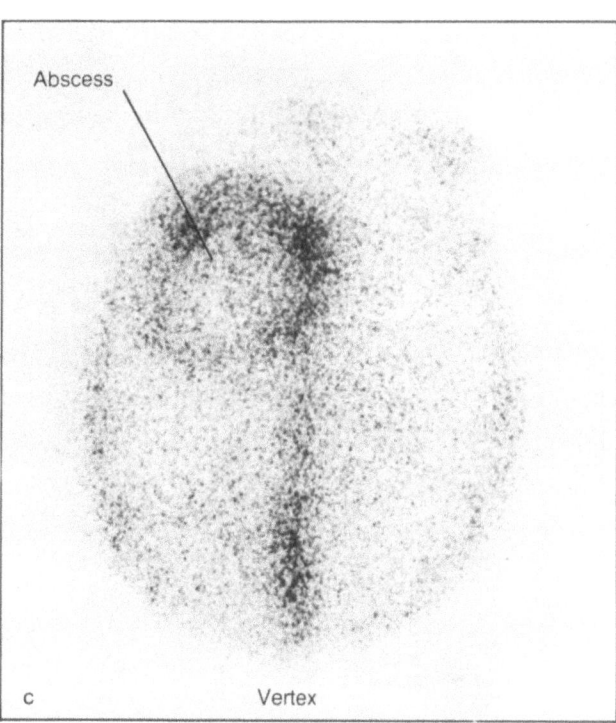

Abscess

c   Vertex

Figure 3.11 a, b and c *Brain scan showing a cerebral abscess in a child with a congenital cyanotic heart disease.*

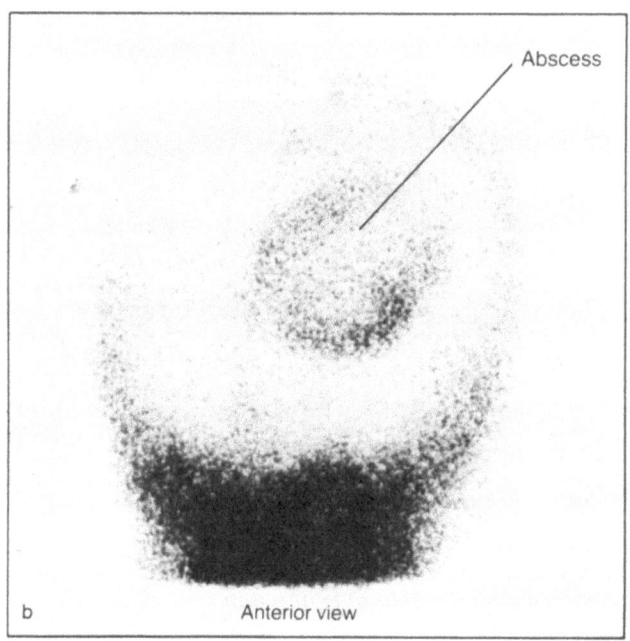

Abscess

b   Anterior view

CT scan is definitely the investigation of choice unless there are particular features to suggest a frontal lobe tumour.

2. Early subdural haematomas, which occur within a day or two of the injury, may be missed (particularly if no dynamic study is performed).

3. A cerebral infarct, if small and if the scan is performed within a day or two of the onset, may not be detected. This, of course, can be a positively useful feature in the differentiation between a cerebral infarct and a neoplasm, as the latter will almost always be positive on the brain scan.

4. Oligodendrogliomas (particularly in the posterior fossa or mid-brain), which are very slow growing, may not be detected because of their small size and low vascularity.

5. The brain scan is not the investigation of choice for pituitary tumours because these will only be detected when there is marked suprasellar extension.

Conclusion

The radionuclide brain scan, preferably performed with the appropriate dynamic blood flow study, is the investigation of choice for most intracranial space-occupying lesions. The majority of problems can be solved by this method, and those which need further investigation can be more clearly defined. The assessment of the brain scan, in association with the clinical findings, cannot be over-emphasized. The final relationship of radionuclide brain scanning with radiographic techniques is, as yet, not clearly defined, but future exciting developments are likely to be found in the field of functional metabolic imaging of the brain using Positron-emitting radioisotopes of carbon, oxygen and hydrogen to study glucose and amino acid metabolism etc.

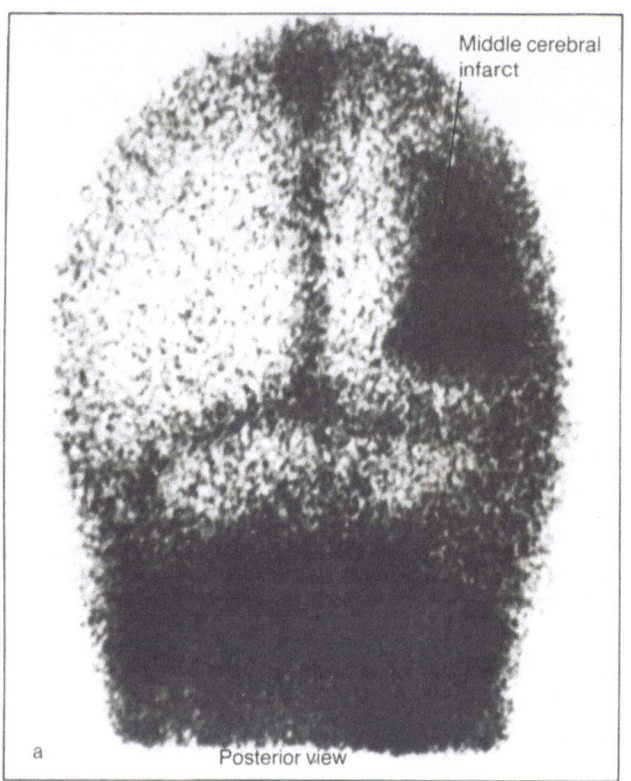

Middle cerebral infarct

a   Posterior view

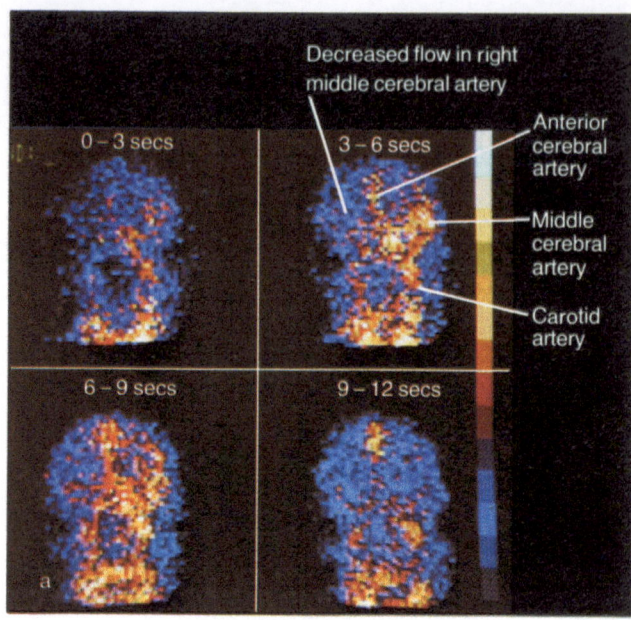

Decreased flow in right middle cerebral artery

Anterior cerebral artery

Middle cerebral artery

Carotid artery

0 – 3 secs

3 – 6 secs

6 – 9 secs

9 – 12 secs

a

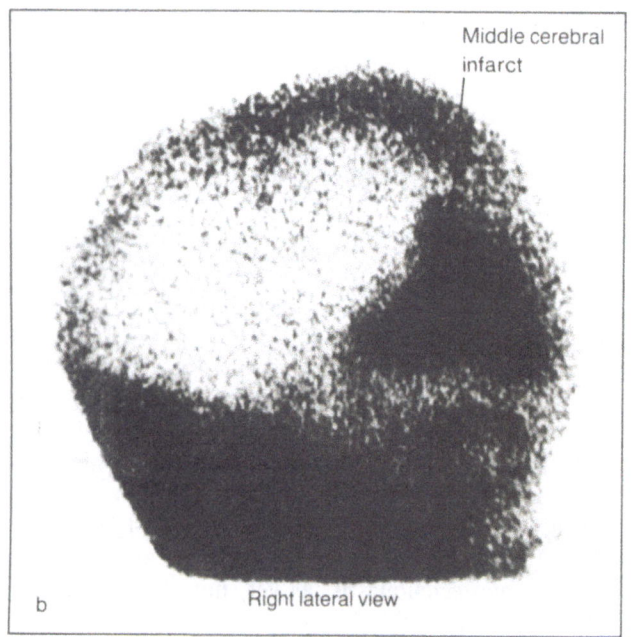

Middle cerebral infarct

b   Right lateral view

Figure 3.12 a and b *Middle cerebral artery infarct (posterior branches) showing the characteristic anatomic distribution with sparing of the posterior cerebral distribution.*

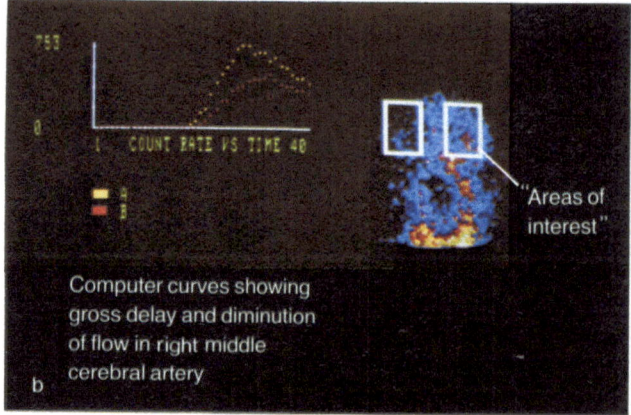

COUNT RATE VS TIME 40

"Areas of interest"

Computer curves showing gross delay and diminution of flow in right middle cerebral artery

b

Figure 3.13 a and b *Shows the dynamic blood flow study from the patient in Figure 3.12, demonstrating decreased flow due to the infarction.*

Further Reading for Chapter 3

Gilday, D. L. and Ash, J., *Radiol.*, 1975, **117**, 93.

Heck, L. L., Gottschalk, A. and Hoffer, P. B., *Static and Dynamic Brain Imaging (Diagnostic Nuclear Medicine)*, Gottschalk, A. and Potchen, E. J. (Eds.), Williams and Wilkins, Baltimore, 1976.

James, A. E., *Cisternography (Diagnostic Nuclear Medicine)*, Gottschalk, A. and Potchen, E. J. (Eds.), Williams and Wilkins, Baltimore, 1976.

Semin. Nucl. Med., 1977, **7** (2), 129.

▷

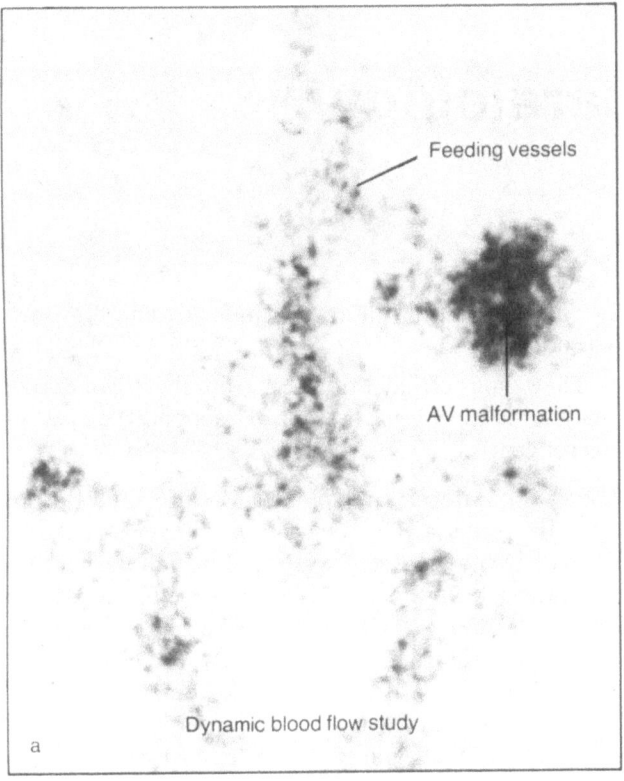

Figure 3.14a *Dynamic anterior view showing a highly vascular AV malformation presenting as epilepsy.*

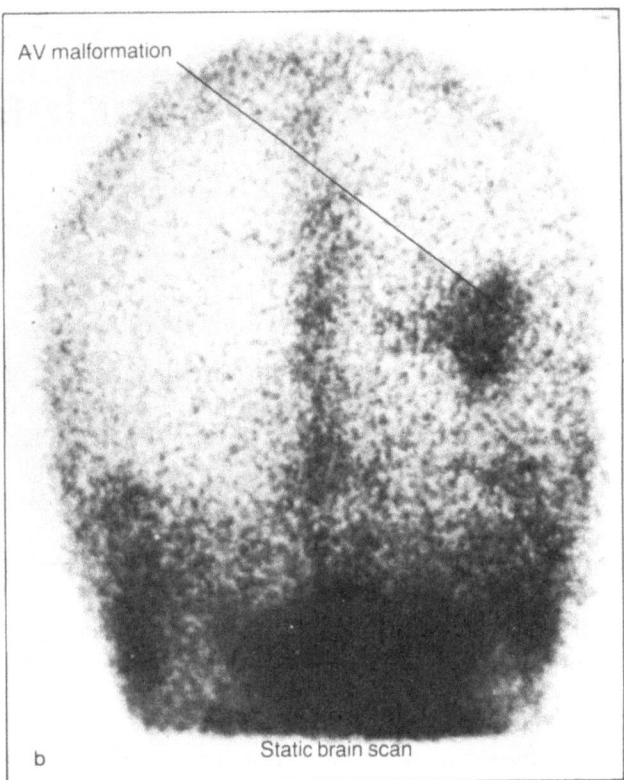

Figure 3.14b *Static anterior view showing a highly vascular AV malformation presenting as epilepsy.*

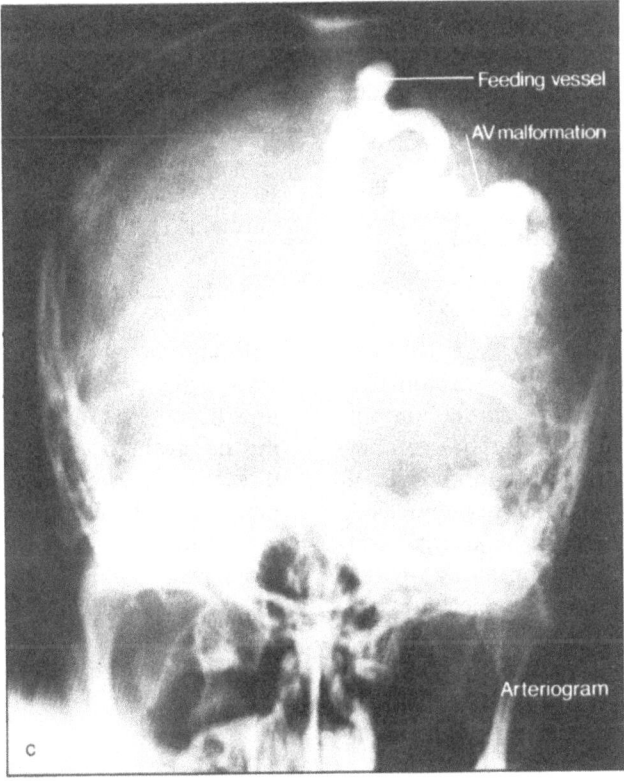

Figure 3.14c *Arteriogram confirming the vascular AV malformation, with large feeding vessel. (The same patient as a and b.)*

4. Nuclear Cardiology

Myocardial Perfusion Scintigraphy

A new dimension in the non-invasive investigation of cardiac disease has emerged from the developments in radiopharmaceuticals and from the progress which has been made within nuclear medicine over the last decade. The alliance of cardiology and nuclear medicine to form a new discipline, cardiovascular nuclear medicine, has ensured that these technical advances are widely applied to relevant problems encountered in clinical practice. Today, the cardiologist can be offered a detailed and accurate analysis of regional myocardial perfusion and ventricular wall motion in patients with a wide spectrum of cardiac disease.

The information which is obtained by myocardial scintigraphy is often complementary to that provided by conventional cardiac catheterization and angiography, but frequently it is unique. The techniques which are used now in cardiovascular nuclear medicine include:

1. Exercise thallium-201 (^{201}Tl) myocardial scintigraphy.

2. The first pass isotope angiogram.

3. Multiple gated acquisition of the cardiac blood pool using technetium-99m (^{99}Tc^m) labelled erythrocytes.

Physiology of Tracer Localization

Following a peripheral intravenous injection, radioactive monovalent cations (e.g. potassium-43, rubidium-81, caesium-129 and thallium-201) are distributed throughout the body (including the myocardium) in proportion to the fraction of the total cardiac output they receive. Similarly, the distribution of tracer concentration within any individual organ is proportional to the regional flow of blood within that organ. Therefore, regions of myocardial ischaemia or necrosis will fail to accumulate tracer and will appear as uptake defects or 'cold spots' on scintigrams which are obtained with these radionuclides.

Theoretically, certain criteria should be fulfilled before the regional concentration of a tracer within an organ can be considered a measure of its regional blood flow.

1. The tracer should be completely mixed with blood and streaming artifacts should be absent.

2. The distribution of tracer should be entirely flow-dependent.

3. The venous effluent of tracer from the organ during analysis should be nil (i.e. an extraction efficiency of 100 per cent).

The cationic tracers are soluble indicators and do not meet these criteria. They concentrate in oxygenated cells by an active transport across the cell-membrane which is determined by the Na$^+$/K$^+$ ATPase pump, a process which does not extract all the indicator from the circulating pool during its first transit. Therefore, these tracers differ from insoluble indicators, such as the labelled microspheres used in perfusion lung scanning. The latter are biodegradeable particles which are physically large enough to become completely enmeshed in the first capillary bed they encounter after injection (i.e. 100 per cent extracted) and which have a distribution determined by regional blood flow rather than regional metabolism.

In practice, when studying regional myocardial blood flow, labelled microspheres can only be administered by intracoronary injection because they are completely extracted by the lungs after an intravenous injection. However, many of the monovalent cations have a myocardial extraction efficiency which is high enough to provide useful information about regional myocardial perfusion.

Thallium-201

Although potassium-43 (^{43}K) is the prototype tracer for myocardial perfusion imaging, thallium-201 (^{201}Tl) has now become established as the imaging agent of choice in the evaluation of patients with ischaemic heart disease. Despite being chemically different from potassium, the hydrated ionic radius of thallium-201 is very similar in size to that of potassium and is biologically analogous. It has a high myocardial extraction efficiency (greater than 80 per cent) and more suitable imaging properties than the other monovalent cations.

Exercise Thallium-201 Myocardial Scintigraphy

Exercise myocardial scintigraphy comprises a routine

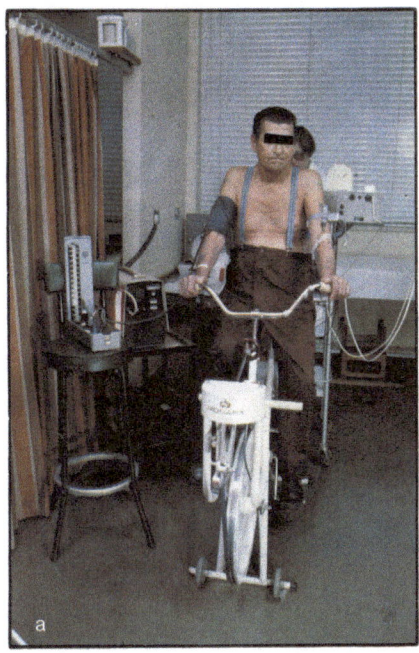

Figure 4.1a *Exercise test performed on a bicycle ergometer with monitoring of the ECG and blood pressure. The indwelling intravenous cannula is positioned before exercise and the portable defibrillator is ready for emergency use.*

stress electrocardiogram (using a bicycle ergometer or treadmill) and the addition of administration of an intravenous injection of ²⁰¹Tl at the time of maximal exercise (Figure 4.1a). Whenever possible, cardio-active drugs should be discontinued before the study, particularly drugs which act on cell-membrane transport systems.

At the onset of exercise limitation by angina pectoris (or whichever symptom limits exercise), 1.5 mCi of ²⁰¹Tl are administered through an indwelling intravenous cannula. The patient is instructed to continue exercise at

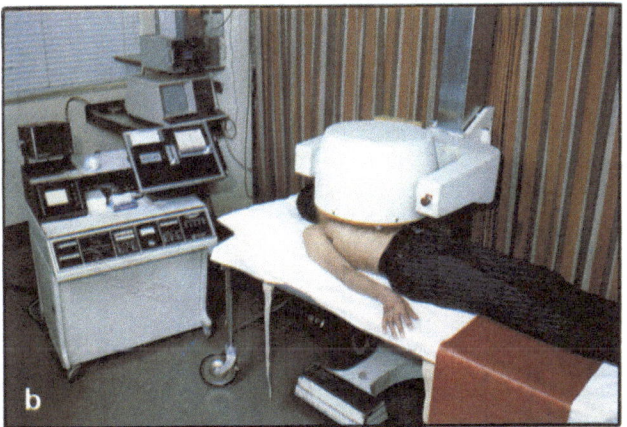

Figure 4.1b *The patient is positioned supine under a scintillation camera ready for cardiac imaging. Myocardial centering is checked with the persistence oscilloscope, which is seen on the upper right of the control console.*

this end-point for at least one to two minutes, then to stop gradually. The ECG is monitored throughout the procedure and during a 10 minute recovery phase. Resuscitation equipment, including a DC defibrillator, should be available if required.

The patient then reclines supine on a trolley, under a scintillation camera which is set to detect the 72.5 keV x-ray peak emitted from the mercury decay product of thallium-201 (Figure 4.1b).

Myocardial scintigrams are obtained routinely in four views: anterior, left anterior oblique (LAO) 45° and 55°, and left lateral projections. The images are simultaneously acquired on transparency film and stored on magnetic disc after digital conversion. Subsequent analysis of the image with simple enhancement and quantitation is then possible. These images, therefore, are the functional equivalent of the anatomical information derived from the coronary arteriogram.

The Normal Thallium-201 Myocardial Image

The myocardial image which is obtained with ²⁰¹Tl depends on tissue mass as well as myocardial blood flow and the extraction efficiency of the cation. Thus, the moderate reduction of activity, normally seen at the apex of the left ventricle in an anterior thallium scintigram, is caused by true thinning of the myocardium in this region and is not a pathological defect. Similarly, the atria are not visualized and the right ventricle is poorly seen in relation to the left ventricle because of the normal differences in myocardial mass seen in these regions.

The relatively even distribution of tracer found within the myocardium of a normal left ventricle is shown in Figure 4.2. The left ventricular chamber is seen particularly well in the LAO projection as a central cavity containing little tracer and surrounded by the septal, inferior and postero-lateral myocardial walls.

Segmental analysis of the myocardial count profile is possible, using the computer facility known as 'area of interest' analysis. The myocardial scintigram can be divided into regions which are outlined free-hand with a light-marker which is controlled by the investigator who uses a joy-stick at the computer console. The count rates in each region or area of interest are then displayed immediately. Normal segmental confidence limits can be established from data obtained in patients with no evidence of heart disease and used to assess suspected image defects more objectively (Figure 4.2e).

The Scintigraphic Anatomy of Ischaemic Heart Disease

Although the thallium-201 scintigram is a functional image of myocardial perfusion, coronary artery

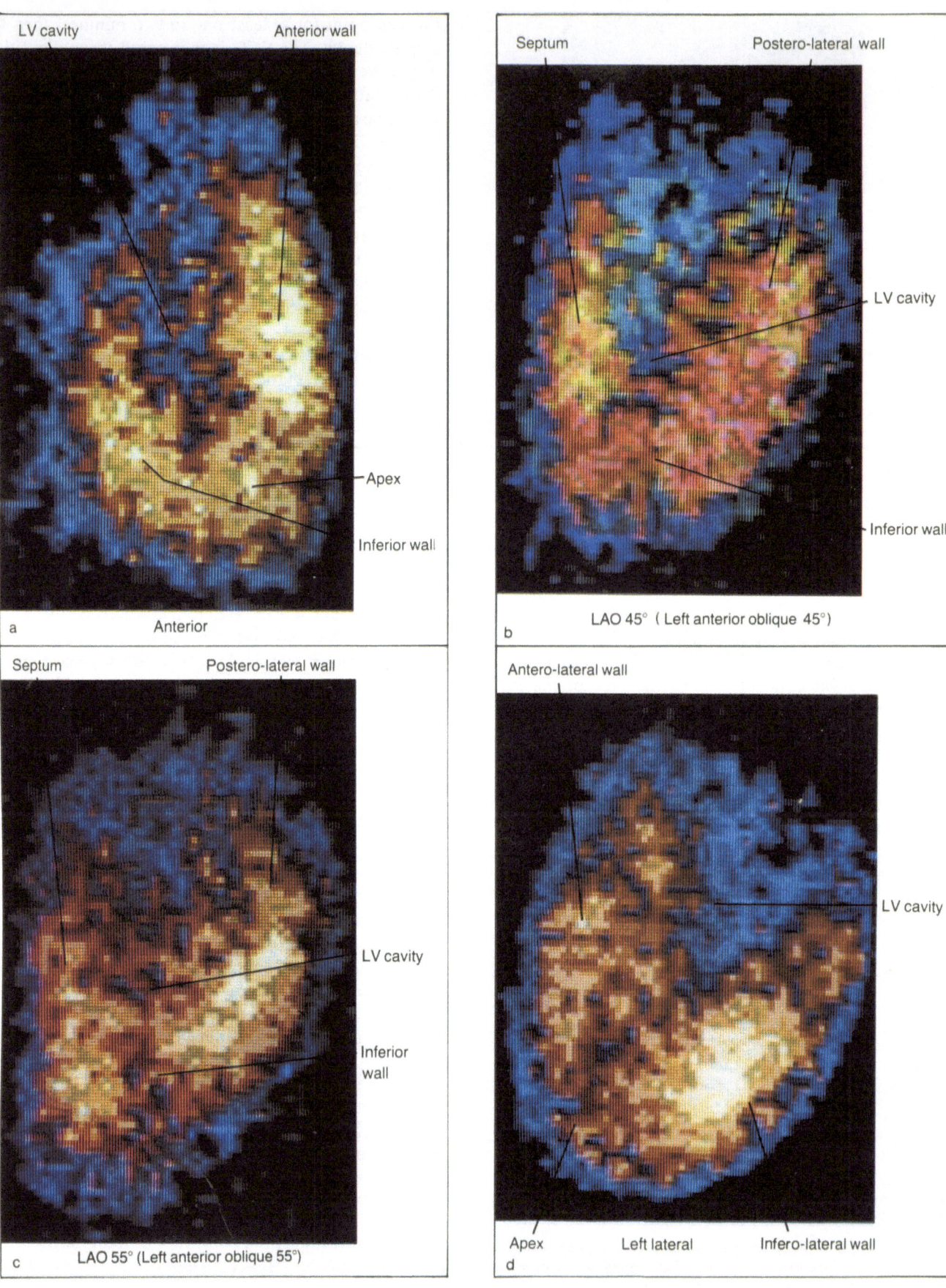

Figure 4.2a, b, c and d *Colour digital images of a normal left ventricle containing ^{201}Tl administered during exercise. The right ventricle and atria are not visualized.*

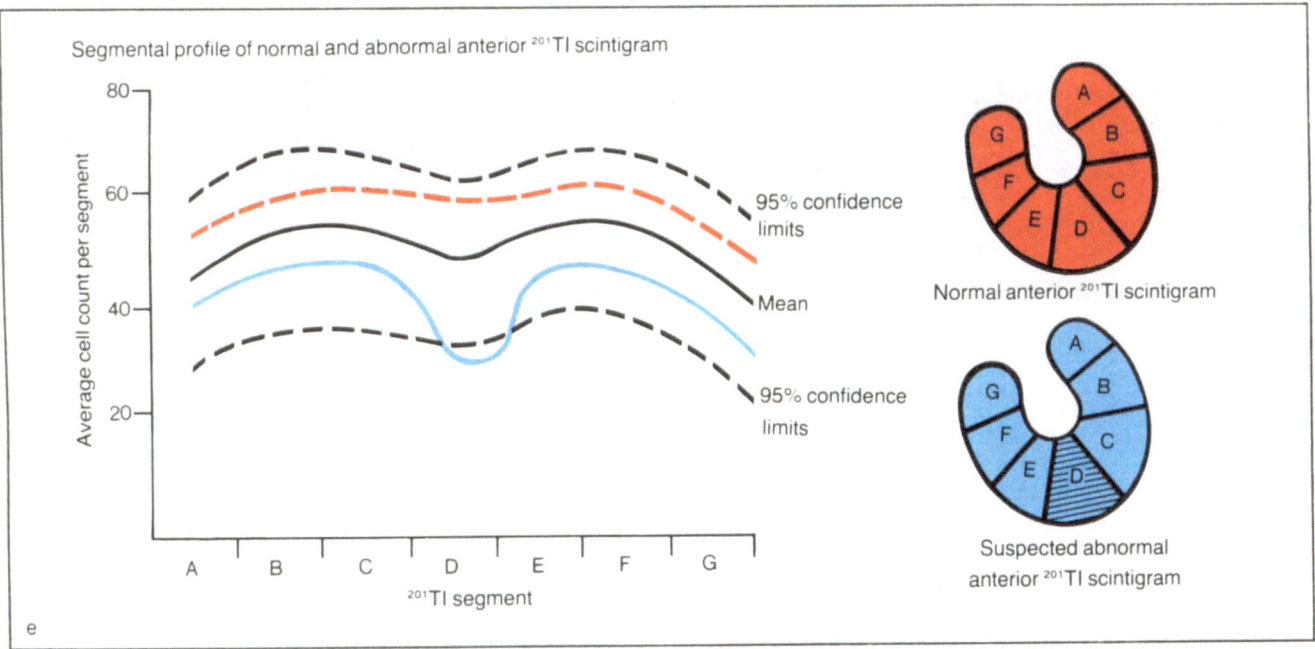

Figure 4.2e *Segmental regions of ²⁰¹Tl activity in the normal left ventricular myocardium can be used to establish a normal myocardial count profile, and confidence limits can be defined. Suspected abnormalities, such as in the apex of the left ventricle, can then be judged more objectively.*

stenoses or total occlusions cause corresponding deficits of tracer uptake in regions of the myocardial perfusion bed which is supplied by diseased vessels. Characteristic patterns of regional tracer deficit are found where there is disease in individual coronary vessels, and it is possible to predict lesions in these coronary arteries by observing the pattern of uptake defects seen in all four views of the myocardial scintigram.

Figure 4.3 provides the key to the interpretation of scintigraphic anatomy and shows that the LAO view is

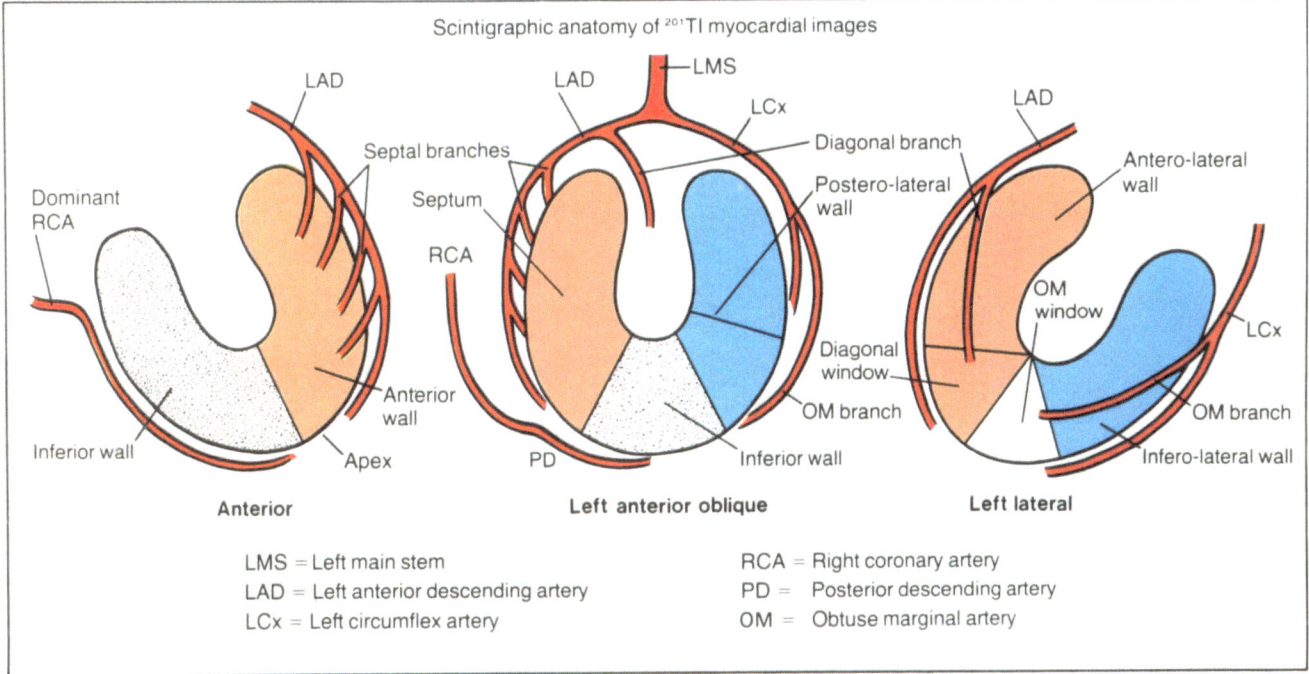

Figure 4.3 *Scintigraphic areas in different projections are delineated according to the major perfusion beds of the left ventricle supplied by specific coronary arteries. Coronary disease can cause any combination of scintigraphic uptake defects.*

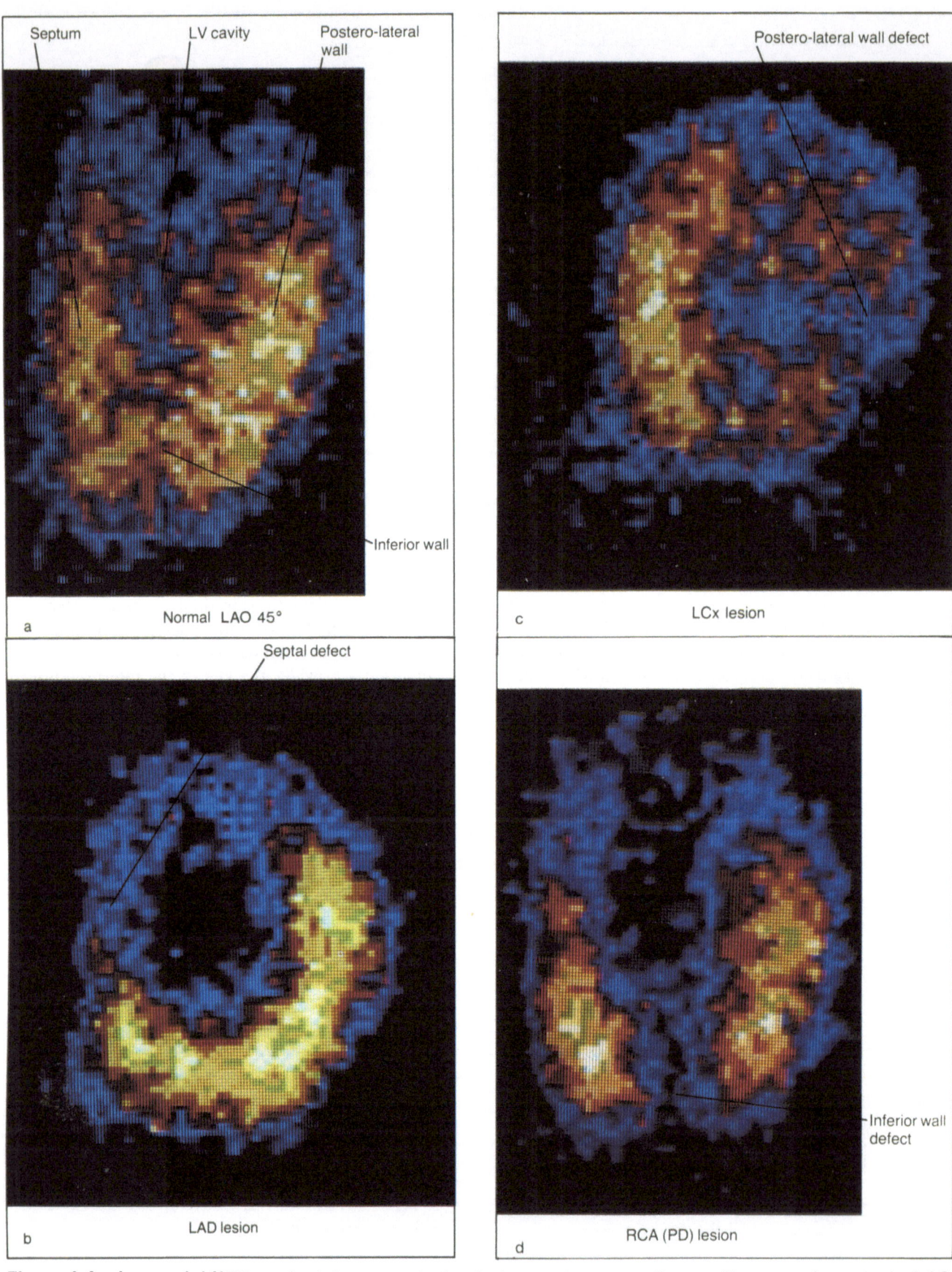

Figure 4.4a, b, c and d ^{201}Tl *uptake defects seen in the single vessel coronary disease. These are shown in the LAO views.* **(a)** *Normal LAO (45°) view,* **(b)** *decreased uptake in the septum due to a LAD lesion,* **(c)** *decreased uptake in the postero-lateral wall due to a left circumflex lesion, and* **(d)** *posterior wall defect due to posterior descending lesion.*

most useful for lesion localization. This is a useful view because the perfusion beds of all three major coronary vessels are maximally separated in this projection. The ventricular septum is supplied by descending septal branches from the left anterior descending (LAD) coronary artery; the inferior myocardial wall is supplied by the posterior descending (PD) artery, which is a branch of the right coronary artery (RCA) in over 80 per cent of subjects (right dominant system), while the postero-lateral wall is supplied by the left circumflex (LCx) vessel and its major obtuse marginal (OM) branch. Several examples of uptake defects caused by lesions in these individual vessels are shown in Figure 4.4.

Some uptake defects denote disease even in third generation coronary arteries, e.g. the diagonal branch of the LAD, and may have important localizing value within the coronary tree.

Delayed Imaging

Profound uptake defects in exercise ^{201}Tl myocardial scintigrams may be attributable either to regions of severe ischaemia or actual myocardial necrosis. In the absence of exercise-induced ischaemia, ^{201}Tl, when in-jected at rest, will be taken up by both normal myocardium and by myocardium which may be abnormal but which is not ischaemic at rest. However, ^{201}Tl will not be taken up by necrotic tissue as this causes a fixed uptake defect in a scintigram, under all conditions.

A similar differentiation can be accomplished more economically by abandoning separate rest and stress injections, and instead re-imaging the myocardium several hours after the initial administration of ^{201}Tl when significant intramyocardial redistribution of tracer has occurred (Pohorst et al. 1977).

An initial septal uptake defect which is seen shortly after exercise (Figure 4.5) may completely disappear during the reperfusion phase five and a half hours later and may be attributed to LAD coronary artery is-chaemia. The uptake defect in the inferior wall, which may be caused by inferior myocardial necrosis, may still be present at this late stage.

Clinical Uses of Thallium[201] Scintigraphy

Detection of Coronary Disease

Coronary disease affecting the proximal coronary arteries has a worse prognosis than disease affecting distal vessels. Similarly, multiple vessel disease has a

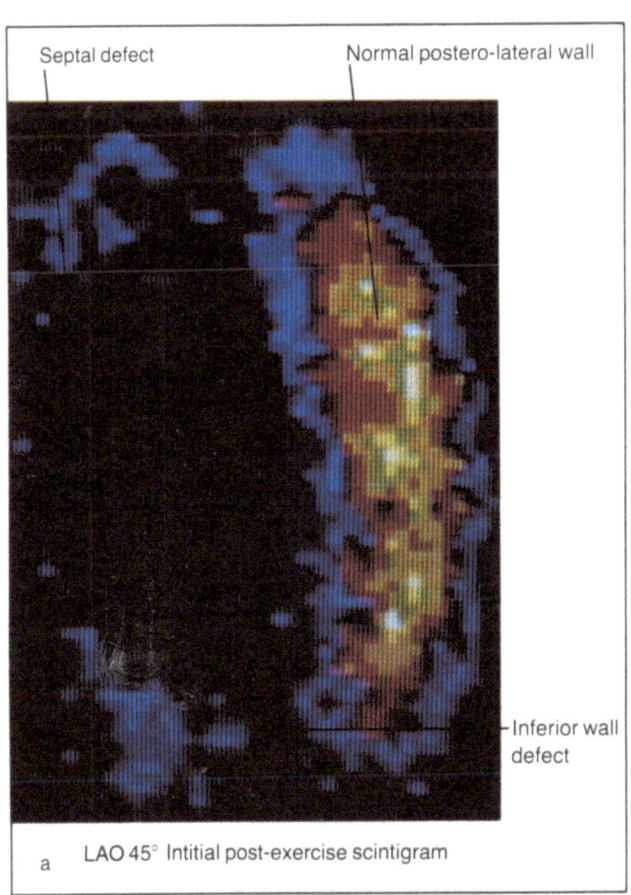

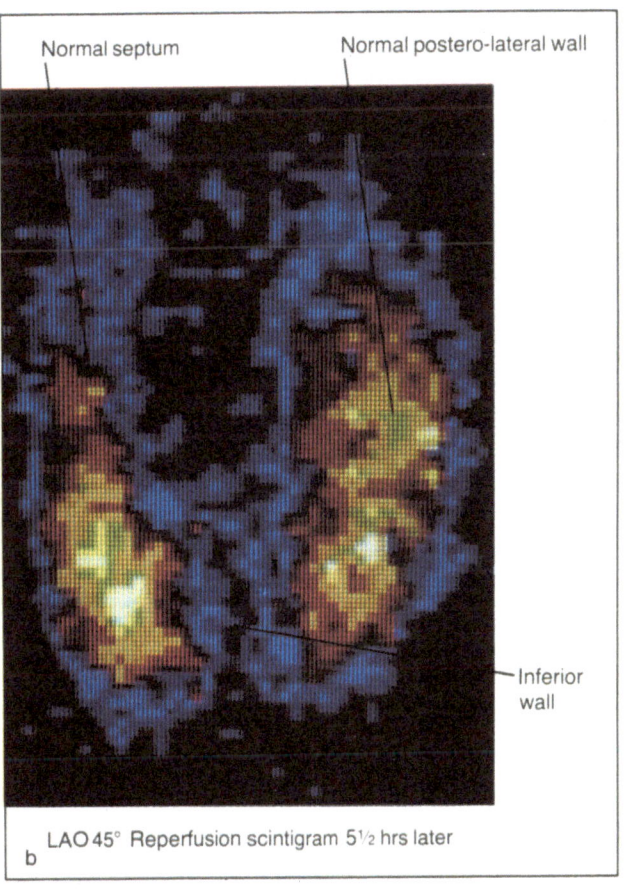

Figure 4.5 *The initial exercise ^{201}Tl scintigram* **(a)** *shows severe uptake defects in the septum and inferior myocardial wall, and* **(b)** *re-imaging some hours later indicated that the septal defect (due to reversible ischaemia) was no longer apparent but the inferior wall defect (due to fixed necrosis) remained unchanged.*

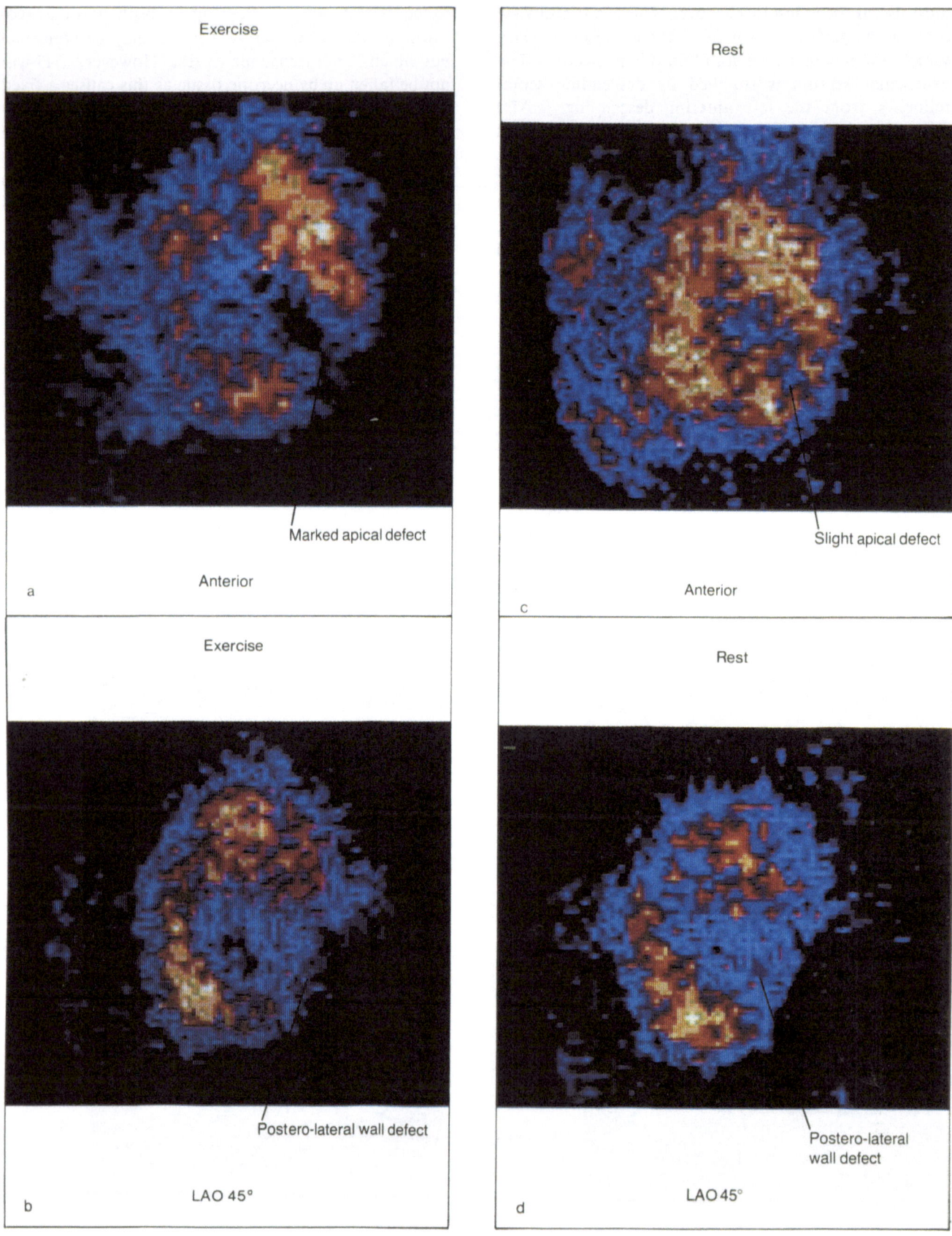

Exercise

Marked apical defect

a   Anterior

Exercise

Postero-lateral wall defect

b   LAO 45°

Rest

Slight apical defect

c   Anterior

Rest

Postero-lateral wall defect

d   LAO 45°

Figure 4.6 *Exercise* ^{201}*Tl scintigraphy demonstrates a reversible apical wedge defect in the anterior view, present on exercise but not rest (i.e. ischaemic defect). The left anterior oblique projection shows another defect in the postero-lateral wall which is unchanged in rest and exercise images (i.e. necrotic defect). Angina is thus attributable to the left ventricular apical region in this patient.*

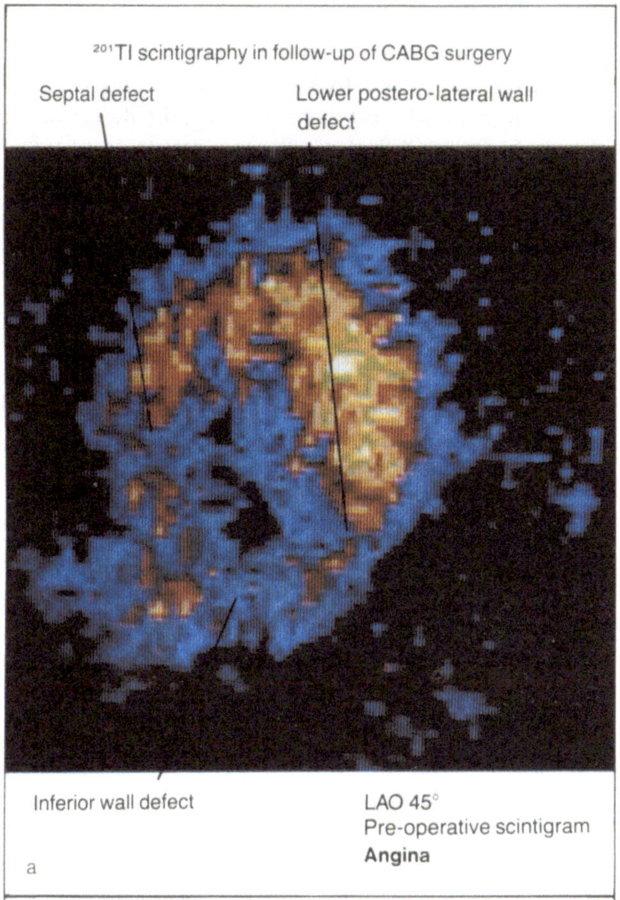

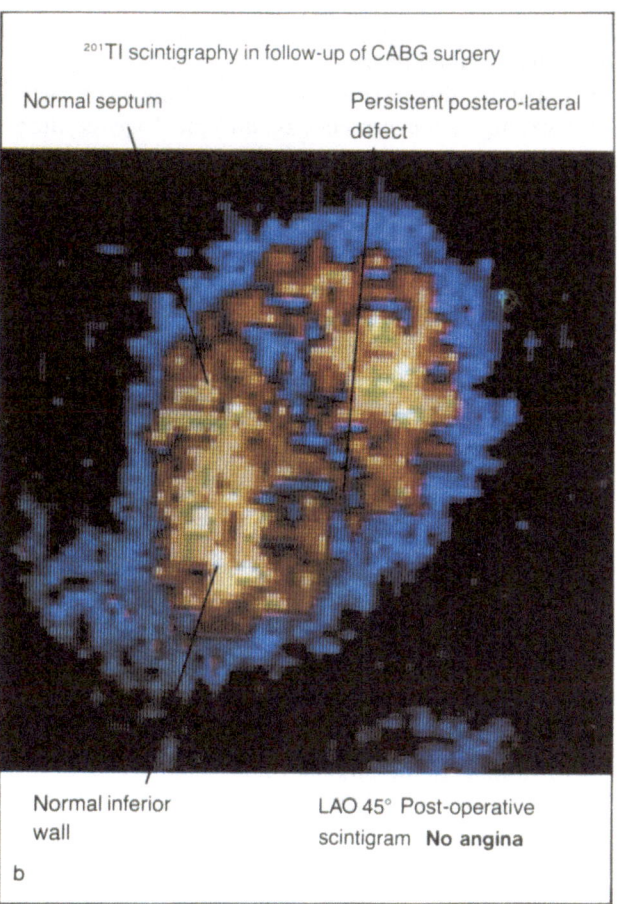

²⁰¹Tl scintigraphy in follow-up of CABG surgery

Septal defect

Lower postero-lateral wall defect

Inferior wall defect

LAO 45°
Pre-operative scintigram
Angina

a

²⁰¹Tl scintigraphy in follow-up of CABG surgery

Normal septum

Extensive inferior and postero-lateral wall defect

LAO 45°

Post-operative scintigram
Angina

c

²⁰¹Tl scintigraphy in follow-up of CABG surgery

Normal septum

Persistent postero-lateral defect

Normal inferior wall

LAO 45° Post-operative
scintigram **No angina**

b

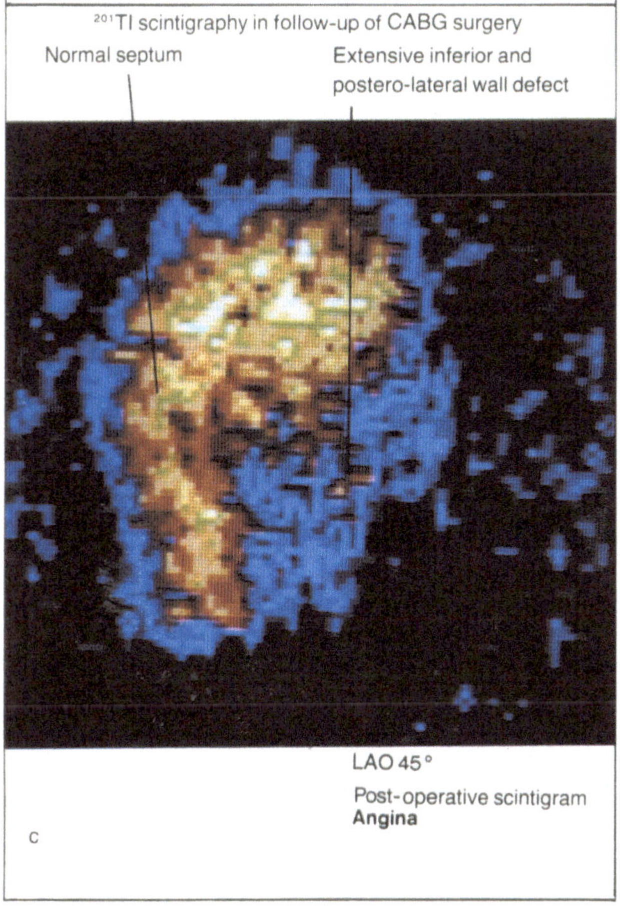

Figure 4.7 (a) *Regional uptake defects in a preoperative ²⁰¹Tl scintigram attributable to proven LAD, RCA and OM coronary disease. **(b)** Normalization of septal and inferior wall defects but persistence of postero-lateral wall defect following triple vessel CABG surgery. This degree of revascularization was associated with the disappearance of angina pectoris. **(c)** Second follow-up ²⁰¹Tl scintigram shows preservation of tracer uptake in the septum (LAD graft patent) but extension of the defect in the postero-lateral wall (RCA and OM graft occlusion). Angina returned despite the single patent graft.*

worse prognosis than single vessel disease. Recent reports confirm that coronary artery by-pass grafting (CABG) not only improves the quality of life in patients with ischaemic heart disease but also prolongs life in certain subgroups, particularly patients with left main coronary disease. It is vital to identify patients with life-threatening coronary anatomy who may present with unimpressive symptoms or no symptoms at all, e.g. referral of a patient whose exercise ECG is strongly positive for myocardial ischaemia in the absence of angina. Coronary arteriography cannot be recommended in every patient with chest pain, nor could it be realistically implemented. Exercise ²⁰¹Tl scintigraphy could be a useful screening test to select patients for definitive coronary arteriography. Knowledge of scintigraphic anatomy enables the investigator to predict, with a high degree of accuracy, both the presence of coronary disease and the affected coronary artery. For example, the presence of an apical wedge defect, septal tracer reduction and diagonal window means proximal LAD disease is highly probable and referral for coronary arteriography would be the right course of action. By contrast, in our laboratory a normal ^{201}Tl scintigram after maximal exercise means that a stenosis greater than 50 per cent in the major proximal coronary arteries is highly unlikely and further investigation is probably unwarranted.

In summary, exercise ^{201}Tl scintigraphy is a safe and non-invasive technique, more sensitive than the exercise ECG in the detection of coronary artery disease (Bailey et al. 1977), and provides prognostically significant information about specific coronary lesions.

The Assessment of Patients for Coronary Artery By-pass Graft (CABG) Surgery

The ability to distinguish regions of myocardial ischaemia from necrosis, by using ^{201}Tl scintigraphy, may be invaluable to the surgeon who is planning myocardial revascularization. Figure 4.6 shows uptake defects appearing on exercise in two regions of the myocardium supplied by different vessels—the LAD and LCx coronary arteries. Repeat rest scintigraphy no longer demonstrated the apical wedge defect which had been apparent on exercise, but the defect in the postero-lateral wall was persistent, i.e. the defect was caused by necrosis, and the postero-lateral wall is a region which is unlikely to benefit from coronary by-pass grafting. Thus, the apex of the left ventricle has been localized by this technique as an angina-producing segment of the myocardium, and an area relevant for surgical revascularization.

Postoperative Assessment after CABG Surgery

Recurrent chest pain following CABG surgery may be typical of angina pectoris, but it is frequently atypical; either situation may be associated with graft closure. A reliable non-invasive method of predicting this event would be extremely helpful in the management of these patients and is provided by ^{201}Tl scintigraphy. Figure 4.7 shows a sequence of ^{201}Tl images which were obtained from a patient who had triple vessel disease—the images were taken before and after CABG. In the first panel, defects are seen in the septum, inferior wall and postero-lateral wall, which correspond to coronary disease in this patient's LAD, RCA and OM vessels respectively. The first postoperative image (Figure 4.7 b) shows a significant improvement in tracer accumulation in the septum, but a defect persists in the lower postero-lateral wall despite by-pass grafting to all three vessels, i.e.

revascularization has been incomplete. Nevertheless, the patient remained free of angina and was discharged well. Angina recurred two months later and a repeat scintigram showed a new extensive uptake defect in the postero-lateral wall, but excellent preservation of tracer accumulation in the septum. From this appearance it was predicted that the LAD graft was patent but that the RCA and OM grafts were probably occluded, an interpretation which was later proved to be correct by coronary arteriography.

At the present these are the three most clinically relevant uses of this technique. However, Table 4.1 summarizes a number of valuable applications and potential applications of ^{201}Tl myocardial scintigraphy, many of which remain incompletely explored.

Thallium-201 myocardial scintigraphy has provided a significant step forward in the assessment of myocardial disease. It provides the necessary functional equivalent to the coronary arteriogram, and it is probably the most sensitive method for the detection of myocardial ischaemia. Thallium-201 myocardial scintigraphy should be the initial method of choice in the assessment of ischaemic heart disease.

Radionuclide Angiocardiography

The clinical importance of radiotracers which are taken

Table 4.1 Applications of Exercise ^{201}Tl Scintigraphy.

1. Detection of specific coronary artery disease, e.g. LAD disease, especially in public transport personnel, such as airline pilots, and in patients without symptoms but strongly positive exercise electrocardiograms.
2. Distinction of myocardial necrosis from myocardial ischaemia, e.g. in the preoperative assessment of CABG patients.
3. Follow-up of CABG patients—non-invasive detection of graft closure.
4. Assessment of patients with anginal pain and normal coronary arteriograms.
5. Investigation of chest pain in patients with hypertrophic cardiomyopathy.
6. Evaluation of the functional importance of the human coronary collateral circulation.
7. Monitoring changes in regional myocardial perfusion during physical training programmes and cardiac drug regimens.
8. As an independent aid to the interpretation of coronary arteriography.
9. Detection of intramyocardial masses, e.g. sarcoid granulomas, tumours etc.
10. Estimation of right ventricular mass in the prediction of pulmonary hypertension.
11. Prognosis of myocardial infarction related to extent of myocardial ischaemia and necrosis.

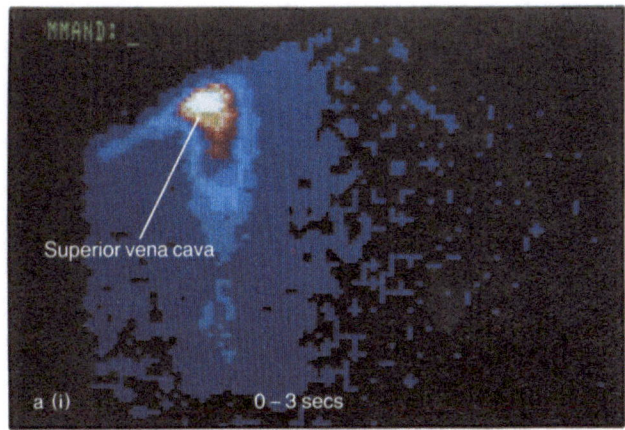

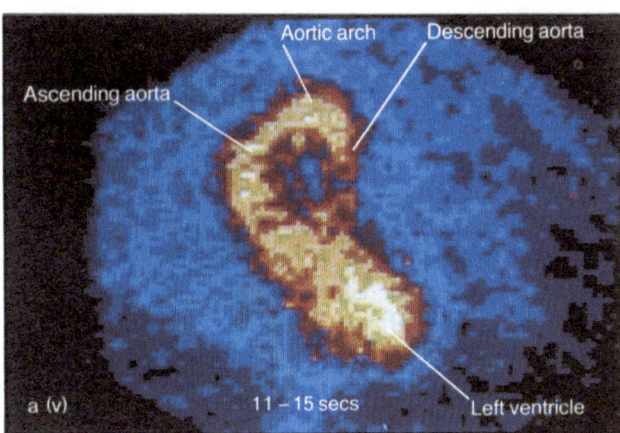

Figure 4.8a *Serial frames of the first pass of $^{99}Tc^m$-labelled red cells through the central circulation. Normal study showing distinct dextro-, pulmonary and laevo-phases in the correct temporal sequence.*

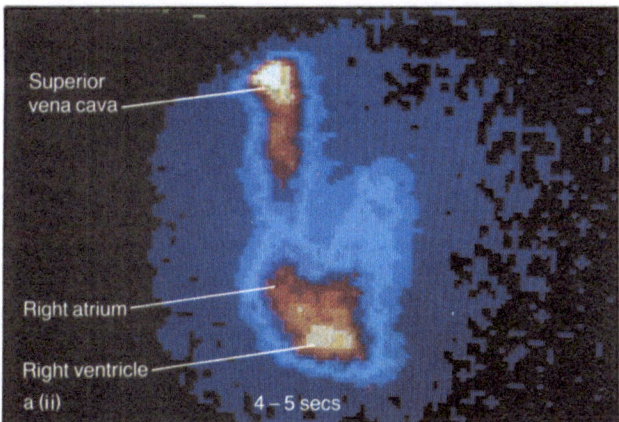

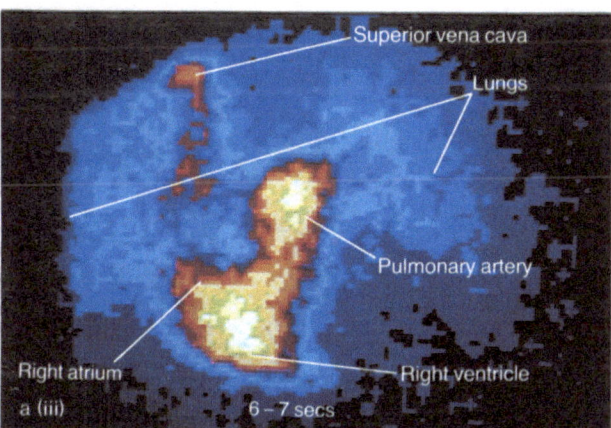

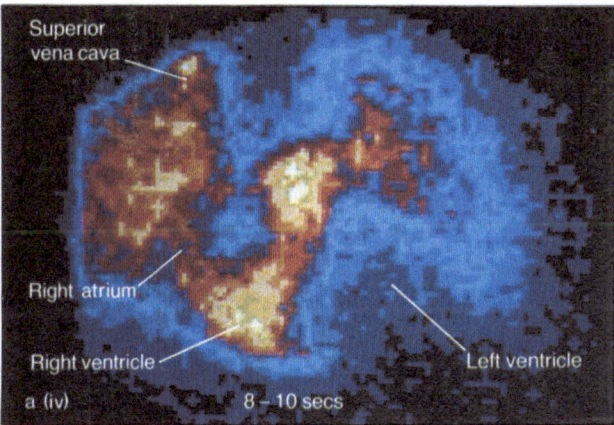

up into the myocardial muscle principally to assess regional abnormalities of perfusion in ischaemic heart disease has been discussed. Another important area is the use of tracers which stay within the cardiac blood pools. These may be imaged as a bolus of radiotracer makes its first passage through the heart (first pass isotope angiogram) for the assessment of functional cardiac anatomy and systemic-to-pulmonary shunting. Alternatively, the cardiac blood pool can be imaged at equilibrium, several minutes after the injection, during different phases of the cardiac cycle for the assessment of regional and total ventricular function.

First Pass Technique

The passage of a radionuclide bolus through the central circulation, after a simple intravenous injection, can be followed by rapid sequence imaging of the praecordium with a scintillation gamma camera. Technically, it is important to achieve a discrete bolus of radionuclide by rapidly injecting a small volume of tracer with high specific activity. In practice 10 to 12 mCi (0.5-1 ml) of technetium-99m ($^{99}Tc^m$), either as pertechnetate or labelled to human serum albumin, or autologous red cells, is injected into a peripheral arm vein and followed immediately by a flushing volume of saline as a 'chaser'. The rate of radionuclide delivery can be increased by leaving a venous tourniquet inflated on the right arm for five minutes, rapidly decompressing the cuff and then injecting tracer during the phase of reactive hyperaemia. Routinely, injections are made into right forearm veins because the venous return from this limb has a shorter and less tortuous course to the right atrium than does the venous return from the left arm. Advantage can be taken of central venous pressure lines already positioned in the superior vena cava, but routine use of these lines detracts from the minimally invasive nature of the standard technique.

The scintillation camera and data processing system are triggered by the detection of a preset minimal count rate and events are then recorded continuously by the computer in list mode (event-by-event) or in predetermined timed frames (histograms) for about 30 seconds. This information is conveniently stored on magnetic disc or tape and can be analysed immediately. Analogue images direct from the gamma camera may also be obtained by using an appropriate imaging device.

Qualitative Analysis

The physician notes the arrival of radionuclide in the superior vena cava and follows its transit through the right heart (dextro-phase), lungs and left heart (laevo-phase) by displaying sequential frames of the study on a TV monitor (Figure 4.8a). These are best displayed continuously, smoothly and repetitively to allow for maximal visual assessment.

This simple technique is helpful in the preliminary assessment of cyanotic congenital heart disease, e.g. in pathological right-to-left shunts, tracer appears prematurely in the laevo-phase of the study (i.e. visualization of the left ventricle and descending aorta) in relation to dextro-phase or pulmonary phase activity.

Conditions such as pulmonary atresia (Figure 4.8b) or tricuspid atresia are demonstrated when radionuclide transit terminates at the site of the absent valve.

In Fallot's tetralogy there is delay in pulmonary filling with early appearance of the ascending aorta, but

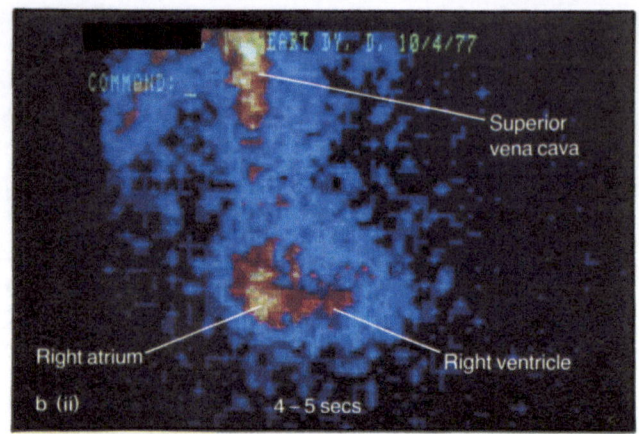

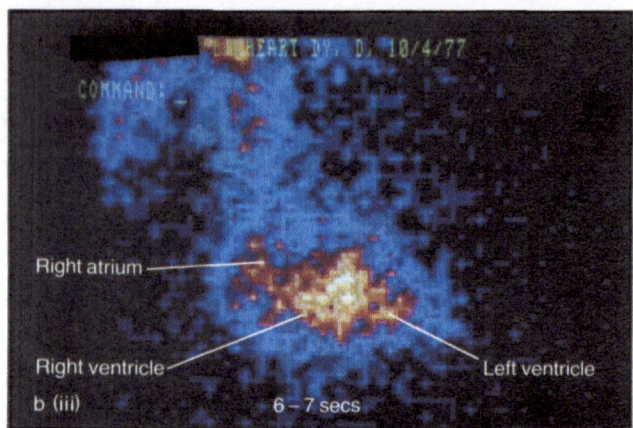

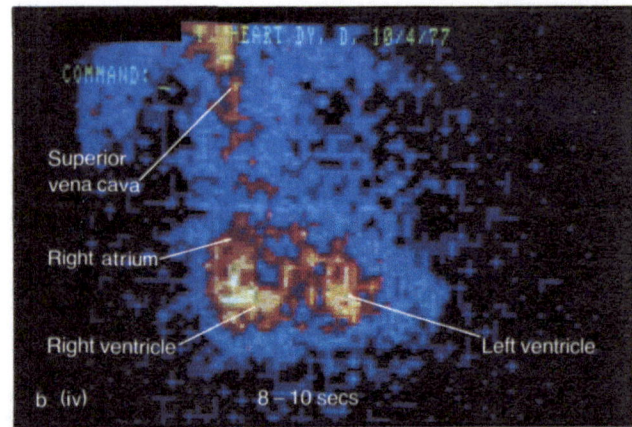

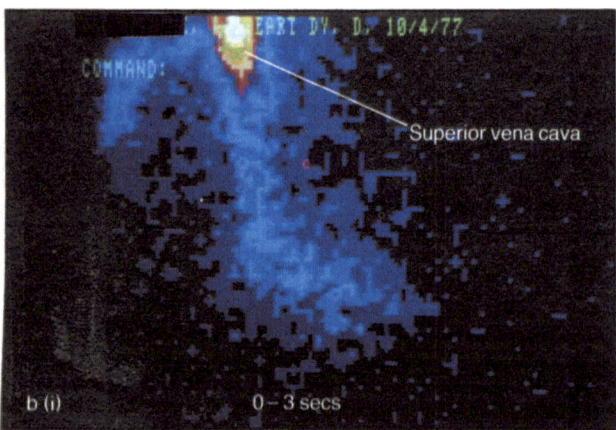

Figure 4.8b *Serial frames of the first pass of $^{99}Tc^m$-labelled red cells through the central circulation. In pulmonary atresia the pulmonary conus is not visualized at all and pulmonary phase activity appears late and is asymmetrical (left lung activity greater than right lung activity). The left ventricle and ascending aorta are seen early in relation to pulmonary activity (premature laevo-phase) indicating an intracardiac right-to-left shunt.*

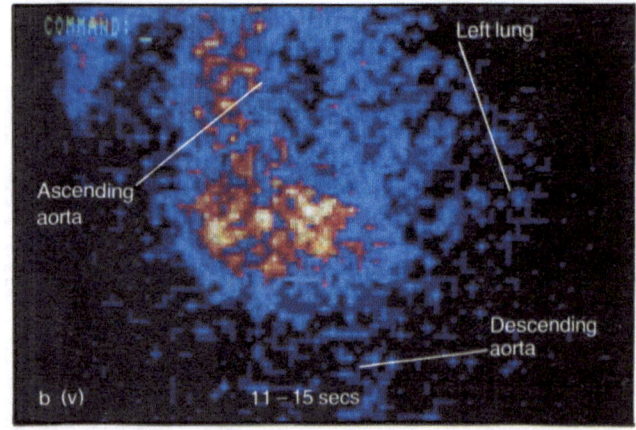

the anatomical resolution of the first pass technique does not allow its accurate differentiation from functionally similar conditions, e.g. double outlet right ventricle with pulmonary stenosis.

Intracardiac left-to-right shunts with rapid intracardial recirculation of the radioactive tracer (the magnitude of which is visually recognized by persistence of high levels of radionuclide activity in the lungs and an indistinct laevo-phase) can be measured using suitable simple dedicated data processing systems.

Quantitative Analysis

By selecting 'areas-of-interest' with the computer light marker, the investigator can divide the radionuclide angiogram into several curves of activity against time. The quality of the tracer bolus is checked by the sharpness or 'spike function' of an activity-time curve which is obtained from the superior vena cava, and the absence of a left-to-right intracardiac shunt can be confirmed by the normal shape of a pulmonary activity-time curve (Figure 4.9). Early recirculation (e.g. via a VSD) prolongs the rate of decline of this curve in proportion to shunt magnitude and, thus, enables an estimate of shunt size. This method of detection is more sensitive than the Fick method, using oxygen saturation analysis, and accurately quantitates shunts which are not at either extreme of flow.

During the first passage of the radioactive bolus through the cardiac chambers, very fast analysis of the changes in activity within the left ventricular cavity demonstrates systole and diastole and enables the ejection fraction to be calculated. (Figure 4.10.) The peaks and troughs of activity inscribed in the main curve derive from counts at ventricular end-diastole and end-systole respectively. A correction for background activity must be made and the ejection fraction is computed as:

$$EF = \frac{\text{Diastolic counts} - \text{Systolic counts}}{\text{Diastolic counts} - \text{Background counts}} = \frac{\text{Stroke volume}}{\text{End-diastolic volume}} \times 100 \text{ per cent}$$

It is an advantage in ischaemic heart disease that in this method there are no assumptions made about ventricular geometry in the calculation of the ejection fraction.

Although ejection fraction is a useful overall estimate of left ventricular function this measurement may vary with both preload and afterload, independent of changes in myocardial function. However, changes of ejection fraction in response to intervention, e.g. drugs, exercise or cold stimulation, are a better means for detecting abnormalities of ventricular function. Segmental wall motion of the left ventricle is a sensitive additional measure of ventricular function, and can also be determined. Single pass radioisotope angiography can be used to provide this information but multiple

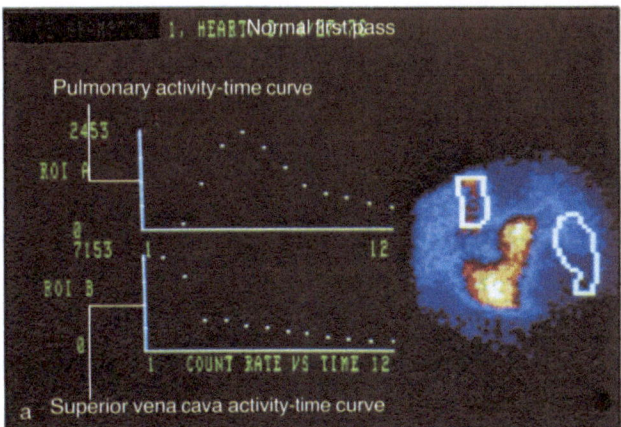

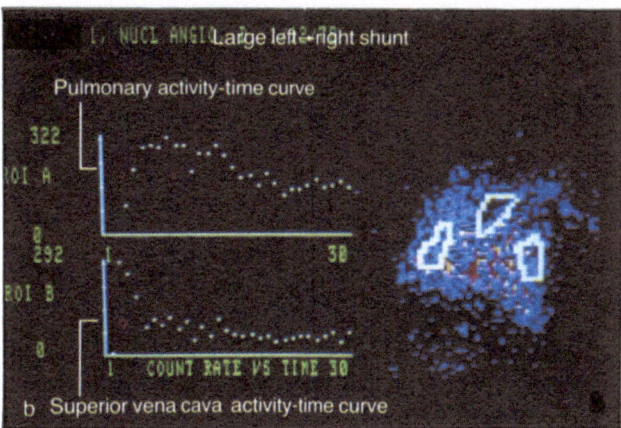

Figure 4.9a and b *Activity-time curves from the pulmonary area (upper curve) and superior vena cava (lower curve) in (a) a normal subject and (b) a patient with a large left-to-right intracardiac shunt. The SVC curve is sharp in both cases, indicating a good bolus of tracer, but there is marked prolongation of the peak activity and rate of decline in the pulmonary curve of the patient with the left-to-right shunt.*

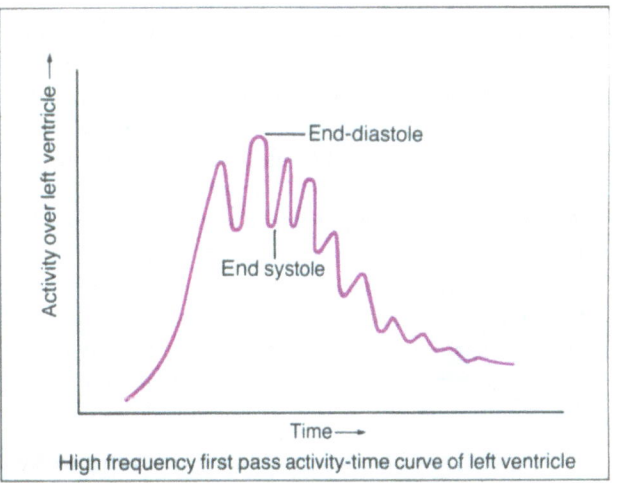

Figure 4.10 *High frequency analysis of the first pass of tracer through the left ventricle shows peaks and troughs of radioactivity representative of end-diastolic volume and end-systolic volume respectively.*

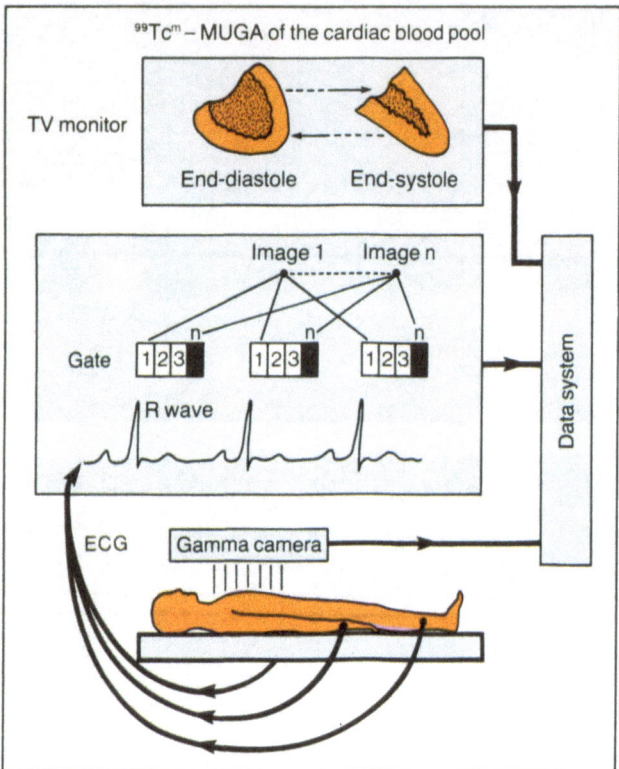

Figure 4.11 *Activity in serial time periods (gates) following the R wave of the ECG is algebraically summated to produce corresponding images of the cardiac cycle which can be displayed in movie mode on a TV monitor.*

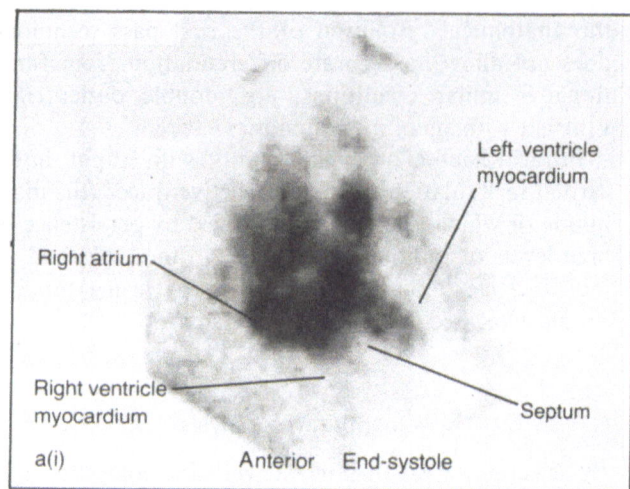

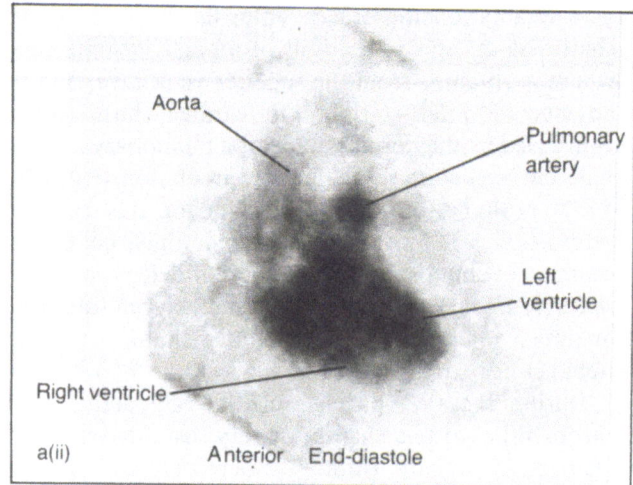

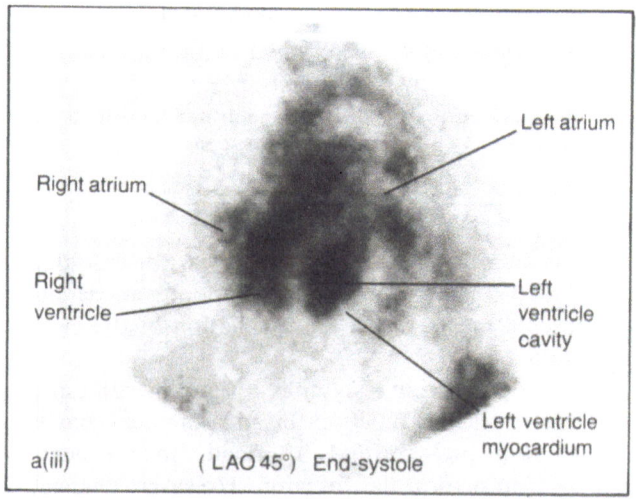

gated imaging at equilibrium is probably superior (discussed later).

No information about arterial pressure can be derived from this technique, and this is an important limitation in the follow-up of patients with moderate left-to-right shunts who are treated conservatively. Thus, a net left-to-right shunt at ventricular level may diminish due to spontaneous anatomical closure of the septal defect or result from the development of pulmonary hypertension with equilibration of right and left ventricular pressures. In both situations a pulmonary activity-time curve will show a reduction of the left-to-right shunt thereby providing false reassurance in the latter instance.

Nevertheless, in the paediatric patient with a systolic murmur it is extremely useful to have a simple, sensitive, minimally invasive screening technique to detect left-to-right intracardiac shunts. A completely normal result enables the paediatric cardiologist to reassure the parents and forego further invasive investigation.

Multiple Gated Radionuclide Ventriculography and the Evaluation of Myocardial Function

Technique

Some of the limitations of the first pass technique have

been overcome by imaging the praecordium after tracer has equilibrated in the cardiac blood pool, then physiologically triggering the scintillation camera to record certain phases of the cardiac cycle (gated cardiac blood pool acquisition). Initially, two images of the

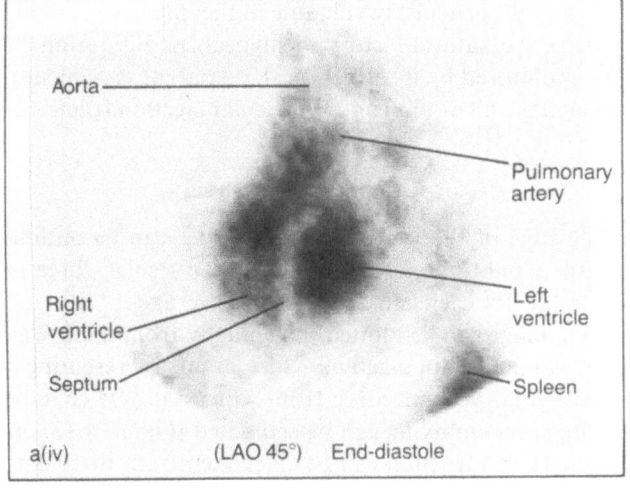

a(iv)   (LAO 45°)   End-diastole

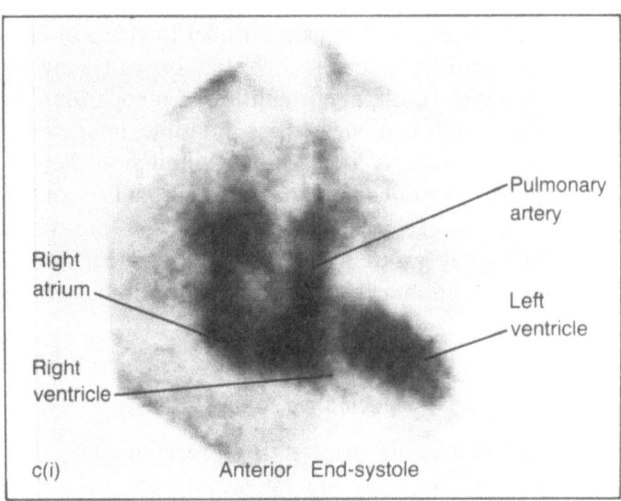

c(i)   Anterior   End-systole

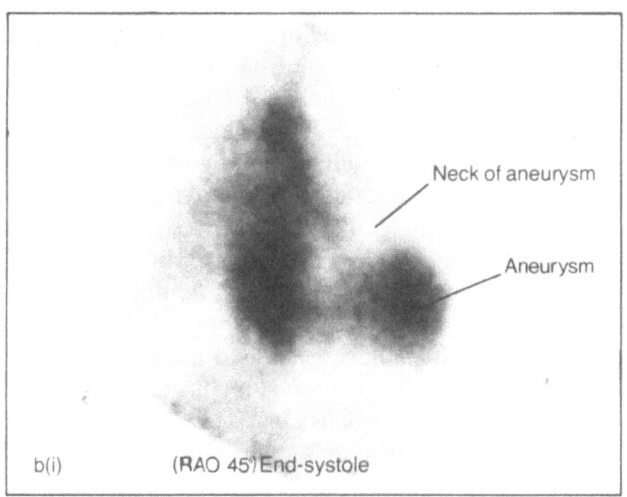

b(i)   (RAO 45°) End-systole

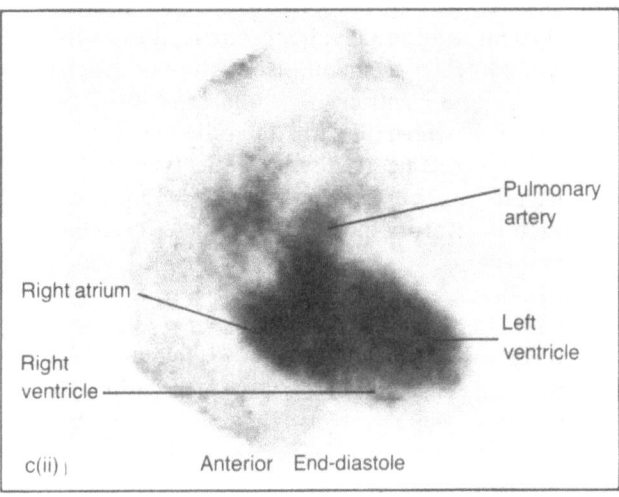

c(ii)   Anterior   End-diastole

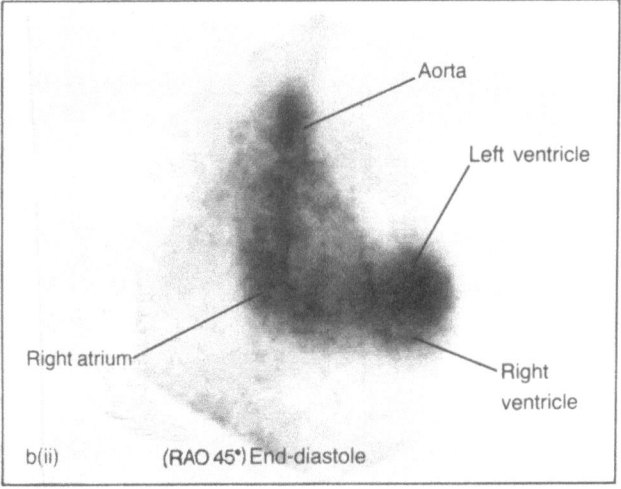

b(ii)   (RAO 45°) End-diastole

Figure 4.12a, b and c (far left, left and above) $^{99}Tc^m$ *MUGA cardiac blood pool scintigraphy showing* (**a**) *normal end-diastolic and end-systolic left ventricular silhouettes in comparison with those seen in* (**b**) *left ventricular aneurysm. Regional paradoxical wall movement in aneurysmal ventricles is readily appreciated during cine-movie display and* (**c**) *congestive cardiomyopathy. The large, poorly contracting ventricle is clearly appreciated.*

during these short phases or 'gates' of 50 to 70 msec duration (Figure 4.11). A stable cardiac rhythm (i.e. a regular R-R interval) is necessary for the selected delay intervals of the gates to correspond to exactly the same phase of wall motion in each cardiac cycle. Separate summation of the counts in each gate over several hundred cardiac cycles eventually produces two radionuclide images corresponding to end-systole and end-diastole (Figure 4.12a).

Recent developments, using more elaborate computer-based techniques, enable multiple (10 to 60) gates to be spanned serially over the cardiac cycle with the production of corresponding multiple images, i.e. multiple gated acquisition (MUGA). This increase in

cardiac chambers were obtained by using the R wave of the electrocardiogram (ECG) and the downslope of the T wave to signal periods of ventricular end-diastole and ventricular end-systole respectively. In each cardiac cycle the scintillation camera acquired counts only

39

temporal resolution brings a parallel increase in functional resolution and the investigator can now appreciate quite subtle abnormalities of myocardial wall movement. He can view these multiple images in a continuous ('endless loop') movie, similar to the cine-angiogram obtained by conventional contrast angiography, except that both ventricles are visible simultaneously as well as the atria and great vessels. (Table 4.2 summarizes current applications of this technique).

Qualitative Analysis

In congenital heart disease this procedure may be a valuable preliminary investigation to select the projection in which certain cardiac structures are optimally defined so that definitive angiography can be planned more accurately. For example, the resolution of the radionuclide technique is sufficient to detect the presence of a ventricular septum and to define the projection in which this structure is best profiled.

In ischaemic heart disease patients with localized ventricular aneurysms (Figure 4.12b) can be differentiated from those with diffuse ventricular hypo-kinesis (Figure 4.12c) and recommended for further cardiac investigation and possible surgery.

Ventricular images of good spatial resolution can be acquired for several hours after a single dose of $^{99}Tc^m$-labelled red cells and the effect of interventions, such as exercise or nitroglycerine therapy, on global and regional ventricular wall function can be assessed. This facility is particularly valuable in the intensive care unit where the natural history of myocardial infarction can be monitored by its effect on the serial measurement of regional wall motion and ventricular ejection fraction.

Quantitative Analysis

The edge of the ventricular silhouettes can be outlined with a light-marker to define a ventricular 'area-of-interest' for each gated image. The average count rate in each image can be plotted sequentially from the R wave to obtain a time-activity histogram representing a ventricular volume curve from which rates of chamber filling and emptying can be estimated (Figure 4.13) and the ejection fraction can be calculated from these data. A correction for background activity is essential to achieve an accurate estimate of the ejection fraction. This is usually obtained by drawing a C-shaped area of interest around the end-diastolic frame close to the ventricular edge. This choice of background area has inherent limitations and may include right ventricular activity and left atrial activity during different phases of the cardiac cycle, e.g. the ventricular end-systolic count rate may be falsely inflated by overlying left atrial activity (maximal in this part of the cardiac cycle), with overestimation of the end-systolic volume and under-estimation of the ejection fraction. Recently, semi-automatic methods have been used to outline the edge of the ventricle and to subtract a constant background area, before the left ventricular activity time curve is plotted and the ejection fraction has been calculated.

Table 4.2 Applications of multiple gated acquisition ($^{99}Tc^m$ MUGA) of the cardiac blood pool.

Detection of patients with ischaemic heart disease
Acute myocardial infarction (casualty and intensive care unit)
Chronic obstructive coronary disease

Assessment of patients with ischaemic heart disease
e.g; Determination of ejection fraction:
Differentiation of reversible and irreversible regions of ventricular asynergy in preparation for coronary artery saphenous vein by-pass grafting
Detection of ventricular aneurysm
Effect of drugs and other interventions such as exercise and physical training.

Assessment of right ventricular function
e.g; Right ventricular infarction causing:
Cardiogenic shock
Cor pulmonale (recurrent pulmonary emboli, etc.)

Detection of congestive cardiomyopathy and hypertrophic cardiomyopathy

Assessment of congenital heart disease
such as; discovering whether there is one ventricle or two

Detection of left atrial myxoma

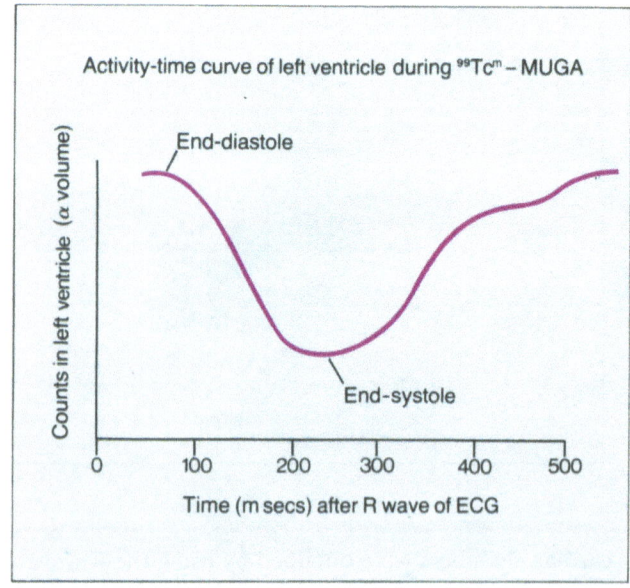

Figure 4.13 *Left ventricular volume time-curve can be plotted from the variation in counts over the ventricle during systole and diastole. Ejection fraction and rates of chamber filling and emptying can be estimated.*

This method has excellent observer reproducibility and comparison with biplane contrast angiography gave a correlation coefficient of 0.93 for ejection fraction determination.

In contrast to patients without ischaemic heart disease, Borer et al. (1978) have shown that patients with coronary artery disease tend to reduce their left ventricular ejection fraction on exercise and to develop abnormalities of regional myocardial wall motion which, in some instances, are prevented by treatment with prophylactic nitroglycerine. Exercise $^{99}Tc^m$ MUGA cardiac blood pool scintigraphy seems to be a sensitive method to detect those patients with coronary artery disease who are asymptomatic.

Combined ^{201}Tl and MUGA Scintigraphy

At present, it is not known whether exercise ^{201}Tl myocardial scintigraphy is more sensitive than $^{99}Tc^m$ MUGA cardiac blood pool scintigraphy in the detection of patients with ischaemic heart disease, and this remains an issue that future comparison will resolve. Both techniques are now established assets and can be suitably combined as one sequential procedure in individual patients. This dual-nuclide scintigraphy must begin with ^{201}Tl myocardial imaging before studies with the $^{99}Tc^m$ label, because the higher energy of the latter precludes sequential studies in the reverse order.

The information which is obtained by both techniques is complementary in that disturbances of regional myocardial perfusion cause corresponding alterations of ventricular wall movement. Severe uptake defects of ^{201}Tl on exercise, which correspond with regional akinesis or dyskinesis at rest, are liable to be caused by myocardial necrosis, whereas a similarly severe ^{201}Tl defect on exercise, which is associated with a region of reversible asynergy at rest, suggests severe ischaemia as the basis for both abnormalities.

Conclusion

The advances in the non-invasive assessment of cardiac wall motion and regional myocardial perfusion in man are a tribute to the successful integration of nuclear medicine and cardiology in a union that is progressing rapidly. The emphasis has been placed on the contribution already made by ^{201}Tl scintigraphy and $^{99}Tc^m$ MUGA cardiac blood pool imaging, but the limitations of both techniques operate continuously and challenge improvement.

References
Borer, J. S., Bacharach, S. L., Green, M. V., Kent, K. M., Johnston, G. S. and Epstein, S. E., *Circ.*, 1978, **57**, 314.

Further Reading
Bailey, I. K., Griffiths, L. S. C., Rouleau, J., Strauss, H. W. and Pitt, B., *Circ.*, 1977, **55**, 79.
Pohorst, G. M., Zir, L. M., Moore, R. H., McKusick, K. A., Gruiney, T. E. and Beller, G. A., *Circ.*, 1977, **55**, 294.
Prog. Cardiovasc. Dis., 1977, **20** (Nos. 1 and 2).
Strauss, H. W. and Pitt, B., *Circ.* (Editorial), 1978, **57**, 645.
Strauss, H. W., Pitt, B. and James, A. E. (Jr) (Eds), *Cardiovascular Nuclear Medicine*, C. V. Mosby Co., St. Louis, Mo, USA, 1974.

5. Imaging the Skeleton with Radionuclides

The use of radionuclide bone scanning has increased more rapidly in recent years than the other nuclear medicine investigations. This has resulted in a dramatic change in the approach to the investigation and study of bone disease. This growth is almost entirely due to the work of Subramanian and his co-workers (1971) when they labelled polyphosphate with technetium-99m and demonstrated that it could be used to depict accurately the activity of bone disease. Until then, bone scanning was being performed infrequently due to the limitations imposed in the use of the available radionuclides.

Initially, isotopes of strontium were used, but these had poor imaging characteristics and often resulted in a high radiation dose to the patient, thus limiting the value of the investigation and restricting the number of patients for whom it could reasonably be used. Subsequently, the use of fluorine-18 began, but this also had a number of significant drawbacks. The gamma ray

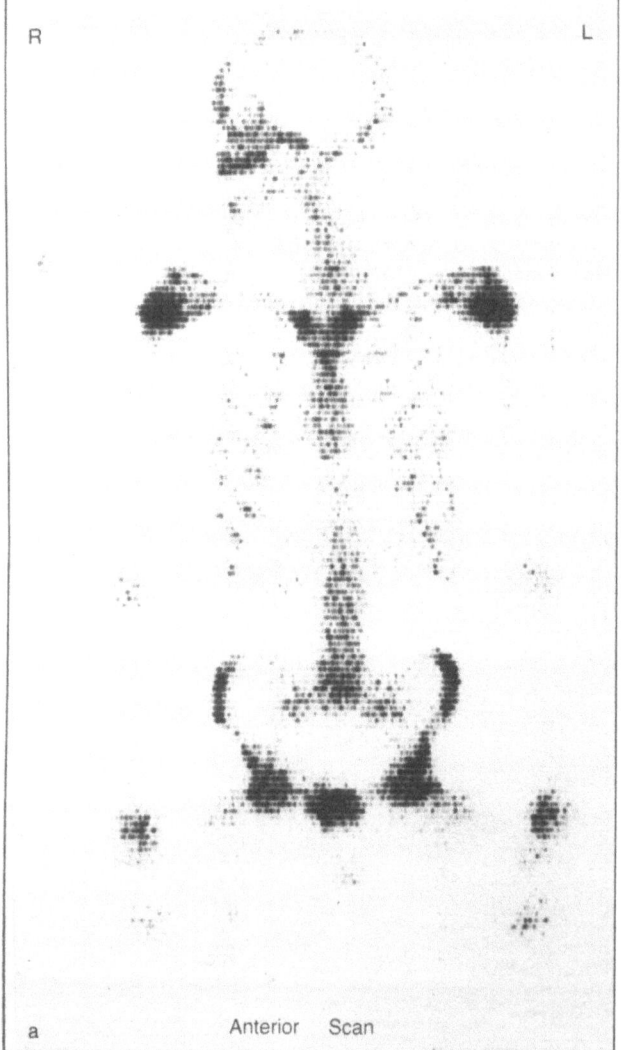
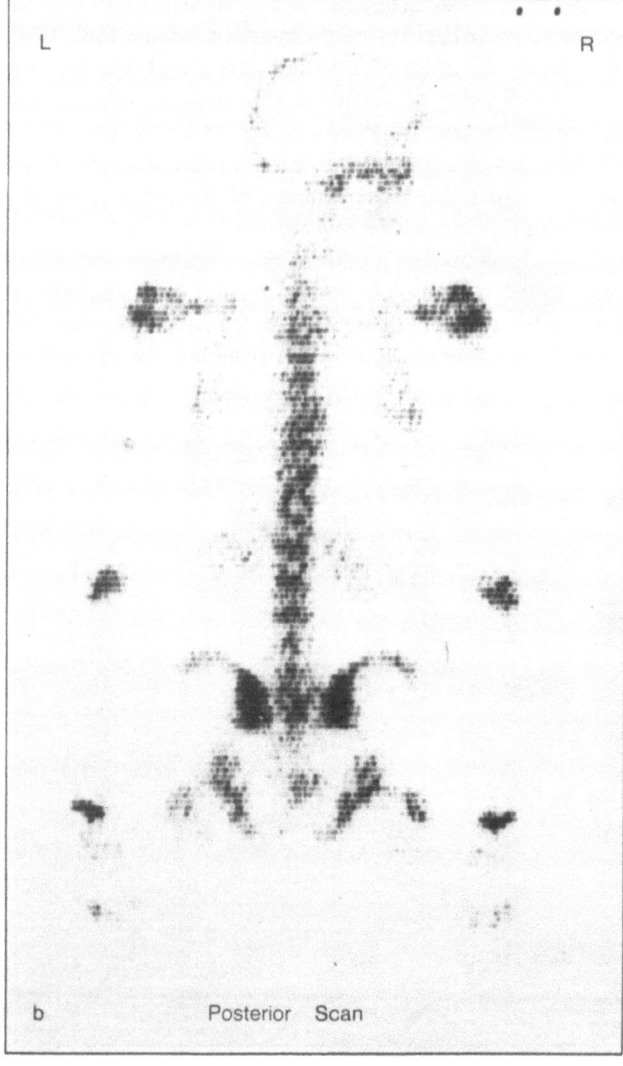

Figure 5.1a and b *Normal rectilinear bone scan showing that the distribution of radiopharmaceutical corresponds to functional skeletal mass, as shown by a high uptake of tracer in the spine and sacro-iliac joints and large joints. There is a low uptake in the ribs and shafts of the long bones. (Note the symmetrical uptake in the kidneys.)*

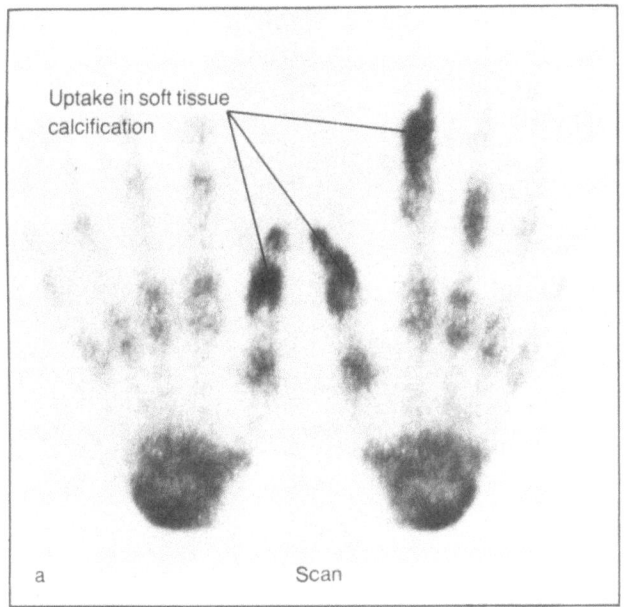

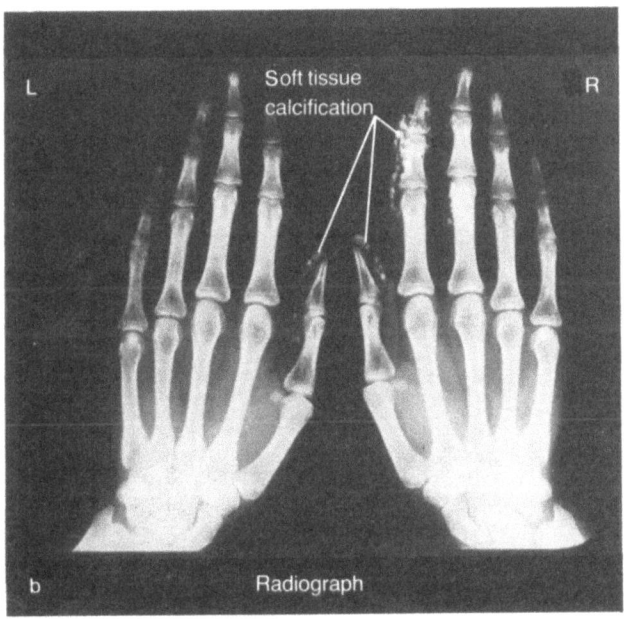

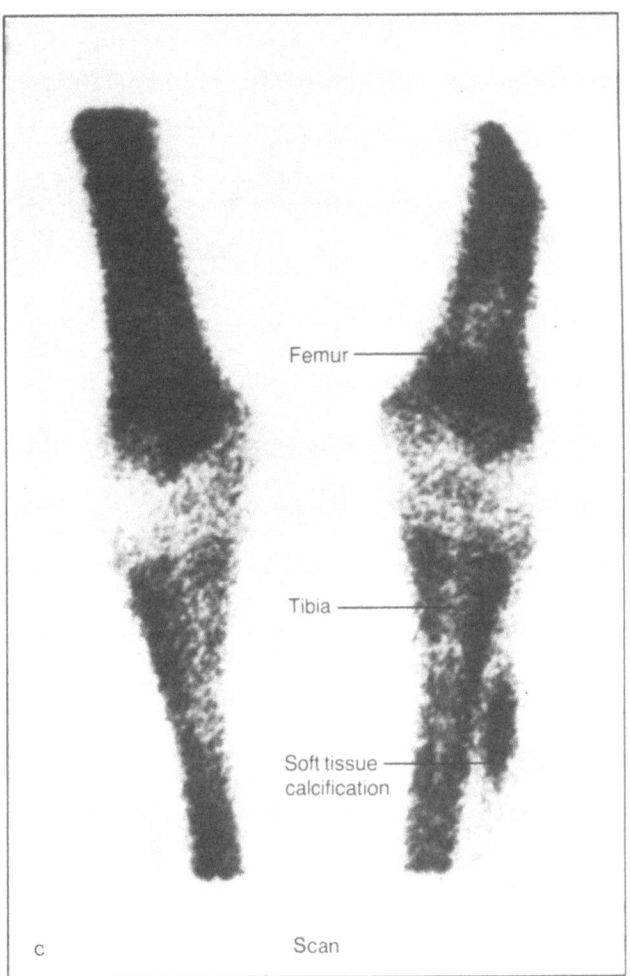

Figure 5.2 *Abnormal uptake of tracer into soft tissue calcification* (**a and b**), *digital calcinosis associated with scleroderma and* (**c**) *Post-traumatic myositis ossificans.*

photon energy was very high (511 KeV) and, although it was suitable for rectilinear scanners, it was not suitable for the new gamma cameras that were becoming more widely used in nuclear medicine. Fluorine-18 was produced in a Cyclotron which made it expensive, and the half-life is only two hours so the logistics of getting the radionuclide from the Cyclotron to the patient were difficult. In spite of these drawbacks, it was used quite extensively and, when easily available, it remains, theoretically, an excellent agent. When technetium-99m, with all its favourable physical characteristics, was attached to polyphosphate, bone scanning rapidly became what it is now: the primary investigation for the detection of regional abnormalities of skeletal function.

It would be fair to say that treating malignant or

skeletal disease without access to modern bone scanning facilities is not offering the patient first rate medical care. It has now been demonstrated unequivocally that bone scanning is many times more sensitive for the detection of local functional changes in bone than is radiology, which requires significant alteration in structure to have taken place before detection is possible. For example, it has been shown that more than 50 per cent of bone in a vertebral body may be destroyed before the change is detectable on a conventional radiograph. However, the radiograph can, of course, be used effectively in certain situations (e.g. to demonstrate changes in pattern associated with specific pathological changes).

The Principles

The technetium-99m phosphate compounds (polyphosphate and more recently developed substances) are actively adsorbed on to the surface of newly formed

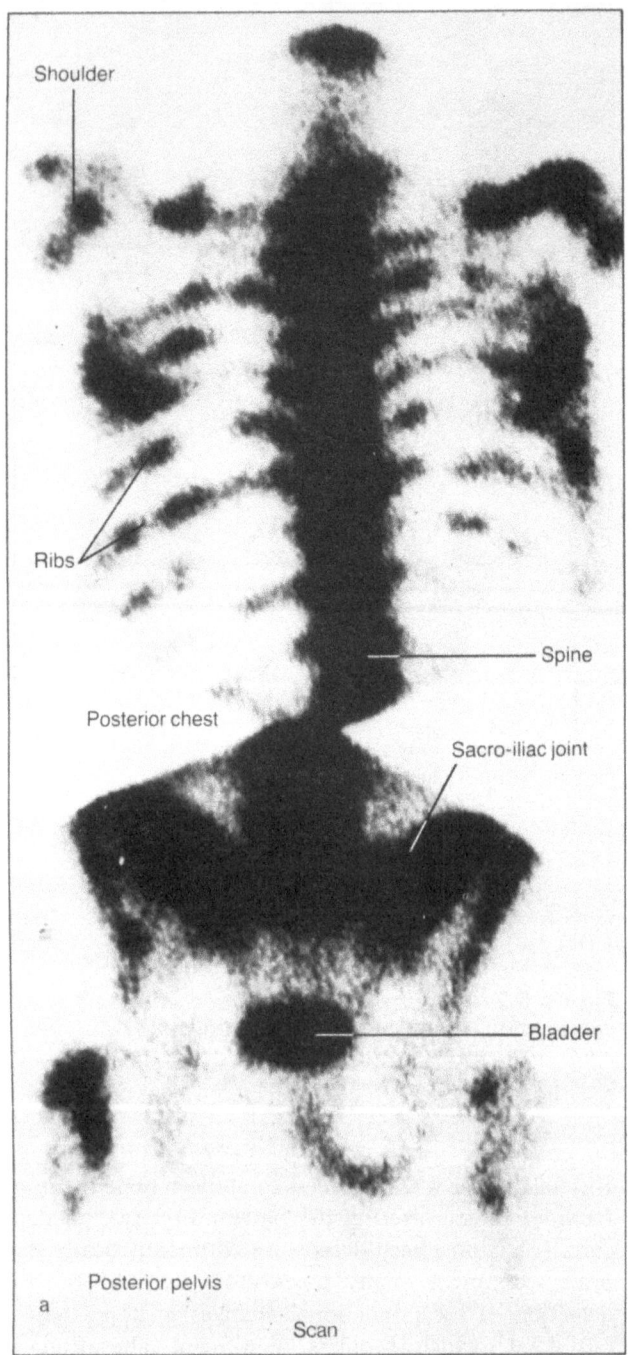

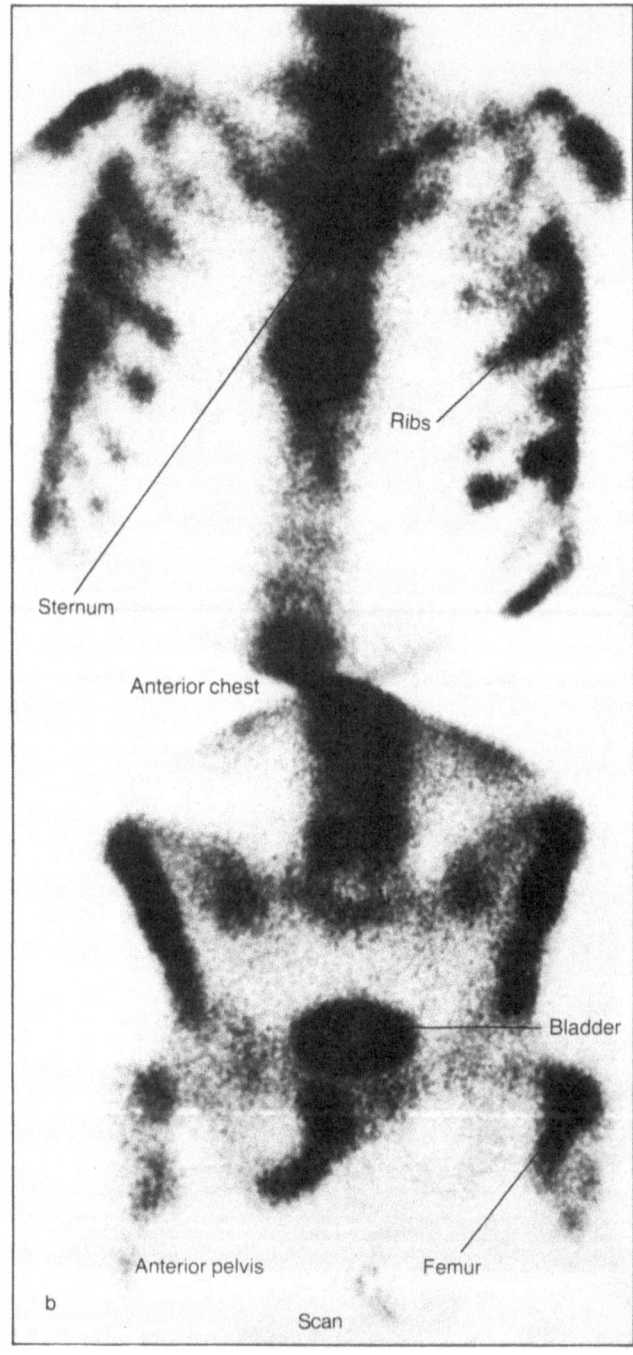

hydroxyapatite crystals and it has been shown that the rate of uptake and the concentration of these materials is related to two factors:

1. The rate of production of new hydroxyapatite crystals, i.e. osteoblastic activity; and

2. The blood flow to the area.

Thus, bone images display a functional picture of metabolic activity and blood flow in bone (Figure 5.1).

This ability to detect functional changes, which occur earlier than any structural change, is the reason why bone scanning is so much more sensitive than conventional radiography. Bone scans are relatively non-specific because almost any disease process in bone results in a change in metabolic function and blood flow, unlike the structural changes which have individual patterns that can be recognized radiographically. Besides being taken up into bone the $^{99}Tc^m$-phosphate compounds are also excreted by the kidneys into the

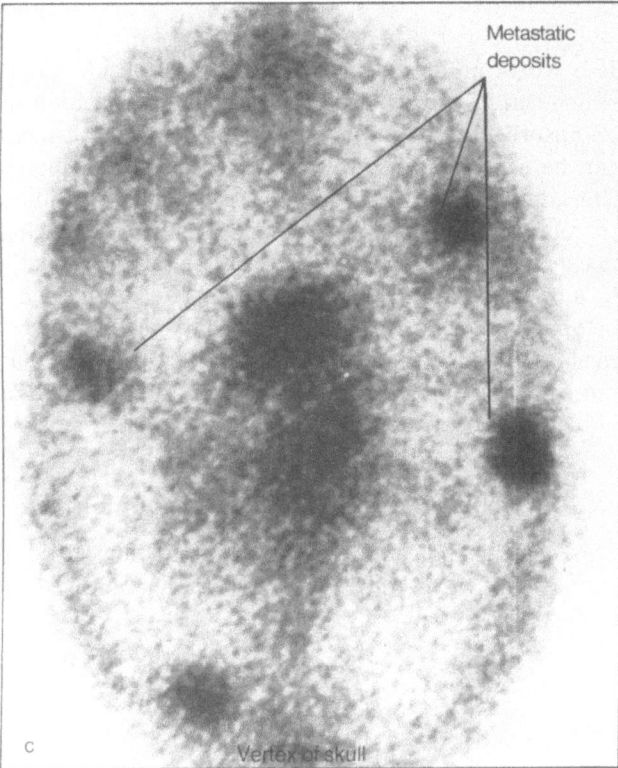

Metastatic deposits

Vertex of skull

Figure 5.3a, b and c (left and above) *Gamma camera images showing multiple active bone lesions due to metastases from carcinoma of the breast, symptom free and undetected on the initial 'routine radiological skeletal survey'.*

urine. Subsequent improvement of the original labelled polyphosphate has been directed towards increasing the rate of blood clearance and uptake into bone. Many agents, such as pyrophosphate, diphosphonate and, currently, the radiopharmaceutical of choice, methylene diphosphonate, have been used. The technetium-99m phosphate compounds are not only taken up by bone and excreted by the kidney but they may be non-specifically taken up by tumours, e.g. breast tumours, bronchial neoplasms and liver metastases, by soft tissue calcification, e.g. myositis ossificans and digital calcification associated with scleroderma (Figure 5.2). None of these have proved to have any clinical value but, more recently, the compound has been shown to accumulate in myocardial infarcts and it may be possible, therefore, to use it effectively in the diagnosis of this condition.

Technique

Patients require no preparation prior to a bone scan. After an intravenous injection of 15mCi of technetium-99m labelled methylene diphosphonate, two to four hours are allowed to elapse, which enables adequate uptake into bone and sufficient clearance from the blood for good images to be produced. Bone scans can be produced with a variety of instruments, including the

whole body rectilinear scanner which has an upper and lower probe and can produce the anterior and posterior views simultaneously; a gamma camera, preferably a large field of view camera (to reduce the number of single images required), or alternatively the newer gamma cameras which have a motorized drive so that they are capable of scanning anteriorly and then posteriorly. There are some instruments which are specifically designed for bone scanning and are a hybrid between a rectilinear scanner and a gamma camera.

An adequate total body survey takes between 30 and 45 minutes and, where possible, the pelvis should be scanned first (after initially emptying the bladder to avoid confusion with radioactivity within that viscus). Although a total body scan is usually necessary, as with any other investigation, the procedure must be tailored to solve the clinical problem most effectively. It may be necessary only to take one or two specific views with a gamma camera, for example, on an incidental radiograph when the question is posed; "is a lesion a bone island or a sclerotic secondary?"—a bone island will be functionally inactive and the metastases functionally active. On a skull radiograph, which was taken for some other reason there may be some doubt about a lesion—it may be a prominent venous lake or a lytic metastasis (again, a venous lake will be functionally inactive and the metastasis functionally active). A fractured scaphoid will be functionally active before radiological changes occur and, naturally, only limited views of the wrist are necessary. In children, a painful hip may be the problem and a total body survey would not be necessary but only careful specific views of the hip.

When the scan is completed and the results are known, the patient is re-examined appropriately—an essential procedure to eliminate possible abnormalities which are irrelevant to the present problem, such as old, badly healed fractures, skeletal deformities, soft tissue tumours, frozen shoulders, etc. The investigations may be completed at this point but, after the clinical examination, further views may be necessary for one of the following reasons:

1. If the previous radiograph was equivocal and the total body scan is negative in that area, a high resolution gamma camera view of the area is a wise precaution.

2. If the problem is one of clinical symptoms suggestive of a skeletal origin and the total body bone scan is negative again, then a high resolution gamma camera view, perhaps with a slightly different projection, is necessary.

3. If the scan is equivocal, a repeat gamma camera view should be performed to resolve this, or if the lesion is definite but the anatomical site is not clear, then a repeat view, perhaps in a different projection, will resolve this.

45

When this has been completed and if it is negative, then no further investigation is necessary, but for at least half of the patients radiographs are essential for the physician to be able to report on the bone scan. This is when the use of the bone scan before the radiograph is particularly helpful. The radiograph is now being used to answer a specific question and, therefore, the radiographic technique can be optimized to answer this particular question and the radiologist can also be 'optimized' to answer this question. Finally, all the clinical bone scan and radiological data are put together in order to answer the question which had originally been asked.

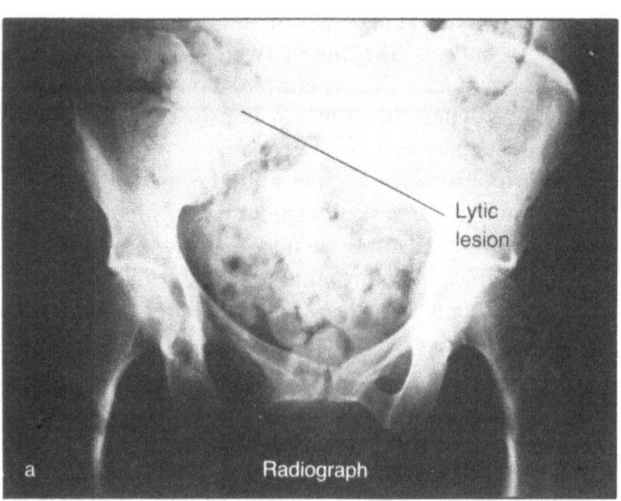

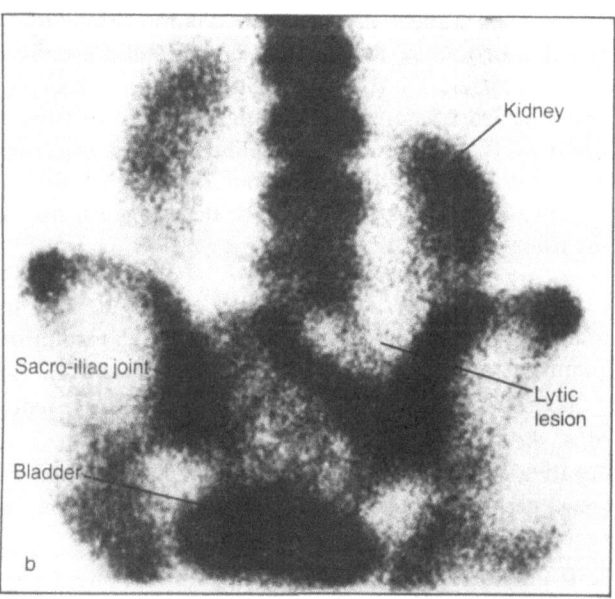

Figure 5.4a and b *Posterior pelvic view showing a large lytic lesion with absent bone and a surrounding osteoblastic reaction. Metastasis from a hypernephroma.*

46

Artefacts

It is worth noting one or two technical considerations which can give misleading results. The interposition of an absorbent material between the patient and camera can be a problem in any nuclear medicine technique. The commonest artefact in bone scanning is the failure to remove a breast prosthesis in a patient following mastectomy. Also, bladder catheters may occasionally be a problem, as may urine bags associated with ureterostomies or nephrostomies and urinary bladder diverticula. Contamination is, again, always a problem, but more so with bone scanning because of excretion by the kidneys.

Clinical Indications for Bone Scanning

The clinical indications for bone scanning are, of course, many and varied, but can be summarized as shown in Table 5.1.

Table 5.1 Clinical indications for bone scanning.

1. Detection of bone metastases, especially breast and bronchus.
2. Assessment of the extent of disease which is defined on the radiograph.
3. Confirmation of equivocal lesions on the radiograph.
4. Assessment of the activity of a radiological lesion.
5. Detection of an active bone lesion in the face of symptoms plus a normal radiograph, e.g. stress lesions.
6. Monitoring the progression or regression of known active disease (e.g. Paget's disease, metastatic breast disease, after oophorectomy).
7. Diagnosis of different functional changes caused by metabolic bone disease.

Total Body Bone Scans for Detection of Metastases

This is the commonest indication for bone scanning and forms approximately 75 per cent of the workload. In most general units where bone scanning is available it has replaced the radiological skeletal survey, and has done so for the following reasons:

1. It is more sensitive.

2. A positive bone scan uptake is much quicker and simpler to detect than an abnormality on a skeletal survey and therefore the error is much less and the time taken to read it is much less.

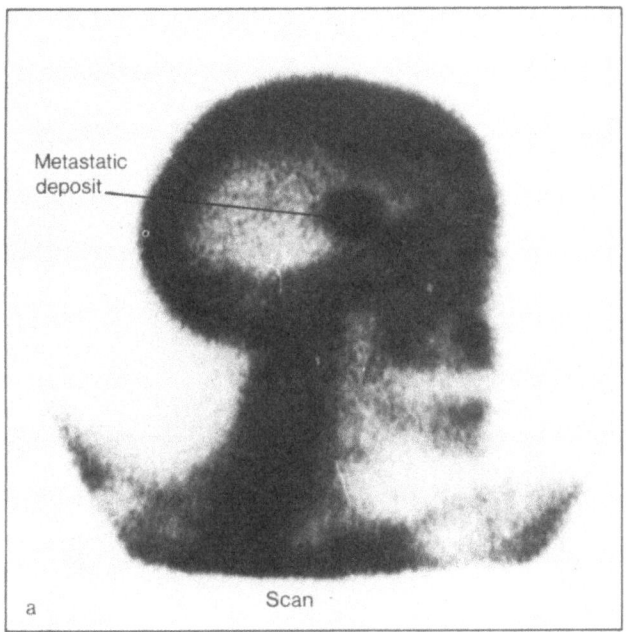

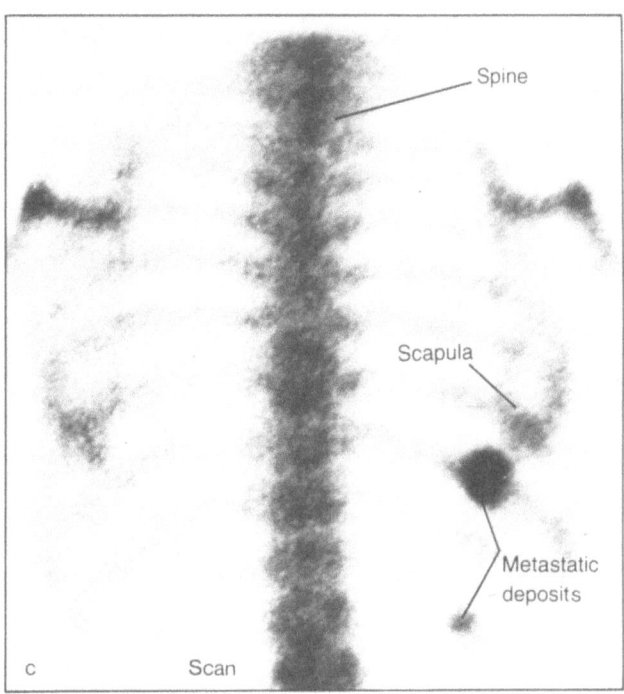

Figure 5.5c *Equivocal cough fractures on the radiograph which were confirmed by bone scan (which demonstrated increased 'activity').*

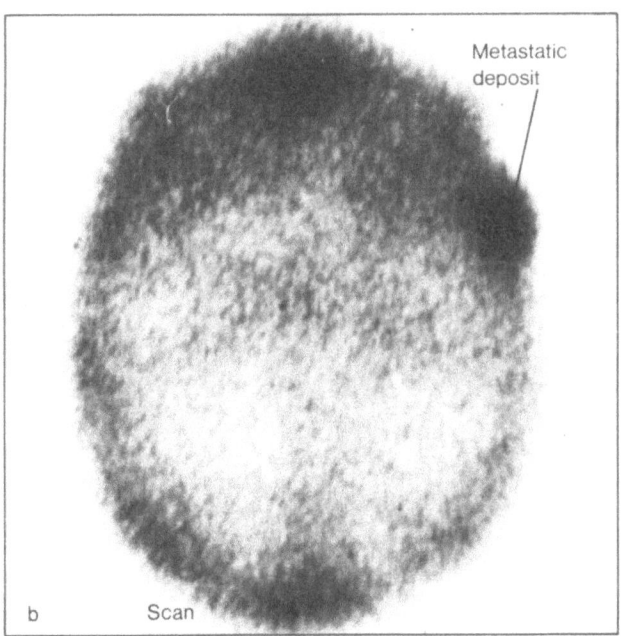

Figure 5.5a and b *Gamma camera views of the skull showing a focal active lesion in a patient radiographed for a head injury. A large 'venous-lake' was noted and a bone scan was performed to confirm this. The activity of the lesion excluded a venous lake and a metastatic breast lesion was diagnosed.*

3. It can be a true whole body survey, whereas most radiological surveys are limited usually to the skull and axial skeleton.

It is now generally agreed that bone scanning is an essential pre-operative investigation in patients with carcinoma of the breast, carcinoma of the bronchus, carcinoma of the prostate and carcinoma of the kidney, but some physicians would argue that it is necessary for staging purposes prior to any form of treatment for any malignancy that may metastasize to bone, including lymphomas (Figure 5.3). Bone scanning may also be used to follow the progress of the disease to detect early recurrence in bone, progression of known bone metastases or regression in response to a particular form of treatment. It should be remembered that some tumours, when they metastasize to bone, produce very little in the way of osteoblastic activity and, therefore, may not produce increased uptake. However, if they are extensive lesions (two classical examples being hypernephroma, where whole bones may disappear with no bony reaction, and myeloma) (Figure 5.4) bone scans can be used to detect this activity. However, the observer must be on his guard to detect areas of loss of functioning bone mass as well as areas of increased functioning bone.

The Equivocal Radiograph

Possibly the second most common indication for a bone scan occurs when a radiograph has been performed, possibly for some unrelated reason, e.g. a chest radiograph in a patient with a cough or a skull radiograph in a patient after a head injury, and a lesion has been noted incidentally. The problem here is usually either:

1. Whether it is a true abnormality or not—a positive

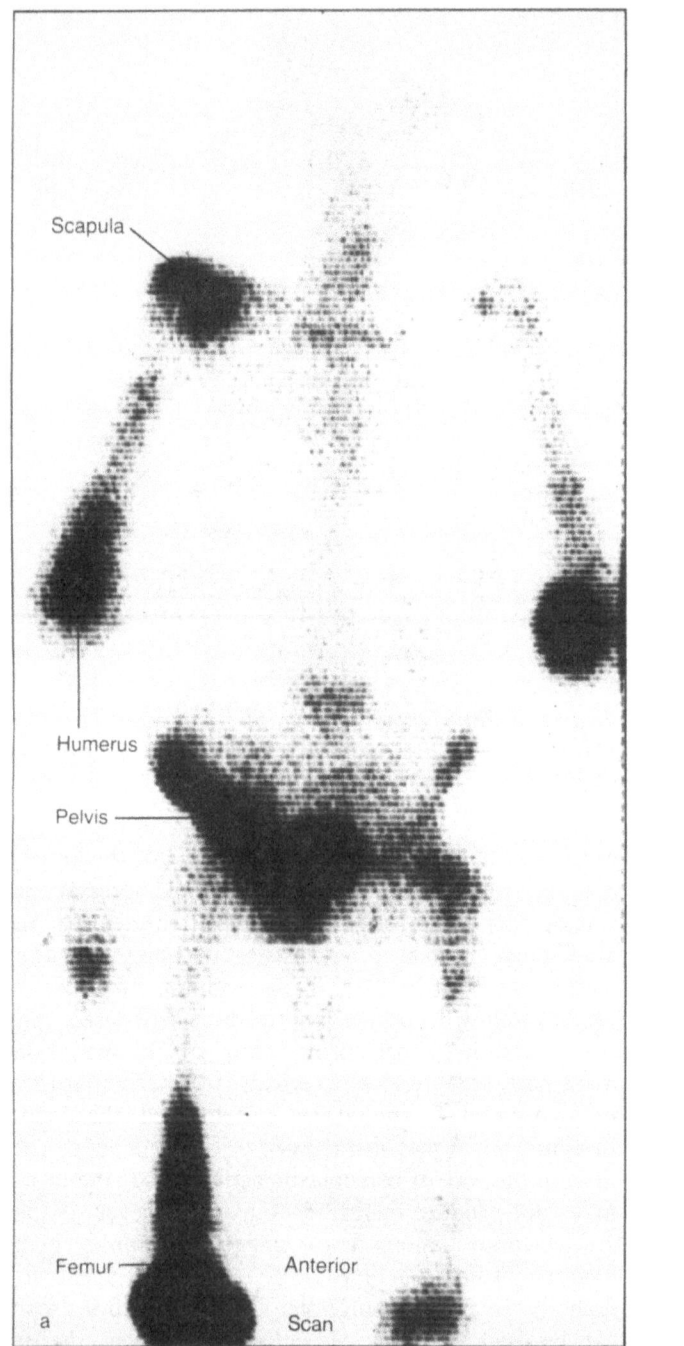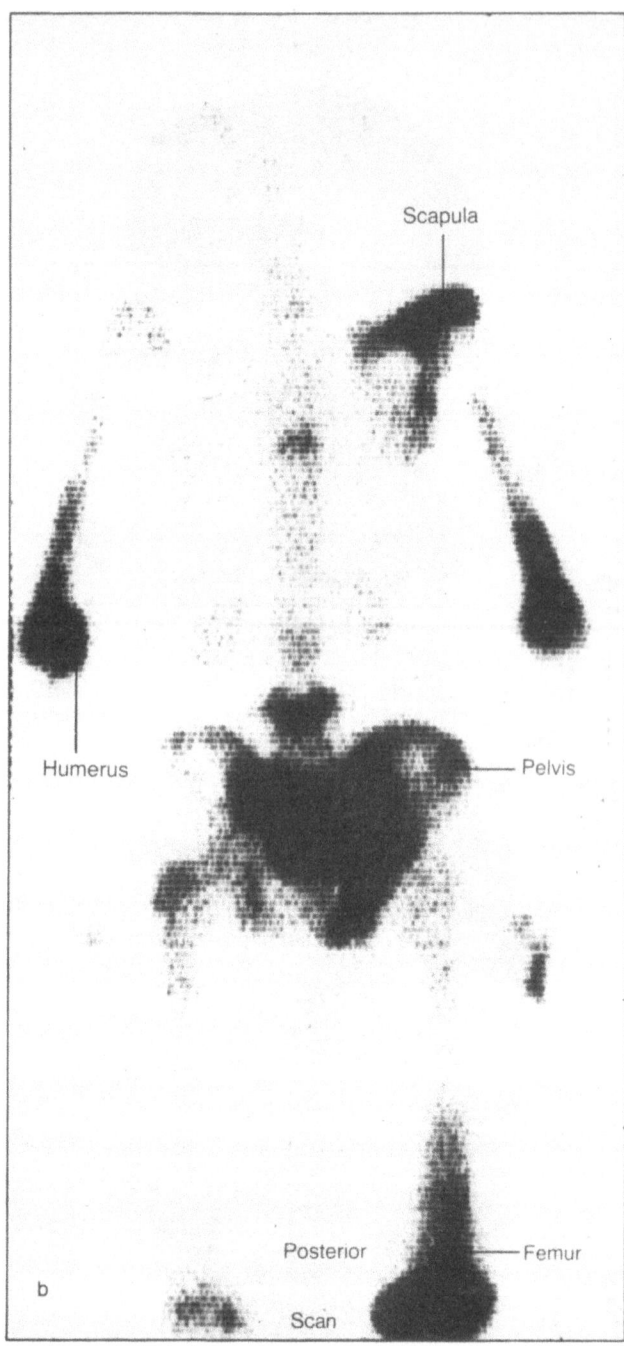

Figure 5.6a and b *The bone scan simply and rapidly identifies the extent of the disease, in this case the extent of active Paget's disease. The scan can be used quantitatively and qualitatively to monitor the response to therapy of this and other widespread bone disease.*

bone scan will support the probability that a true lesion exists (Figure 5.5).

2. When there is a definite lesion detected on the radiograph but the nature of this is uncertain, e.g. with an area of dense bone, the lesion may be a bone island, osteoid osteoma, or a metastatic deposit. A bone island

characteristically will be functionally inactive, an osteoid osteoma characteristically will be very active, single and occurring in a younger age group, and a metastasis would, of course, occur in an older age group and be functionally active and frequently multiple.

3. When a definite bony lesion has been detected on an

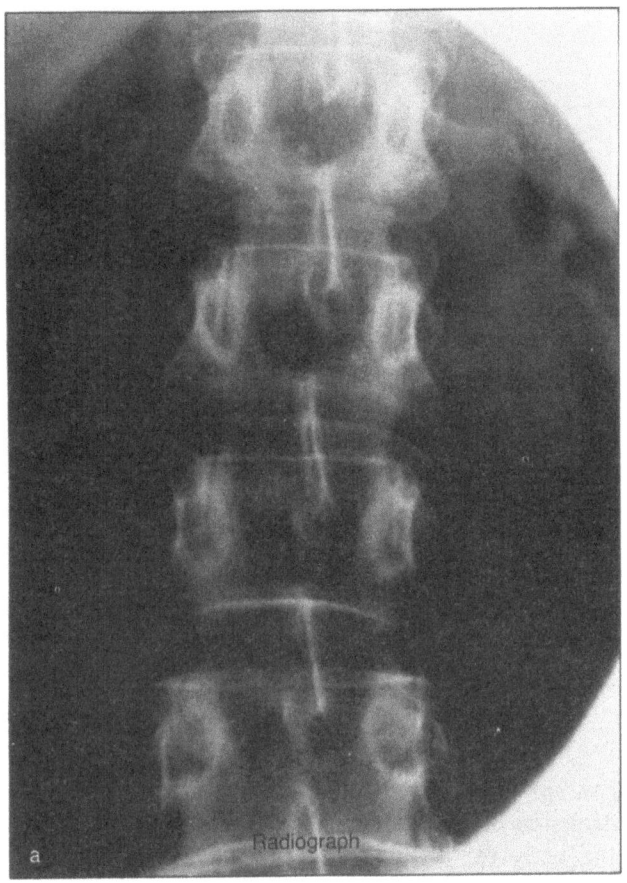

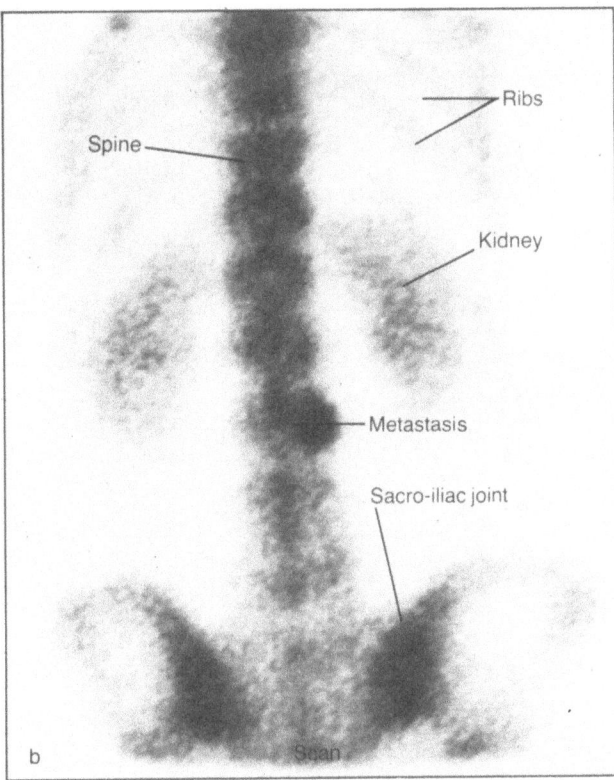

Figure 5.7a and b *This patient presented with low back pain. Routine lumbar spine radiograph (a) was normal. The scan (b) shows an active lesion in the pedicle of L.3. Later tomography confirmed this with subsequent discovery of a bronchial carcinoma.*

incidental radiograph, there may be uncertainty about the extent of the bone lesions. A bone scan would, of course, be more appropriate than a skeletal survey for reasons previously mentioned (Figure 5.6).

Clinical Suspicion of Skeletal Disease with Normal Radiographs

Examples for this category are:

1. The patient with back pain which is non-typical of low back strain, when bone scanning may detect an active metastasis as the cause (Figure 5.7).

2. The child with a painful, irritable hip—bone scanning has been shown to be an effective method of differentiating skeletal abnormalities, e.g. Legg Perthe's disease, from other non-skeletal causes (Figure 5.8).

3. In patients with early osteomyelitis who present with pain and normal radiographs.

4. Stress fractures, e.g. athletes may have stress lesions of the tibia or metatarsals which are often positive before there are radiological changes (Figure 5.9a and b). The situation is similar with fractures of the

scaphoid bone (Figure 5.9c and d).

5. Early detection of unstable hip replacements and chronic infection where scans may be positive in the absence of any radiological changes (Figure 5.10).

Metabolic Bone Disease

Bone scanning is used in the detection of metabolic bone disease, and there are several areas which are under active consideration. These areas include: the detection of the extent of Paget's disease and response to therapy with for example calcitonin, the detection, quantitation and qualitation of activity in diseases, such as parathyroid disease and osteomalacia with fractures. The investigation of their place in the clinical study of metabolic bone disease has not been established.

Summary

Bone scanning has now become an essential part of routine investigation in clinical medicine. Its future appears to be assured because of the fundamental

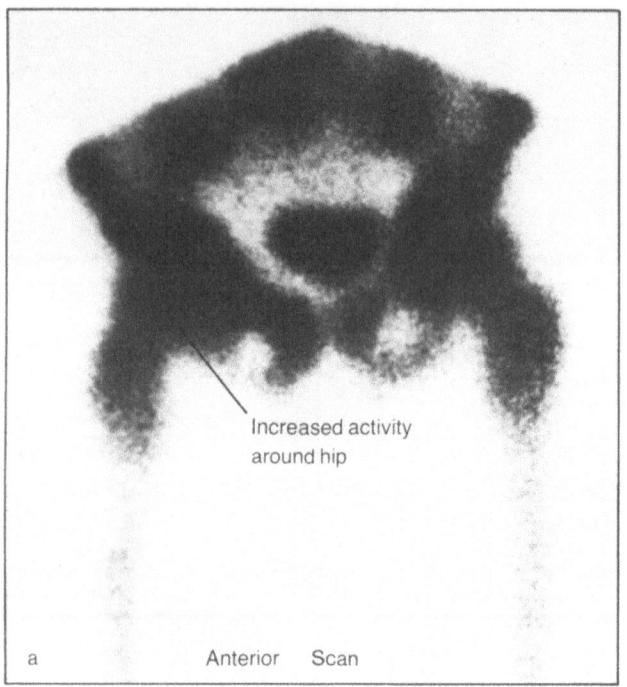

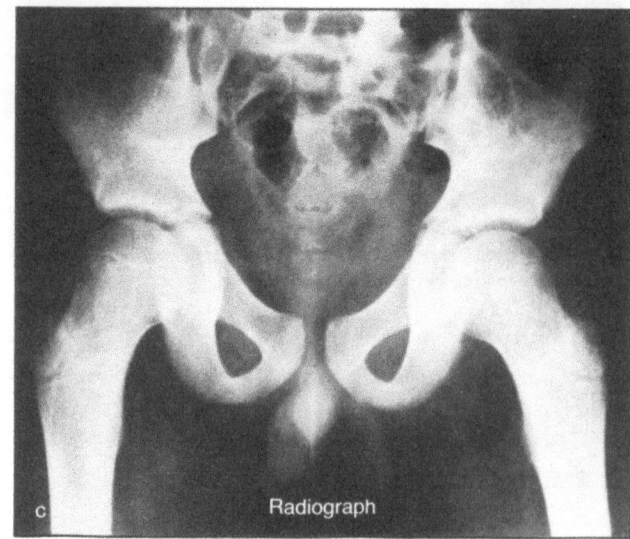

concept on which it is based, which is that of early detection of functional changes and the ability to scan the body rapidly, and this makes it unlikely to be replaced by any of the high resolution radiological procedures. New radiopharmaceuticals will undoubtedly appear and improve sensitivity, and thus increase bone uptake relative to the surrounding soft tissue. Also, there is likely to be increased emphasis on benign bone disease when the place of the functional changes on the bone scan becomes more clearly established. There is likely also to be an increasing emphasis on the quantitation of the functional changes using computers, for example in measuring the speed of resolution of active lesions with chemotherapy and the healing of fractures. It is possible that with the future introduction of Positron detecting gamma cameras we will come full circle and see an increasing use of fluorine–18 bone scanning.

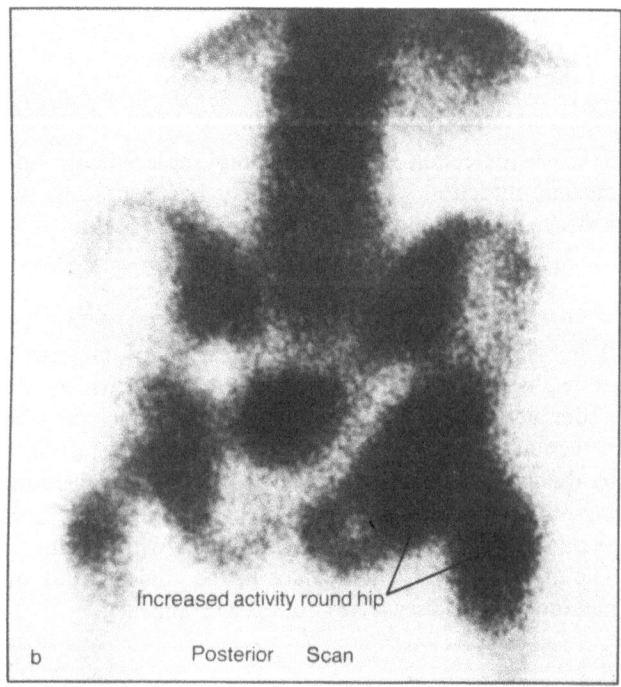

Figure 5.8a and b *Scans of a child with early Legg Perthe's disease showing active uptake around the abnormal hip before the development of the characteristic radiographical changes* (**c**).

Further Reading

Mall, J. C., Beckerman, C., Hoffer, P. B., Gottschalk, M. D., *Radiol.,* 1976, **118**, 323.

Merrick, M. V., *Br. J., Radiol.,* 1975, **48**, 327.

Semin. Nucl. Med., (Benign Bone Disorders), 1976, **7**(1).

Subramanian, G., and McAfee, J. G., *Radiol.,* 1971, **98**, 192.

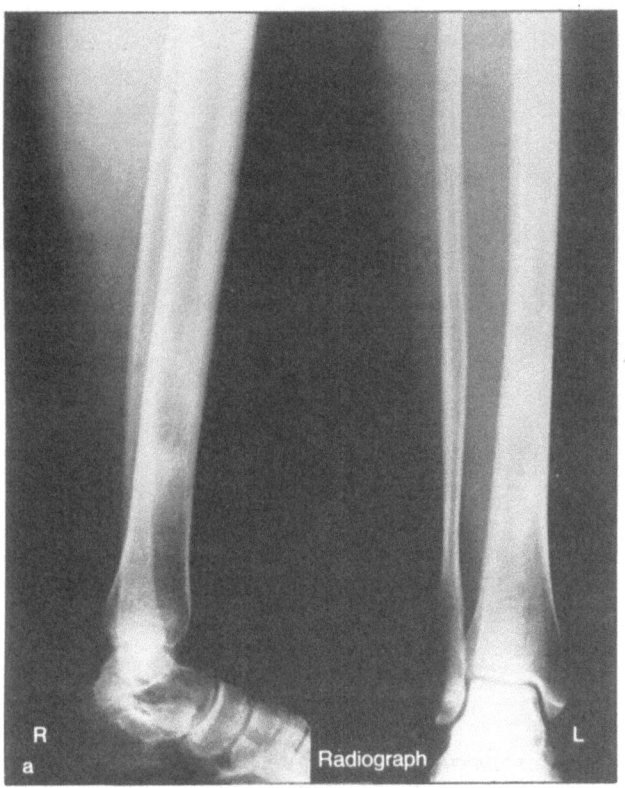

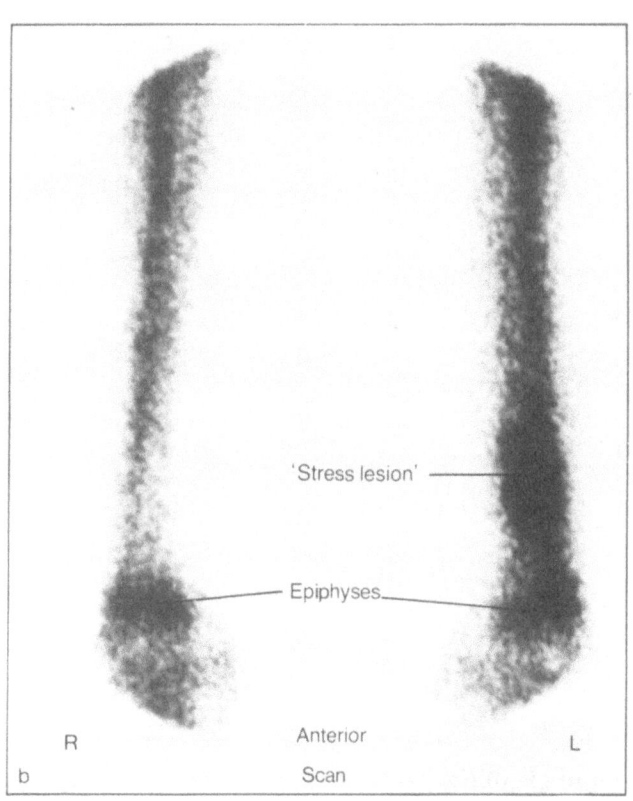

Figure 5.9a and b *Active stress lesion in the tibia of a young athlete. Note also the functional activity of bone around the epiphyses.*

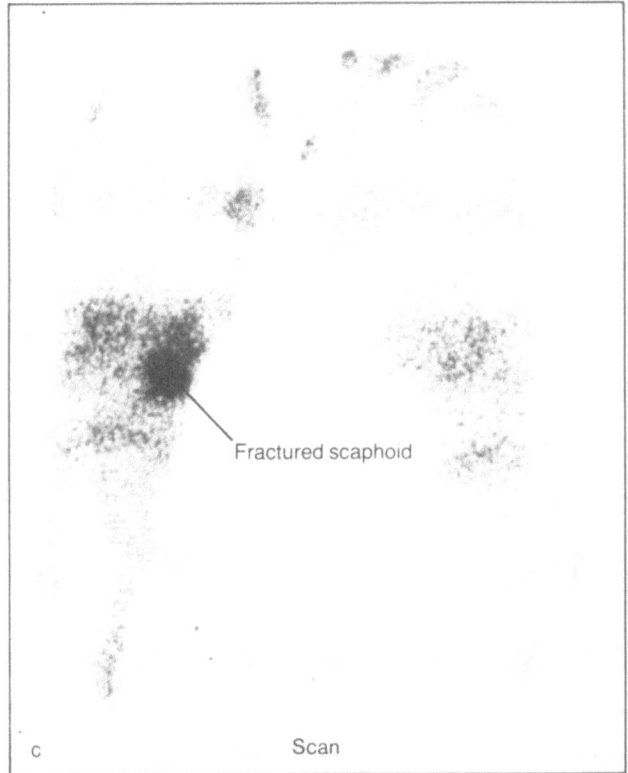

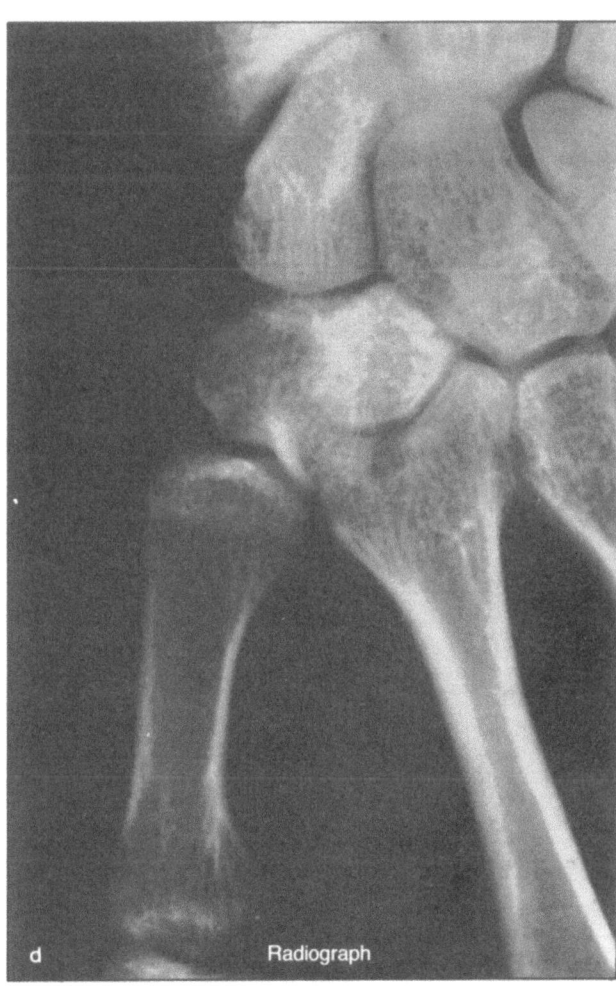

Figure 5.9c and d *Early scaphoid fracture becoming positive on the bone scan* (c) *before the radiograph* (d).

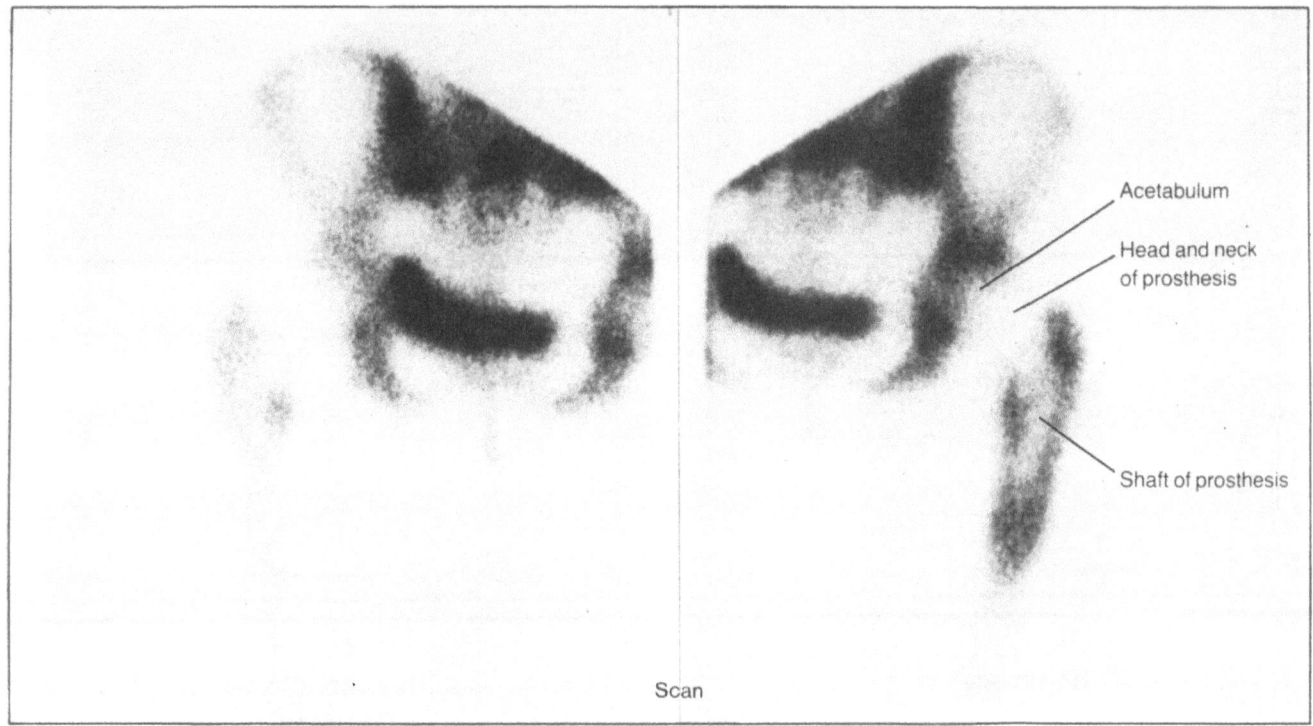

Acetabulum

Head and neck
of prosthesis

Shaft of prosthesis

Scan

Figure 5.10 *Bone scan of a patient with bilateral hip replacement for osteoarthritis. Recent development of pain in the left hip is associated with activity around the shaft of the prosthesis due to loosening and consequent movement.*

6. Ventilation Perfusion Lung Scanning

Clinical interest in radionuclide imaging of the lung began with the work of Knipping et al. (1955) who used the relatively insoluble inert gas xenon-133 in an attempt to diagnose carcinoma of the bronchus. Although unsuccessful in his primary objective, he was able to demonstrate that functional information could be obtained from the gamma ray emission image of xenon-133 within the lung. Initially, this method was used by West and associates who, between 1950 and 1965, used the Cyclotron-produced radioactive gases ^{15}O and $C^{15}O_2$ and demonstrated how factors such as gravity affect the distribution of ventilation and perfusion within the lung. (West 1960.)

The main clinical application of radionuclide imaging of the lung had to await the work of Wagner who reported in 1965 the use of a single intravenous injection of radioactively labelled microparticles to demonstrate regional pulmonary perfusion and to diagnose pulmonary embolism. Refinements in the technique of lung imaging followed with the introduction of the gamma camera and technetium-99m labelled particles.

Pulmonary Functions Visualized with Radionuclides

The lungs function primarily to bring the right-sided cardiac output into close proximity to alveolar gas so as to allow gaseous exchange. At a microscopic and macroscopic level this needs a close balance between the regional perfusion of the pulmonary capillaries and the regional alveolar ventilation. Respiratory diseases may lead to imbalances between these two functions and lung scanning is suited ideally to the study of such disturbance as it requires little cooperation from the patient, and is non-invasive, while providing a topographical comparison between the two areas.

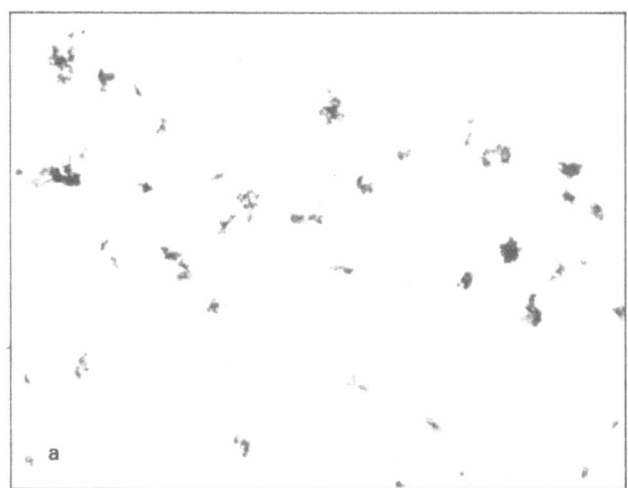

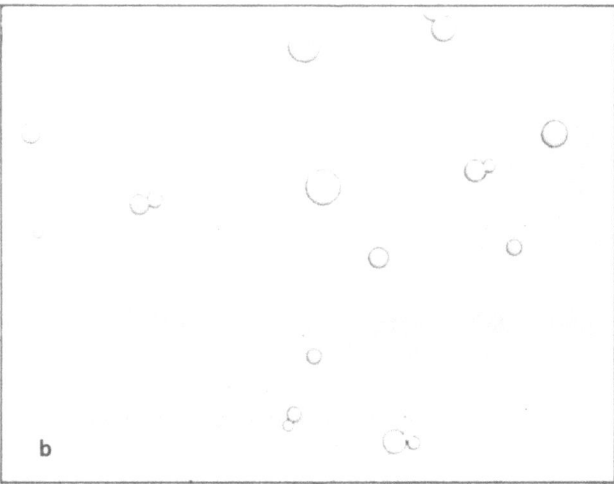

Figure 6.1 *This shows the relative sizes of macroaggregates, microspheres of human albumin and red blood cells at the same order of magnification and concentration.* **a)** *Macroaggregates of human albumin between 200-400,000 particles per ml.* **b)** *Microspheres of human albumin 130,000 particles per ml.* **c)** *Red blood cells 5.9 million per ml.*

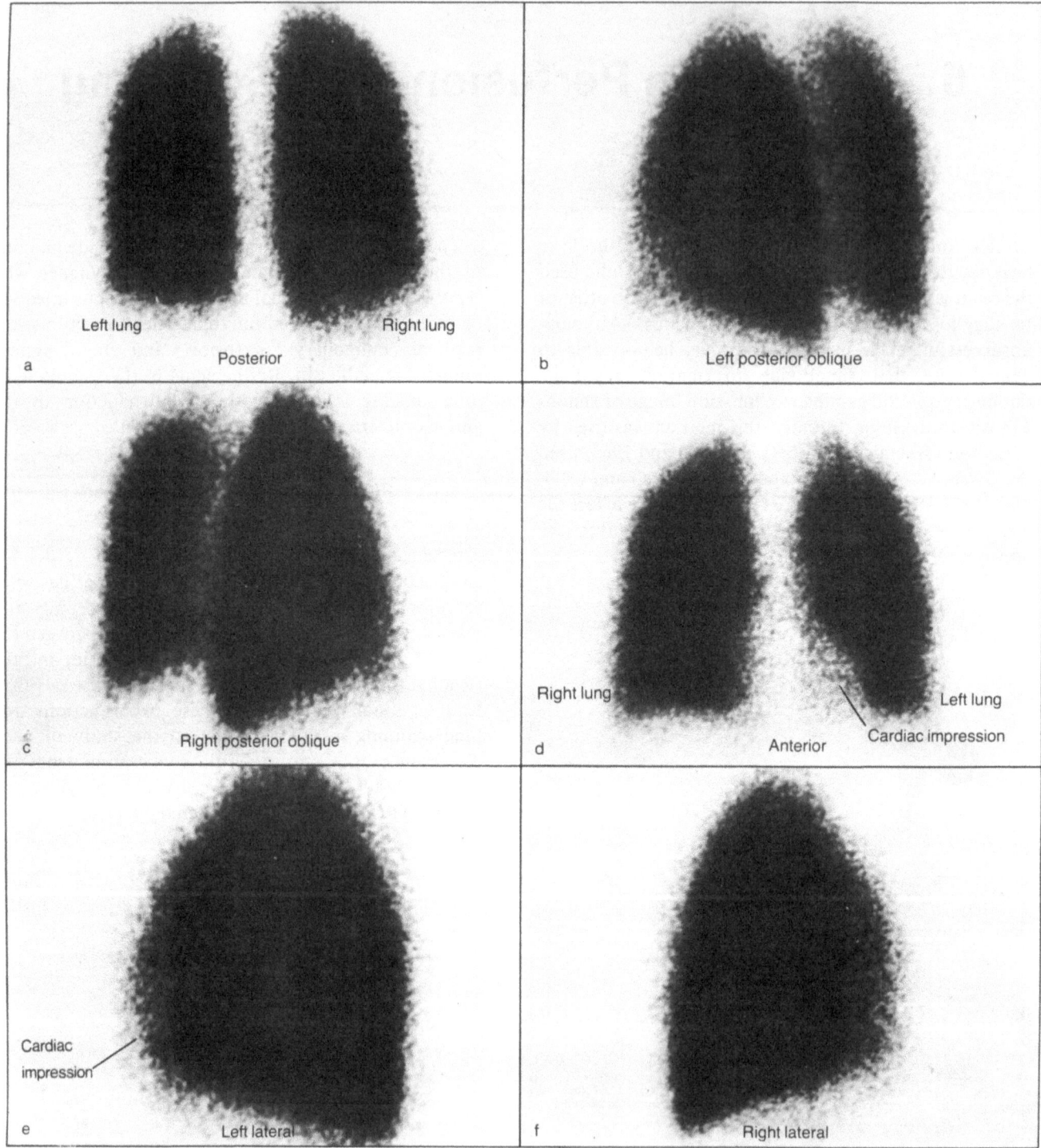

Figure 6.2 *A normal perfusion lung scan obtained with macroaggregates of human albumin labelled with $^{99}Tc^m$. The individual views of the lung are shown:* **a)** *posterior,* **b)** *left posterior oblique,* **c)** *right posterior oblique,* **d)** *anterior,* **e)** *left lateral and* **f)** *right lateral.*

Regional Perfusion of the Lung

Currently, the methods used to visualize regional pulmonary perfusion depend upon the principle of temporarily concentrating a gamma ray emitting nuclide within the pulmonary capillaries.

The most commonly used method involves microparticles labelled with technetium-99m ($^{99}Tc^m$). Two sorts of particles may be used—microspheres or macroaggregates of pyrogen-free human albumin. They both have two important characteristics—a similar density to red blood cells and a range of size between 15 and 70μ (see Figure 6.1). Their density is important as it determines distribution in the pulmonary circulation after mixing in the right ventricle. They have been shown experimentally to follow regional pulmonary perfusion and their size determines where they have become temporarily obstructed in the pulmonary vasculature. The 300 million pulmonary arterioles have diameters between 15 and 30μ, whereas the 280 billion pulmonary capillaries have diameters between 5 and 7μ. As the microspheres or macroaggregates are scattered through the pulmonary circulation, they become obstructed temporarily in a small number of these vessels, in proportion to the regional perfusion. The distribution of gamma ray emission from the $^{99}Tc^m$ labelling is therefore proportional to regional perfusion. This information is obtained from a single intravenous injection of approximately 150,000 of the microparticles labelled with 1-4 mCi of $^{99}Tc^m$.

It is important to obtain anatomical information about regional lung perfusion, in particular the lobar and segmental nature of perfusion defects. Therefore, it is necessary to obtain a number of views of the lung, taken from the different surfaces of the thorax. Usually the anterior, posterior, both lateral views and right and left posterior oblique views (see Figure 6.2) are obtained. The right and left posterior oblique views have the advantage that the most distant lung is 'thrown' to one side of the proximal lung image, thus avoiding obscuring of the detail of the closer lateral surface by the 'shine through' of gamma ray emissions from the distant lung.

Regional Ventilation of the Lung

The same principle (as previously described) applies to obtaining an image of ventilation of the lung, i.e. concentrating a sufficient amount of gamma ray radionuclide in the functioning element of the lung (the distal air spaces) to obtain satisfactory resolution between well and poorly ventilated regions. The problem is that a single breath of the presently available insoluble radioactive gases provides too low a gamma ray emission to enable satisfactory resolution with a gamma camera.

Recently, steady state breathing of the short-life inert gas krypton-81m has been shown to provide an image representing regional ventilation. The principle is that a continuous supply of this isotope is mixed in air which is breathed quietly by the patient. As the half-life of the isotope is only 13 seconds, the amount of radioactive gas in any part of the lung at one time relates to the regional ventilation of that part.

The continuous supply of krypton-81m is provided by a 'generator' in which a product of a Cyclotron, rubidium-81, is adsorbed to a cation resin. This isotope has a half-life of 4.7 hours, decaying to provide krypton-81m which is eluted from the resin by a stream of air.

The ventilation image obtained with $^{81}Kr^m$ is comparable to the perfusion image obtained with the microparticles labelled with $^{99}Tc^m$ in that both are obtained with the patient at rest, and breathing quietly. These radionuclides are suitable for high resolution images using a gamma camera as they have gamma ray emissions of 191 and 140 KeV respectively. Furthermore, using the 'energy window' on the gamma camera the emissions from each radionuclide may be imaged separately, without changing the position of the patient, to obtain successively an image of regional perfusion, and of regional ventilation. This is of particular value when assessing the 'matching' between regional ventilation and perfusion.

Each patient receives a single intravenous injection of microspheres or macroaggregates and is then positioned in front of the gamma camera, either in the sitting or lying position (Figure 6.3). A perfusion image is obtained, then a ventilation image of the same view, with the patient simply breathing the air/krypton mixture from an oxygen mask. The further views of the lungs are obtained by repositioning the patient.

Before the introduction of krypton-81m the ventilation image was obtained using the low energy and relatively insoluble gas xenon-133, which has a half-life of 5.27 days. There were two main difficulties in its use—it has a low energy gamma ray emission of only 80 KeV and a long half-life. When tidally breathed an equilibrium is reached at the point when the concentration of the radioactive isotope in the lung is determined by the lung volume and not by the regional ventilation, as the rate of inflow of the isotope equals the rate of outflow due to the long half-life. The regional ventilation can only be assessed during the short 'wash in' or 'wash out' periods. This contrasts

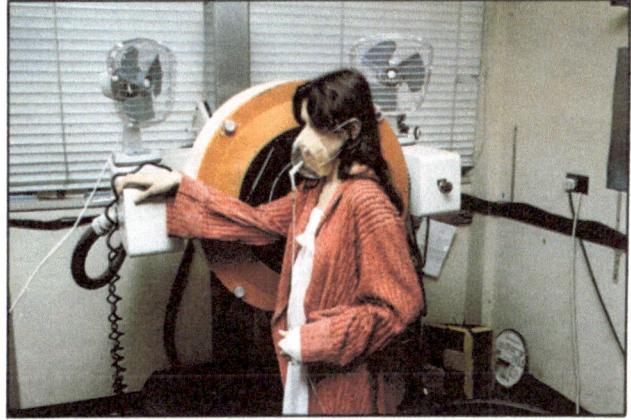

Figure 6.3 *A patient is shown sitting in front of the wide view gamma camera, breathing the air-krypton-81m mixture through a mask. The krypton-81m generator is shown in the foreground with the air cylinder behind the camera. An electric fan behind the patient drives the free $^{81}Kr^m$ away from the camera.*

Table 6.1 Diagnosis of pulmonary embolus.

A high index of suspicion is the primary requirement.

Symptoms Breathlessness Chest pain, often pleuritic Haemoptysis Syncope Fever No symptoms at all *Physical signs* Raised respiratory rate Tachycardia Pleural rub Circulatory collapse No abnormal signs	*Investigations* Chest radiograph — linear shadows ECG — rightward shift in axis, Q_3 T_3 — RSR^1 pattern on V_1 and V_2 *Arterial gas tensions* Reduced $PaCO_2$ Reduced PaO_2 *Respiratory function* Normal FEV_1 and V C Reduced gas transfer factor (TLCO)

with krypton-81m which has a 13-second half-life and remains in a continuing 'wash in' phase. An additional problem with xenon, again attributable to its long half-life, is the fact that, over a period of time, significant amounts dissolve in interstitial fluid and fat so that the total counts obtained from a surface of the thorax represent only in part those from the distal air spaces, the remainder representing the body wall distribution.

Clinical Applications

Pulmonary Embolism

In clinical practice, pulmonary embolism is a common and serious disease. The massive and almost invariably fatal pulmonary embolism, when over 50 per cent of the pulmonary circulation is obstructed by emboli, is usually preceded by premonitory smaller emboli which often go undiagnosed, leaving the patient at risk.

The symptoms of pulmonary embolism are non-specific as are the physical findings (see Table 6.1). Indeed, often, many of the usually recognized features (haemoptysis with a pleuritic pain and a rub) are not present and may occur days after the initial embolism. Breathlessness may be the only symptom. The chest radiograph, ECG and blood gases are often normal.

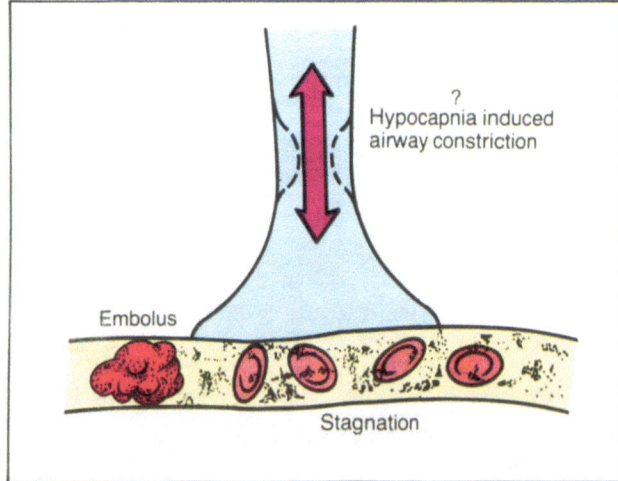

Figure 6.4 *In the presence of an obstruction of the pulmonary arteries, after a pulmonary embolus in man, the ventilation of that region usually remains unaffected. This appears to be the result of collateral ventilation and the weakness of the hypocapnia-induced bronchoconstriction.*

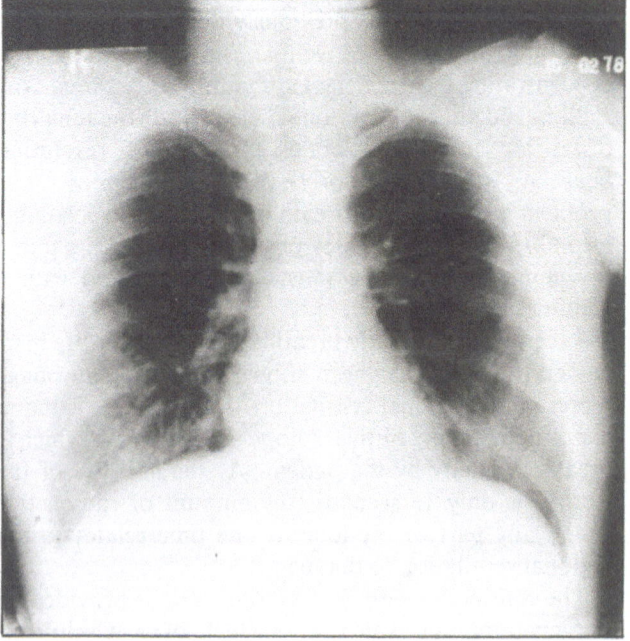

Figure 6.5 *The clear chest radiograph of the patient with glomerulonephritis.*

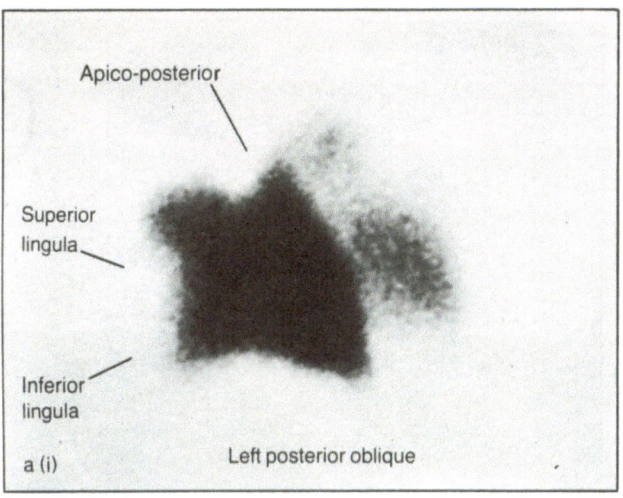

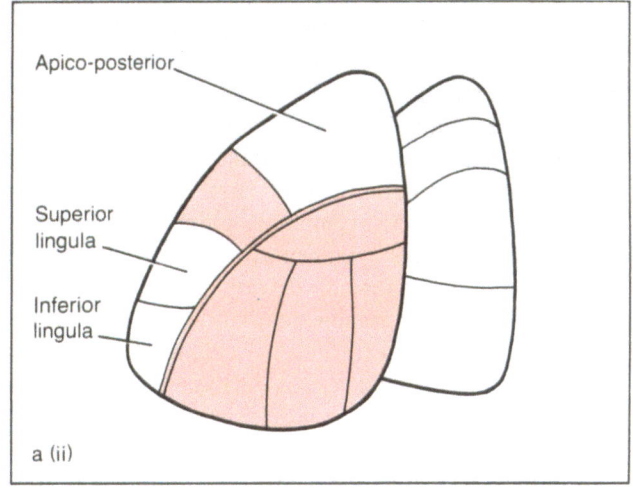

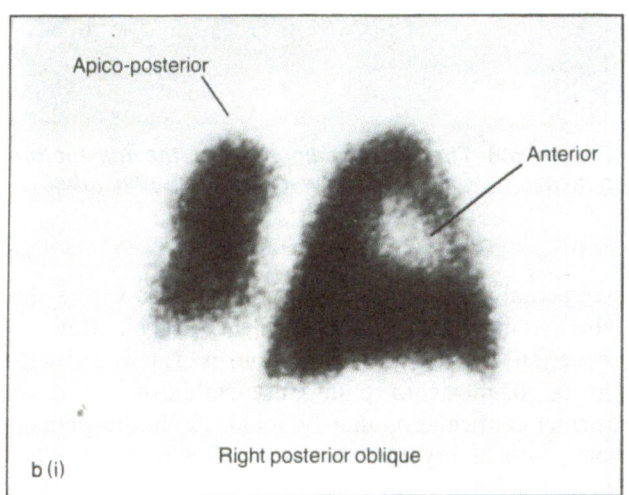

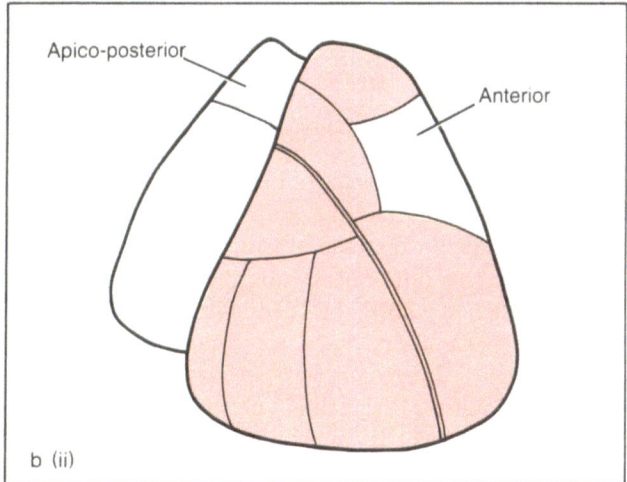

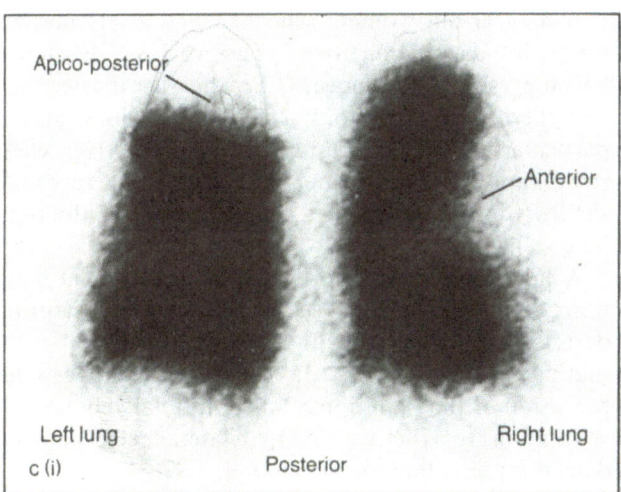

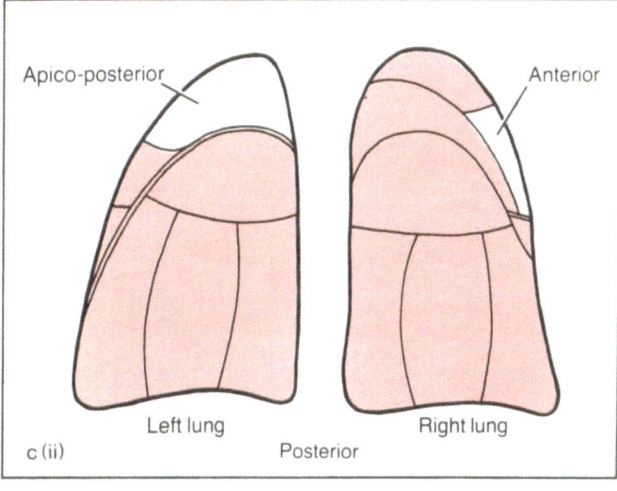

Figure 6.6a, b and c *The left and right posterior oblique views, and the posterior view of the perfusion image in the glomerular nephritic patient. Beside each is the stylized drawing illustrating the segmental pattern of the perfusion defects.*

These observations serve to underline one important consideration; the diagnosis can only be made in the presence of a high index of suspicion. It is in this context that the non-invasive investigation of lung scanning provides a most convenient means of diagnosis. This is particularly important when considering whether or not to anticoagulate the patient with heparin or warfarin as prophylaxis against further and possibly massive pulmonary emboli.

Pulmonary embolism exhibits two features which produce a characteristic disturbance of regional perfusion and ventilation. The first is that emboli frequently obstruct segmental pulmonary arteries producing multiple segmental perfusion defects. Second, these perfusion defects are usually not associated with comparable ventilation defects. This is probably due to the efficiency of collateral ventilation of the lung and the weakness of the hypocapnia-induced bronchoconstriction which is seen in animals following pulmonary artery occlusion (see Figure 6.4). As a result of these two features of pulmonary embolism, it is possible to make a particularly accurate diagnosis when using a combination of ventilation and perfusion images of the lung.

Examples of Pulmonary Embolism

A 32-year-old man developed breathlessness on exercise some six months after the diagnosis of glomerulonephritis. Physical examination, other than a cushingoid appearance (a result of his steroid therapy), was entirely normal. He had a normal ECG and his chest radiograph (Figure 6.5) was clear.

A perfusion lung scan was performed and revealed bilateral multiple segmental perfusion defects (see Figure 6.6). It will be appreciated that using the left posterior oblique view provides evidence of a loss of perfusion of the lingula as well as the apical posterior segment of the left upper lobe. The picture of multiple

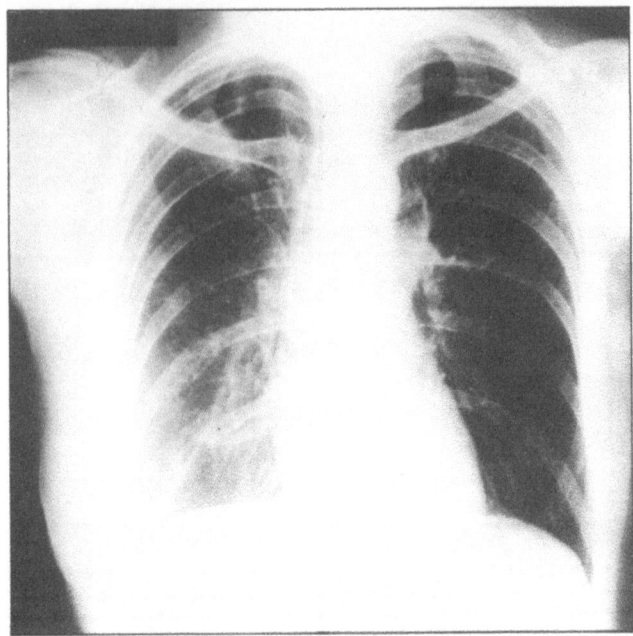

Figure 6.8 *The chest radiograph of the mastectomy patient showing the shadow in the right upper lobe.*

segmental perfusion defects, in association with a clear chest radiograph without evidence of air flow obstruction on clinical examination, is usually sufficient for a diagnosis of pulmonary embolism. However, further confirmation may be sought, as in this patient's case, with a krypton-81m ventilation scan (shown in Figure 6.7) where there are no comparable ventilation defects.

A 42-year-old woman, who had had a left mastectomy for carcinoma two years earlier, developed haemoptysis and dyspnoea. Other than her mastectomy scar there were no abnormal physical findings, and in particular no added sounds in her chest. Her chest radiograph was not normal (see Figure 6.8), revealing shadows in the right upper and mid-zones of the right lung.

A lung scan was performed despite a clinical diagnosis of metastatic lung disease. This revealed perfusion defects in both lungs, with normally distributed ventilation (see Figure 6.9). In particular, there was no perfusion of the right upper lobe, but relatively normal ventilation, together with many bilateral sub-segmental defects representing smaller emboli.

The patient was anticoagulated and remained well with no further symptoms and a clear chest radiograph.

If repeated lung scans are performed, following an embolus, there is often a progressive clearing of the perfusion defects. In this patient a repeated perfusion image showed a complete clearing of the perfusion defects after three weeks. In patients younger than 65 years of age, and without co-existing cardiopulmonary disease, most small emboli clear within three months;

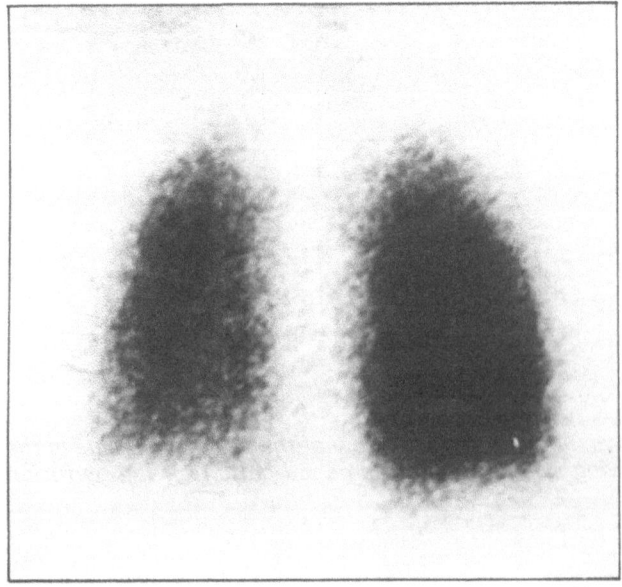

Figure 6.7 *The comparable posterior ventilation image of the same patient (as in Figures 6.5 and 6.6) showing no defects in ventilation.*

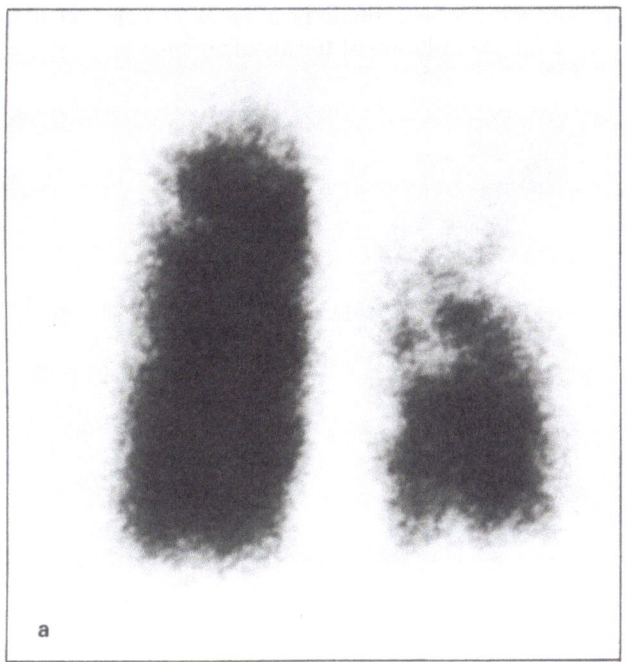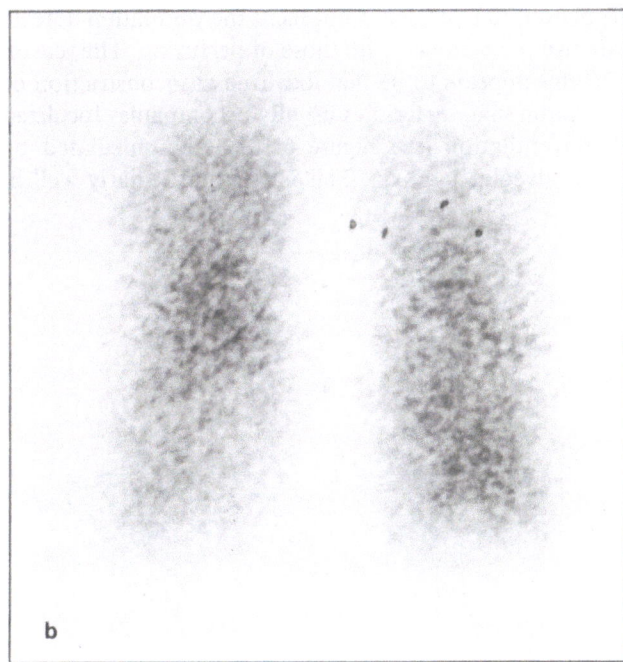

Figure 6.9a and b *The posterior views of* **a)** *perfusion and* **b)** *ventilation of the same patient. As will be seen, the right upper lobe has greatly diminished perfusion but normal ventilation. Throughout both lungs there are many sub-segmental perfusion defects.*

often in young patients they clear within days, which makes it necessary to perform a perfusion lung scan as soon as the diagnosis is considered.

The Use of the Lung Scan in Other Pulmonary Diseases

Particular use is made of the fact that pulmonary embolism results in defects in regional perfusion, without comparable changes in regional ventilation. In diseases of the lung, primarily affecting the ventilatory

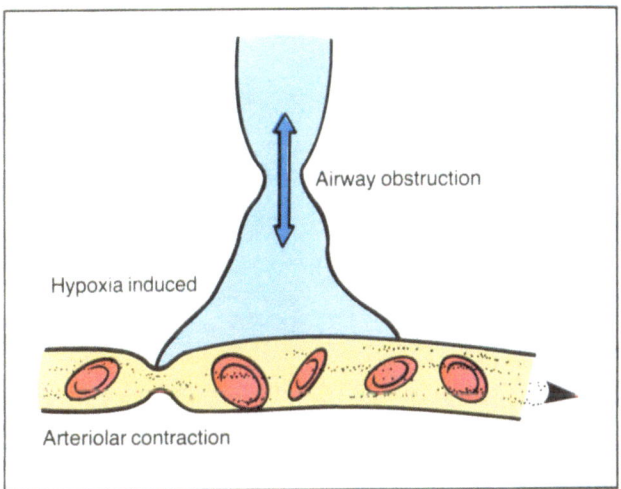

Figure 6.10 *In the presence of a reduction in alveolar ventilation and resultant hypoxia, in man there is a concomitant arteriolar constriction allowing a matching between regional ventilation and perfusion.*

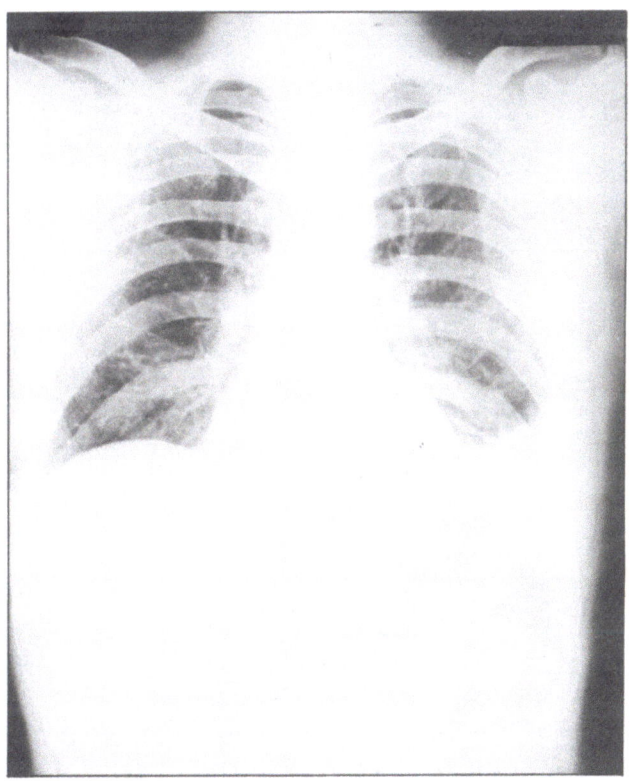

Figure 6.11 *The chest radiograph of a man with a left lower lobe pneumonia.*

59

function, this pattern is not seen; the ventilation defects are usually *matched* with those of perfusion. The reason for this appears to be that localized vasoconstriction of the pulmonary arterioles usually accompanies localized hypoventilation (see Figure 6.10) and is mediated by local alveolar hypoxia. This is seen particularly well in

pneumonia, where there is a local alveolar exudate preventing ventilation of the distal air spaces.

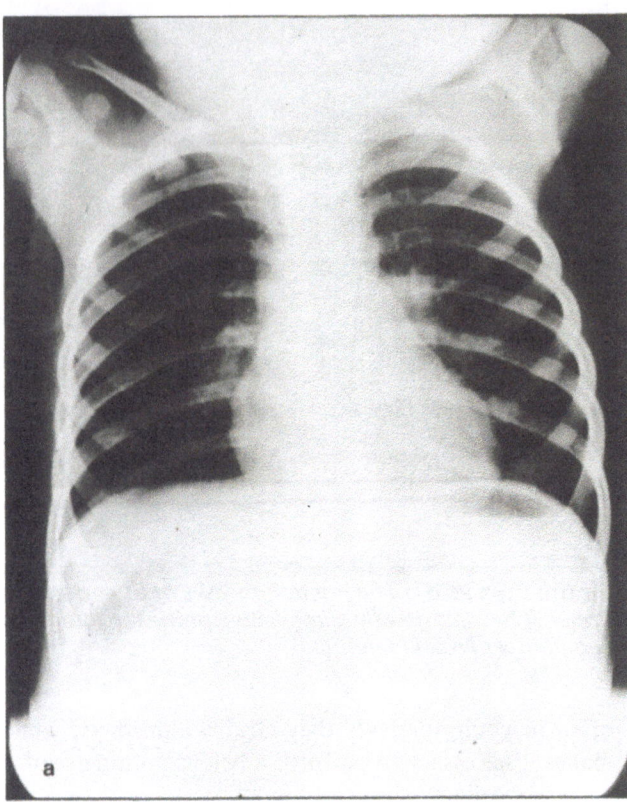

Figure 6.13a *The chest radiograph of the child who had inhaled a peanut. Note the reduction in vasculature on the right side.*

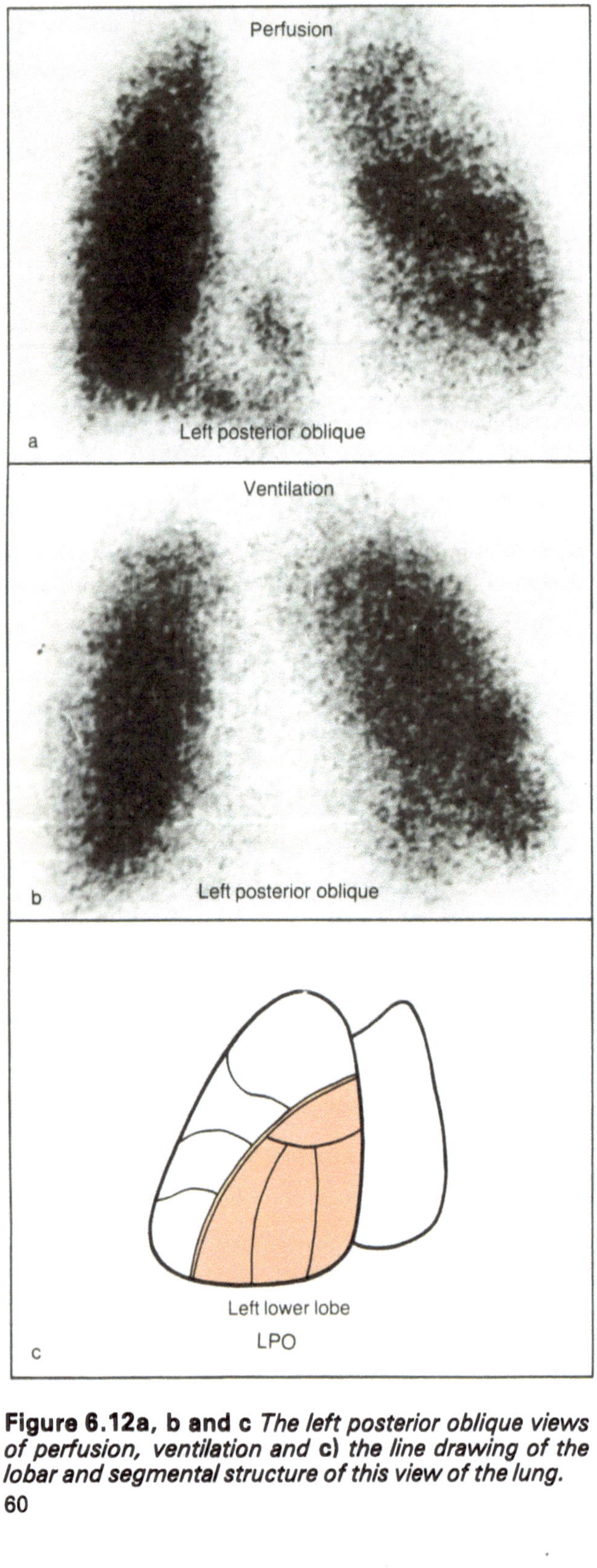

Figure 6.12a, b and c *The left posterior oblique views of perfusion, ventilation and* c) *the line drawing of the lobar and segmental structure of this view of the lung.*

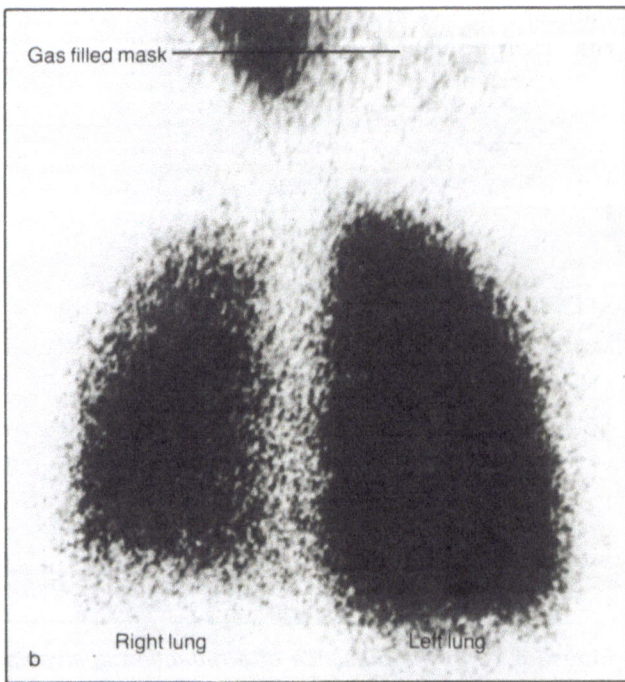

Figure 6.13b *The ventilation image showing how the whole right lung is under-ventilated.*

An Example of Pulmonary Disease

A 32-year-old man presented with a left-sided pleuritic chest pain and a cough with 'rusty' coloured sputum. He had no abnormal physical findings except for a fever (39°C), but his chest radiograph revealed a left lower lobe shadow (Figure 6.11). A white cell count revealed a leucocytosis and a total count of 19,000. His perfusion and ventilation lung scans revealed a matching reduction in perfusion and ventilation of the left lower lobe, seen well on the left posterior oblique views (see Figure 6.12). It is noteworthy that the perfusion is less

affected than ventilation. The continued partial perfusion of an unventilated lobe probably accounted for the patient's lowered arterial oxygen tension of 9.5 kPa, acting as a right-to-left shunt.

The Factors which Influence Pulmonary Regional Ventilation

In addition to those lung diseases, such as pneumonia, in which the distal air spaces are filled with fluid, other primarily ventilatory lung diseases may also result in disturbances of regional ventilation.

Airways Obstruction

Regions of the lung served by large airways are likely to fill early during inspiration, whereas those which are served by relatively narrow airways take longer to fill. During tidal breathing of the krypton-81 m/air mixture, with a relatively fixed inspiratory time, the regions of the lung served by narrow airways receive less krypton-81m than those served by larger airways.

Lung Fibrosis

Regional fibrosis of the lung results in a reduction in regional compliance—that is, it reduces the possible change in lung volume for a given pressure gradient between the pleura and the alveoli. Whilst tidal breathing of the krypton-81m/air mixture with a relatively fixed inspiratory volume and fixed alveolar-pleural pressure gradient, the regions of the lung with lower compliance receive less krypton-81m than the regions with higher compliance.

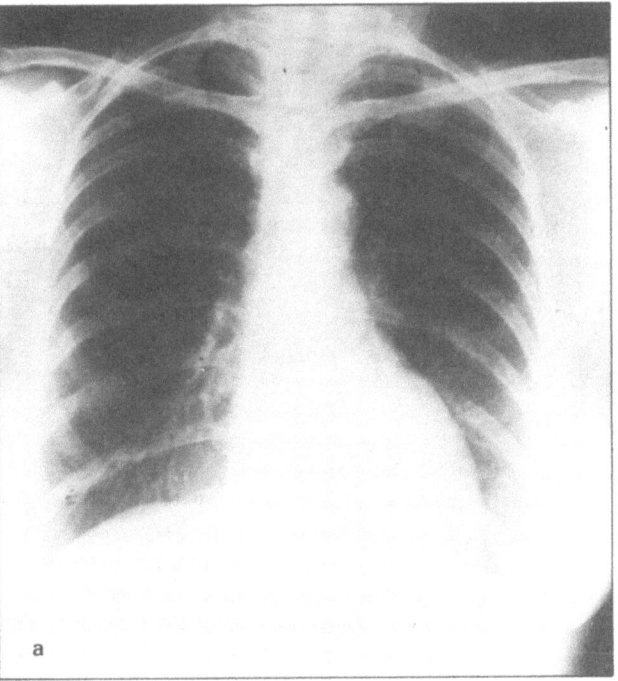

Figure 6.14a *The clear chest radiograph of a woman with acute obstructive bronchitis.*

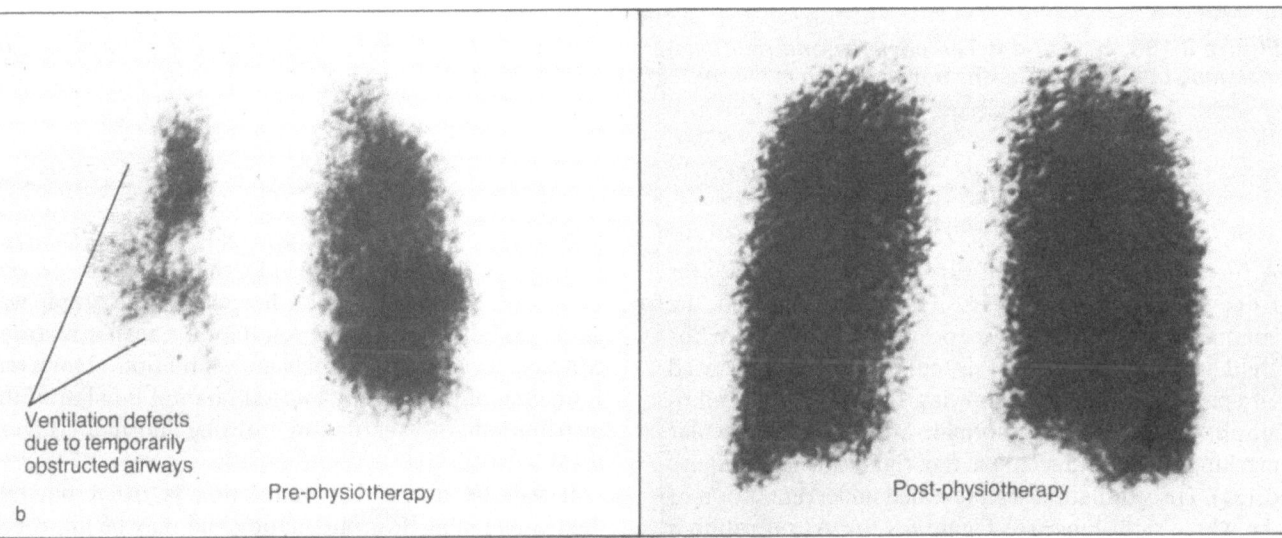

Figure 6.14b *The ventilation images before then after physiotherapy in the same woman (posterior view).*

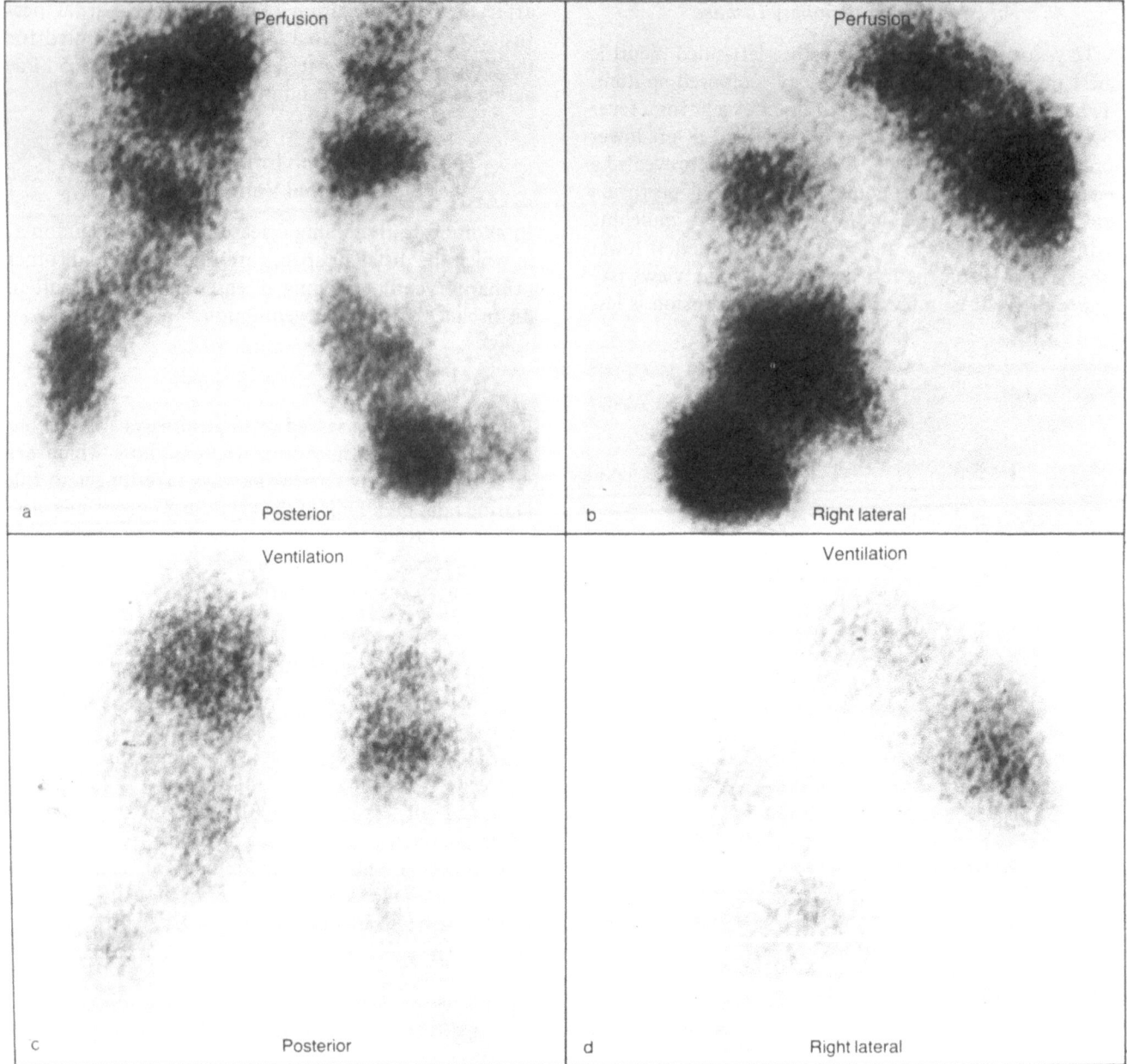

Figure 6.15a, b, c and d *The posterior and right lateral ventilation and perfusion images illustrating the degree of matching between perfusion and ventilation in chronic airflow obstruction.*

Examples of Airways Obstruction

A three-year-old child had suffered for twelve months from wheezy breathlessness. His mother related the commencement of his dyspnoea to a period when the child had eaten a packet of peanuts and had experienced an episode of choking following this. His chest radiograph was regarded as normal, although the vascular markings were reduced on the right side (see Figure 6.13a). His ventilation scan revealed underventilation of the whole right lung (see Figure 6.13b). At operation a peanut was removed from the right main bronchus.

Another patient—a 58-year-old woman, suffered from obstructive bronchitis. During an acute exacerbation of her illness, when her chest radiograph was clear (Figure 6.14a), ventilation scan revealed widespread bilateral defects in ventilation. However, following physiotherapy and salbutamol inhalation the distribution of ventilation became normal (Figure 6.14b).

It will be noted that ventilation is often patchily distributed in airflow obstruction and may be improved by therapy.

The Disturbance of Perfusion in Ventilatory Disorders

The Disturbance of Perfusion in Ventilatory Disorders

In association with ventilatory disturbance there are associated matching perfusion defects as a result of localized arteriolar vasoconstriction.

Examples of Disturbance of Perfusion in

Ventilatory Disorders

A 68-year-old woman suffered from chronic obstructive bronchitis for 20 years, and her primary complaint was one of exercise dyspnoea. She had widespread wheezes on auscultation, but her chest radiograph was clear. Her FEV_1 was only 30 per cent of the predicted value.

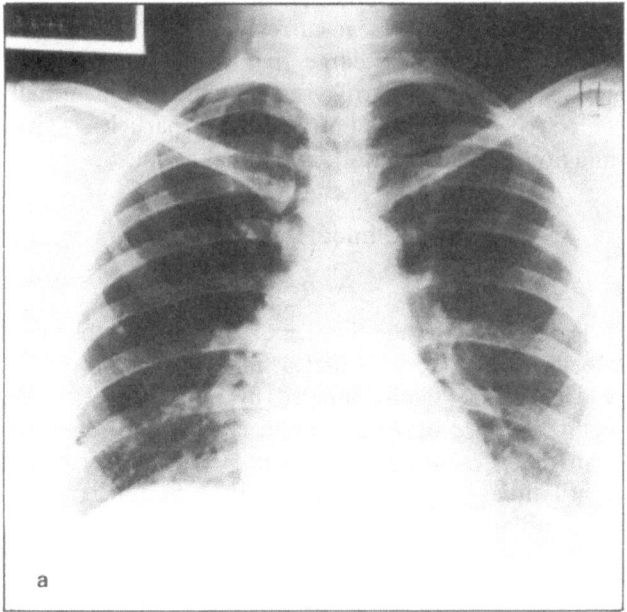

Figure 6.16a *The patient's chest radiograph showing a calcified primary focus in the right mid-zone.*

The ventilation and perfusion scans reveal bilateral multiple matching defects (see Figure 6.15). The perfusion scan, when taken alone, could be interpreted as showing evidence of multiple pulmonary emboli. Therefore, it is of great importance, in the presence of clinical evidence of airflow obstruction, to perform both ventilation and perfusion studies and to determine the degree of matching between the defects in each.

Similar matching perfusion and ventilation defects may be seen in fibrotic lung diseases, an example of this is described in the following case-study. A lady in her sixties complained of a sharp left-sided chest pain but had no abnormal physical signs on examination. Her chest radiograph was clear, but, as will be seen, there was a small calcified primary tuberculous focus in the right mid-zone (Figure 6.16a). Both perfusion and ventilation scans revealed a large defect in the right mid-zone, presumably related to local fibrosis (Figure 6.16b and c).

The Localization of Pulmonary Disease

The last example illustrates the sensitivity of lung scanning in defining the location of disturbances of ventilation when compared with the chest radiograph. Use may be made of this facility in determining the site to which more specific pulmonary investigations should be directed.

An Example of Localization of

Pulmonary Disease

A 34-year-old woman complained of exertional breathlessness, but had no abnormal physical signs and normal respiratory function tests. Her chest radiograph

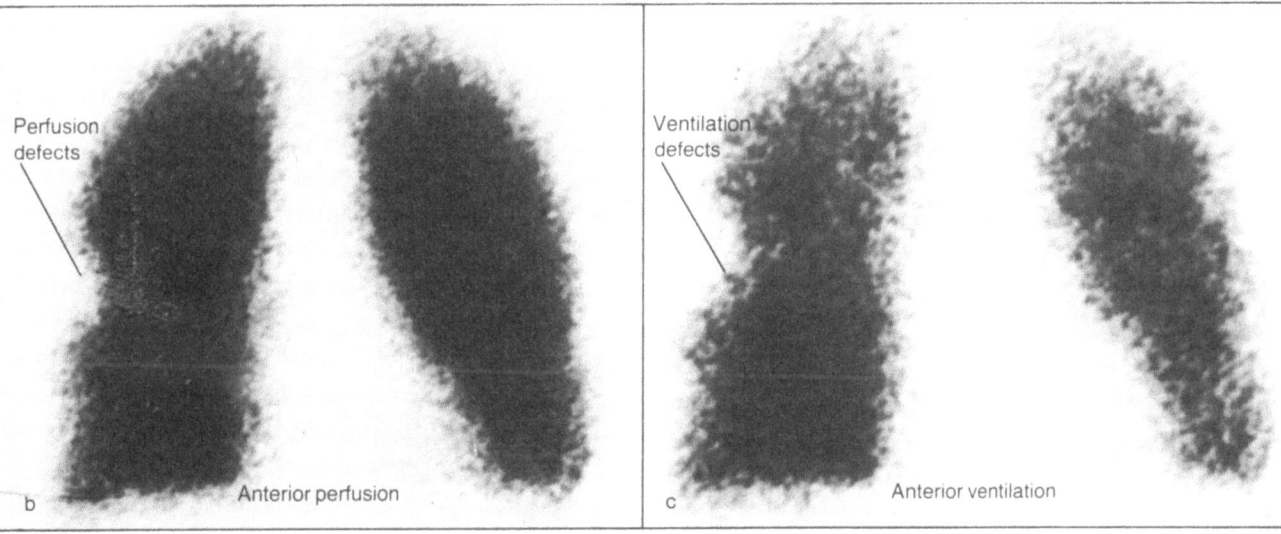

Figure 6.16b and c *The anterior images of perfusion and ventilation from the same patient, showing the large area of reduced perfusion and ventilation in the right mid-zone.*

was not remarkable (Figure 6.17a). The perfusion and ventilation scans of the lung revealed local defects in the right lung (Figure 6.17b and c). Later, a bronchogram was taken, which gave the appearance of an obliterative bronchiolitis. The same principles may be applied to localizing other primary pulmonary lesions, e.g. emphysematous bullae, or carcinoma of the bronchi when a major bronchus is obstructed.

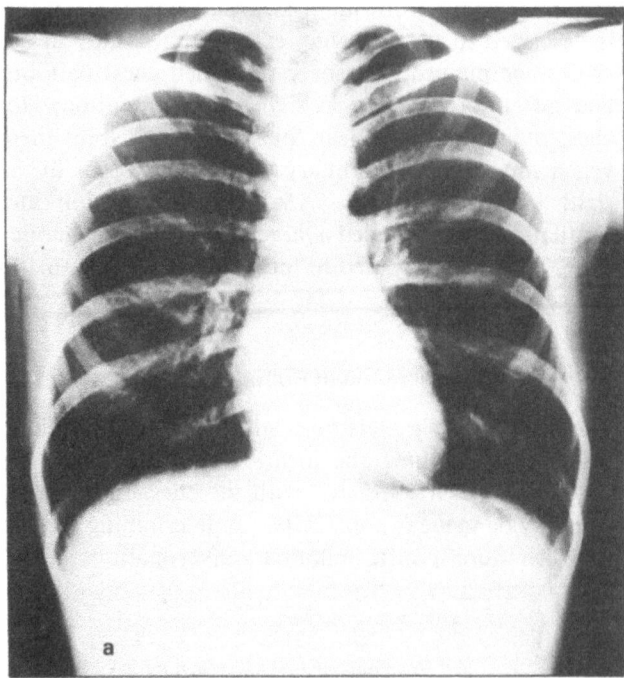

Figure 6.17a *The clear chest radiograph of a woman who was suffering from increasing breathlessness. There is reduced pulmonary vasculature of the right mid- and lower zones.*

Complications and Contraindications

Lung scans can be performed with little inconvenience to patients, and provide not only an accurate diagnosis of pulmonary emboli but also enable the localization of deficiencies in lung function which are not visible on the chest radiograph. This is achieved with a minimal risk to the patient, the hazard being infinitely smaller than with other procedures which are available to demonstrate the same functional impairment.

There is a small risk of causing obstruction to the pulmonary circulation with microspheres or macroaggregates when this is already compromised, as in obliterative pulmonary hypertension. However, only eight fatalities have been recorded over the last 12 years and these were the result of using particles with a greater range of size than those in current use.

In the presence of large right-to-left (intracardiac) shunts there is a risk of systemic microemboli; usually only 50 per cent of the normal dose of particles is given and noticeable complications are thus avoided.

Future Clinical Developments

Aerosols

It is possible to grade the size of albumin microspheres labelled with $^{99}Tc^{m}$, so that a 'mist' may be produced which can be tidally inhaled by a patient. Particles below the size of 7μ appear in normal subjects to be distributed, as with krypton-81m, according to regional ventilation and so provide another means of performing the ventilation scan.

However, in pulmonary disease the particles are distributed less according to regional ventilation than to

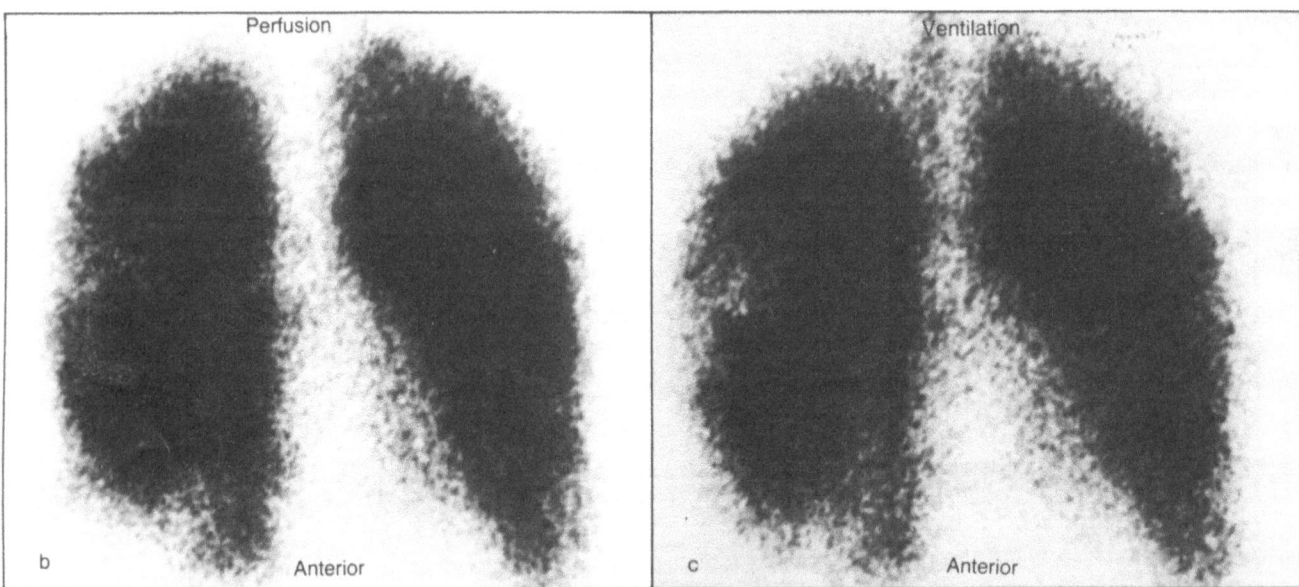

Figure 6.17b and c *The comparable anterior views of ventilation and perfusion in the same patient, showing the reduced ventilation and perfusion of these two zones.*

local areas of turbulence in the airways and sites of mucus concentration. Use has been made of this increased uptake of the labelled particles into mucus to study the clearance rates of mucus from the lungs in diseases such as bronchitis and the syndrome of Kartagener (sinusitis, bronchiectasis and dextrocardia.)

Ventilation, Perfusion Ratios

The introduction of the short half-life isotopes such as krypton-81m, which may be used to study both regional perfusion and ventilation, provides opportunities to study factors which may affect simultaneously both perfusion and ventilation.

In many pulmonary diseases the local balance of perfusion to ventilation can be disturbed, resulting in imperfect gaseous exchange. To visualize these disease processes it is possible, by storing first a perfusion then a ventilation image with a computer, to obtain regional ventilation to perfusion ratios for one view of the lung. This method, although in its infancy, will provide ultimately both scientific and clinical information about many pulmonary diseases.

Further Reading

Fazio, F. and Jones, T., *Br. Med. J.*, 1975, **3**, 673.

Hughes, J. M. B., *Br. J. Dis. Chest,* 1975, **69**, 153.

Knipping, H. W., Bolt, W., Keppath, H., Valentin, H., Ludes, H. and Emllen, P., *Desch. Med. Wachensch.*, 1955, **80**, 1146.

Wagner, H. N., *Am. Rev. Respir. Dis.,* 1976, **113**, 203.

Wagner, H. N. (Jr), Sabiston, D. C. (Jr), McAfee, J. C., Tow, D. and Stern, H. S., *New. Eng. J. Med.,* 1964, **271**, 377.

West, J. B. and Dollery, C. T., *J. Appl. Physiol.,* 1960, **15**, 405.

Williams, O., Lyall, J., Vernon, M. and Croft, D. N., *Br. Med. J.,* 1974, **1**, 600.

7. Renal Scanning

In nuclear medicine, the kidneys have attracted more interest than many other organs in the body. This is understandable when one considers that nuclear medicine is a considerably better technique for the study of function rather than structure. Techniques for the study of renal structure, such as intravenous urography and ultrasonography, are well developed but are extremely poor at the assessment of regional function. Tracer techniques with radionuclides have filled this gap and add the functional component to the other imaging techniques.

Nuclear medicine techniques for the study of the kidneys fall into three groups (Table 7.1). The first group consists of methods for measuring total renal

Table 7.1 Nuclear medicine techniques in renal disease.

1. Tests of total renal function
   Measurement of the glomerular filtration rate
   Measurement of the effective renal plasma flow

2. Probe techniques
   Renography

3. Gamma camera imaging
   a) Static renal imaging
   b) Dynamic renal imaging

function. The second comprises non-imaging methods involving surface counting using probe techniques, which are generally being replaced by the third group, using a gamma camera, with or without a computer, which allows visual and quantitative assessment of the renal tract. This last group can be further divided into those methods used for static imaging and those used for dynamic imaging. Because there is an overlap between the indications for these tests, it is convenient to consider the tests first and then to consider the range of clinical problems in which the various tests may be of value.

Nuclear Medicine Techniques

Tests to Measure Total Renal Function

Following Homer Smith (1951), it may be thought that 'renal function' consists of two discrete entities—glomerular filtration and tubular secretion. These are traditionally estimated by measuring the clearances from the blood of indicators handled by these mechanisms. Inulin is used for the measurement of glomerular filtration rate (GFR), and PAH (p-amino-hippuric acid) for the 'effective renal plasma flow' (ERPF). Unfortunately, it is not simple to measure chemically either inulin or PAH. In practice, the only test used clinically is the estimation of the clearance of endogenous creatinine for the measurement of GFR, but this is time-consuming and inaccurate, the errors increasing with impairment of renal function when tubular secretion of creatinine becomes important. In addition, any clearance technique using urine measurement requires 'complete urine collections'—a theoretical concept in the uncatheterized patient!

Fortunately, many other compounds labelled with radionuclides, which are measured easily and are excreted only by glomerular filtration, are available. A selection of those used in clinical practice is shown in Table 7.2. They can be divided into two groups—

Table 7.2 Agents used for the measurement of glomerular filtration rate (GFR).

Chelates of metallic radionuclides	^{51}Cr-EDTA
	^{99}Tc^{m}-DTPA
	^{169}Yb-DTPA
Radiographic contrast media	^{125}I-Iothalamate
	^{125}I-Diatrizoate

chelates of metallic radionuclides, and radiographic contrast media labelled with radioactive iodine isotopes. In the technique usually used with all these agents, a known amount of the labelled compound is injected intravenously and then serial blood samples are taken, usually at two, three and four hours after injection. Later blood samples are taken when there is evidence of impaired renal function, and the rate of clearance from the blood is determined. Knowing the total activity injected, the absolute clearance of the compound can be determined. This is a technique which is within the capabilities of all nuclear medicine departments.

In a similar approach, the clearance of ^{131}I-ortho-iodo-hippuric acid (OIH, hippuran), an agent which is handled by the kidney in a manner similar to PAH, can be used for the measurement of ERPF by taking serial blood samples over a period of about one hour, following the injection of a known quantity of tracer. However, this has not found a useful place in the routine investigation of renal function.

Renography

The uptake and excretion of tracers which are handled by the kidneys can be measured by using external radiation detectors positioned over the kidneys. In practice, the tracer commonly used for renography is ^{131}I-labelled OIH. The most widely used method involves three probes—one over each kidney and one over the heart. Because the renal probes have a relatively large field of view (necessary to ensure that the whole of each kidney is included), it is necessary to correct for the vascularity of non-renal tissue, such as liver and spleen, which cannot be separated from the kidney. This may be achieved by the prior injection of a small dose of labelled albumin, which gives an indication of the relative sizes of the blood pools within the fields of view of the probes. When the relative vascularity is known, the radioactivity recorded by each renal probe can be corrected in order to remove the effect of the blood pool seen by that probe. This may be performed either by using a simple analogue computer or a general purpose digital computer. The process is known as computer assisted blood background subtraction (CABBS) renography.

CABBS renography may be used to assess divided renal function, and in the investigation of possible renal disease. It is relatively simple and cheap, but is best regarded as a screening test, as an abnormal renogram can be produced by many pathological processes.

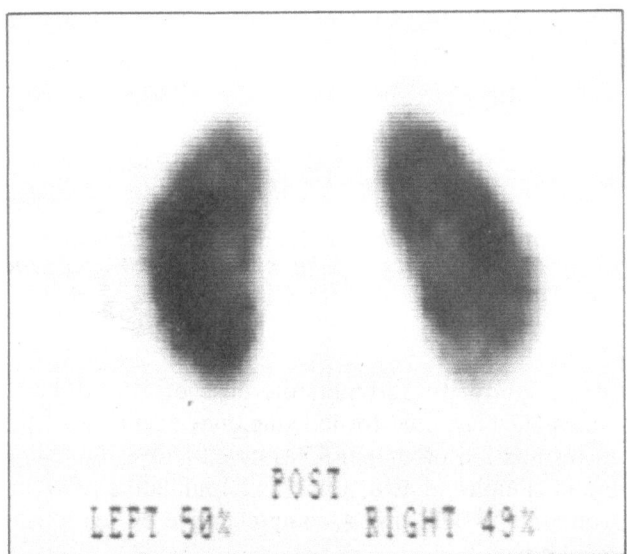

Figure 7.1 *Normal posterior static renal scan ([99]Tc[m]-DMSA) with divided function.*

Imaging Methods

Static Imaging

The principle of the method is to have a radiopharmaceutical which is fixed in the renal parenchyma, so that images may be obtained which show the functional anatomy of the kidney. The earliest attempts at static imaging were performed by using radioactive mercury-labelled ([205]Hg or [197]Hg) chlormerodrin. This procedure showed that the rate of uptake by the two kidneys was an index of divided renal function, but was of little value for imaging.

Static imaging is now usually performed following an intravenous injection of [99]Tc[m]-labelled compound, such as dimercaptosuccinic acid (DMSA, DMS). Approximately two-thirds of the injected radioactivity is taken up in the renal parenchyma, and remains there indefinitely. The remaining activity is excreted in the urine, about 10 per cent of the injected activity being excreted over three hours. The kidneys are imaged after three or more hours to obtain an image which shows the distribution of functional renal tissue. Furthermore, the ratio of DMSA uptake between the kidneys gives the divided renal function, so that if the total renal function is known (for example, by measurement of the GFR), the absolute function of each kidney may be estimated (Figure 7.1). As a further refinement, it is possible to analyse the distribution of function within a kidney.

Dynamic Imaging

With the development of the gamma camera, it was a natural step to image the kidneys following the injection of ^{131}I-OIH as this agent was widely used for renography. However, the physical properties of iodine-131 are not ideal, and it was only with the introduction of [99]Tc[m]-labelled compounds that dynamic renal imaging has become routine. Initially it was hoped that this would give all the information obtained by the IVU, but it should be appreciated that the radiological methods have the advantage of better structural resolution and the place of radioisotopic renal imaging is in the assessment of functional change.

The dynamic imaging agent of choice is [99]Tc[m]-DTPA, which, as has been noted in Table 7.2, is a chelate handled by glomerular filtration (and can be used for the measurement of GFR). The gamma camera is positioned posteriorly over the kidneys and 15 mCi of [99]Tc[m]-DTPA is injected intravenously as a bolus. An image is recorded for the first 30 seconds following this, and shows the major blood vessels, both kidneys, liver and spleen, the amount of activity reflecting their relative vascularity. Following this, an image at two minutes after injection shows the distribution of function within and between the kidneys. By five minutes, activity should be seen in the collecting system. Serial

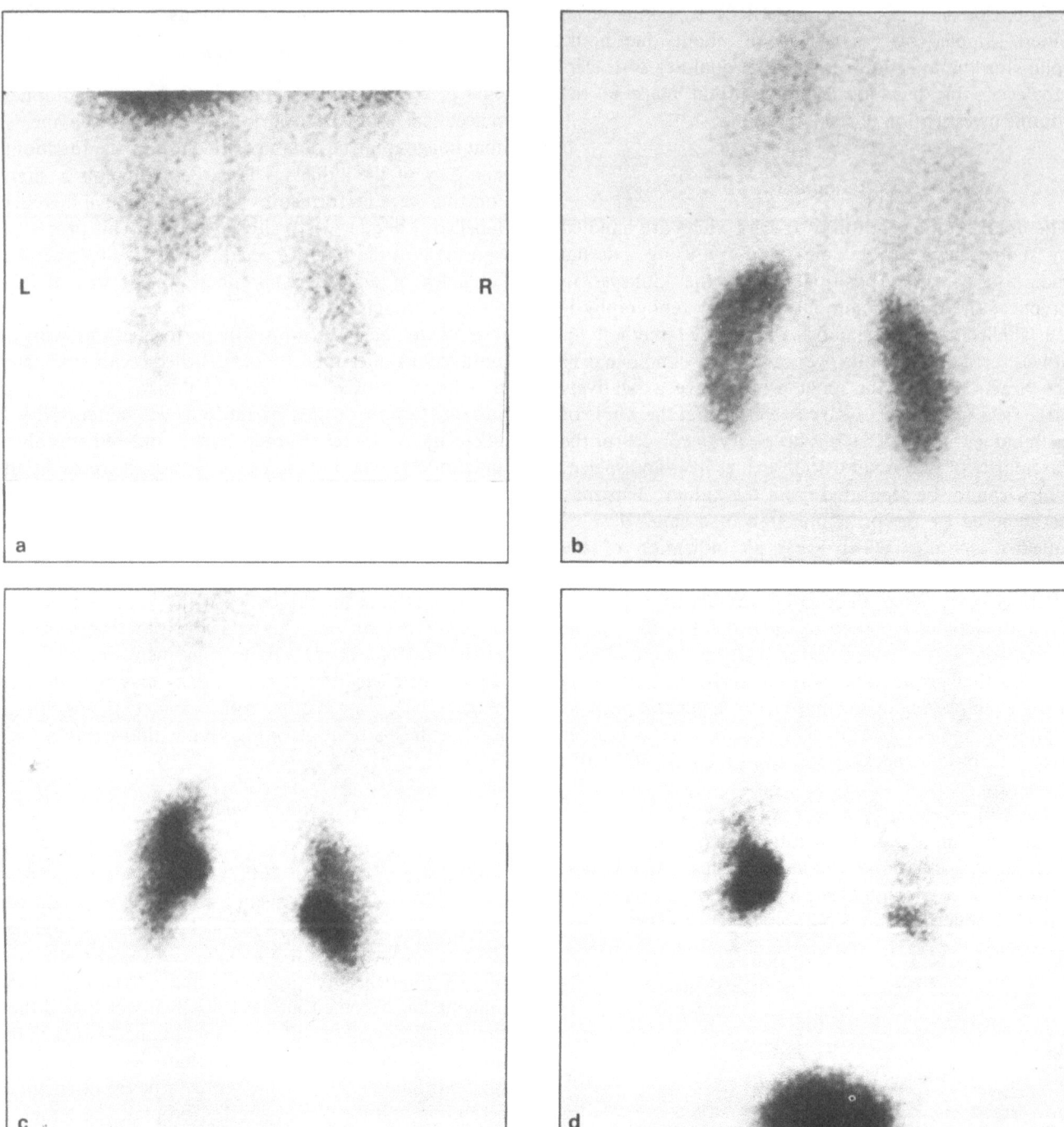

Figure 7.2 *Dynamic renal scan on patient with dilated left kidney and normal right kidney. Vascularity of kidneys is readily assessed on* (a) *0-30 second image;* (b) *at two minutes, distribution of functioning parenchyma is seen, and* (c) *the collecting system is seen at five minutes, and* (d) *at 30 minutes.*

images over 30 minutes show progressive excretion and clearance of the tracer. If there is any possibility of obstruction, further imaging for 15 minutes after frusemide-induced diuresis may be of value (Figure 7.2).

Quantitative assessment using an on-line mini computer allows measurement of relative renal vascularity, overall excretion, and estimation of the degree of obstruction, adding considerably to the value

of the study. In addition, the dose of $^{99}T_{c}{}^{m}$-DTPA, which has been used for imaging, may also be used for the estimation of the GFR (as noted above by taking blood samples at two, three and four hours after injection, thus allowing a comprehensive evaluation of renal function.

The *residual volume* in the bladder is easily determined after a dynamic renal study by recording the

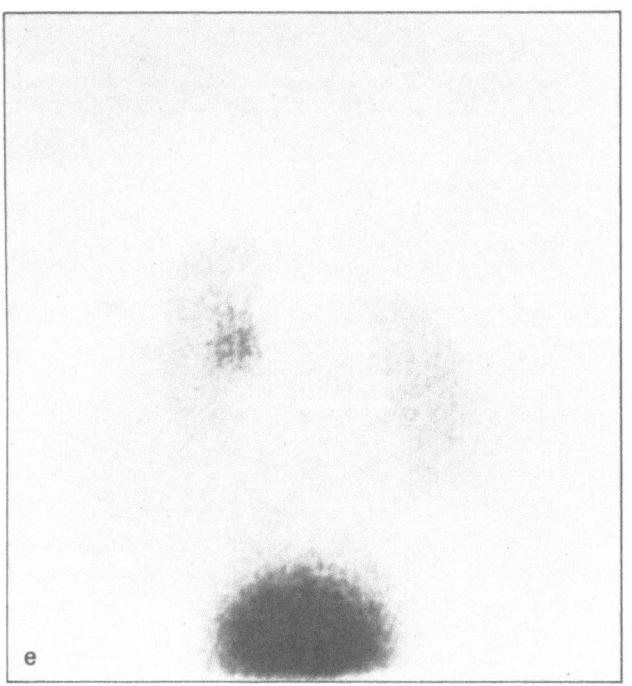

Figure 7.2e and f *Following Frusemide* (e) *35 minutes and* (f) *40 minutes there is rapid washout of* $^{99}Tc^m$-*DTPA from both kidneys, confirming dilatation rather than obstruction.*

difference in bladder count rate immediately before and after voiding. If the volume of urine passed is known, then the count rate per ml of the urine is known, and the residual volume is estimated from the post-voiding count rate. Alternatively, a small amount of activity may be introduced into the bladder by suprapubic puncture, and the same measurements made.

Vesico-ureteric *reflux* can be studied by imaging the ureters and kidneys as the patient voids, using the activity present in the bladder after the dynamic renal study. This has the advantage that it is not necessary to catheterize the patient or to give any further irradiation. However, this 'indirect' method is probably not as sensitive as the 'direct' method in which a tracer, such as $^{99}Tc^m$-pertechnetate, is introduced into the bladder by using a catheter. The bladder is filled, as in the radiological micturating cystogram, and imaging is performed during filling and voiding. In expert hands, this gives excellent results, and the ability to record continuously on the computer allows detection of minor degrees of reflux, as well as quantitation of the volumes at which reflux occurs and the volume of urine refluxing. Possibly the major advantage, however, is the considerable reduction in radiation dose.

Some of the techniques which are available for the study of the kidneys have been discussed, and it is appropriate now to consider the clinical problems in which these may be of value. Indications for static and dynamic renal imaging are set out briefly in Table 7.3.

The measurement of divided renal function and the intra-renal distribution of function is probably the most

Table 7.3 Indications for static and dynamic renal imaging.

Static imaging	Dynamic imaging
Regional distribution of renal function	Renal failure
	Major arterial disease
Divided renal function	Renal perfusion
Evaluation of possible renal masses	Lesion vascularity
	Outflow tract assessment
	Reflux
	Renal transplantation

important contribution of nuclear medicine techniques in renal disease. This is most obvious in the patient with renal calculi (Figure 7.3) or in the patient with a horseshoe kidney (Figure 7.4), where the surgeon wishes to operate with minimum damage to the patient's functioning renal tissue. The use of DMSA static imaging allows easy visualization of the distribution of function, as well as its quantitation (Figure 7.5). A more general use of this approach is in the patient with known renal disease such as pelvi-ureteric junction (PUJ) obstruction, where the indications for surgery are marginal—the patient is not currently having pain or infection. In this case, serial estimations of the function of the affected kidney allow the patient to be followed in the knowledge that any impairment of function will be detected, and surgery can be performed. Similarly, the post-pyeloplasty patient may be readily followed in order to assess progress of renal function (Figure 7.6).

In cases such as these, the approach of choice is to

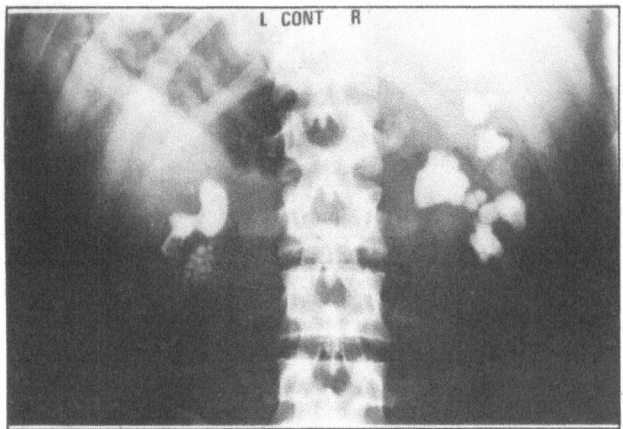

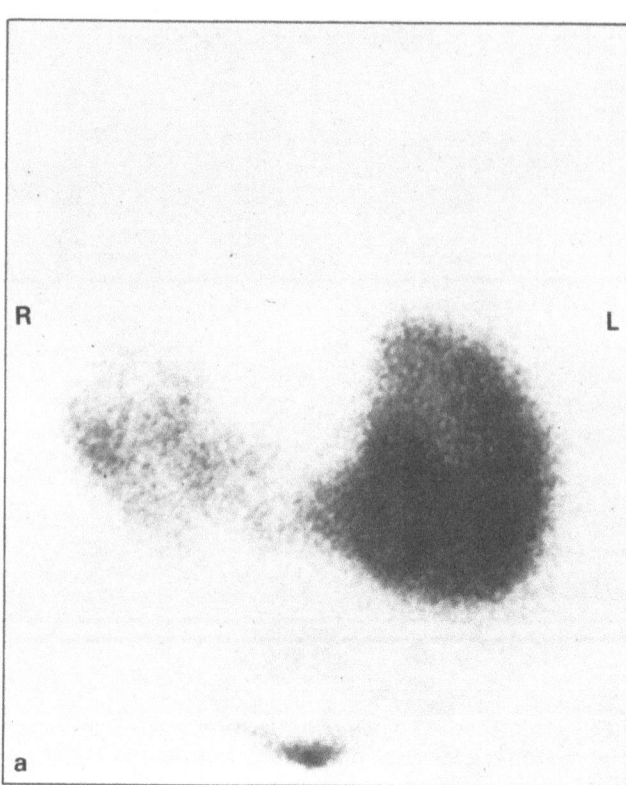

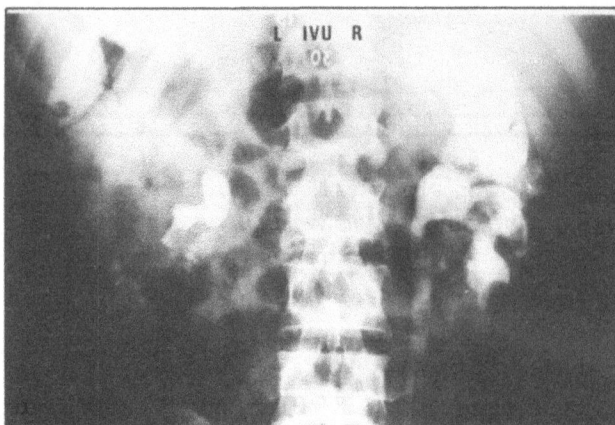

Figure 7.3 *Control film* (a) *and IVU film* (b) *in patient with renal calculi. Where is the functioning renal tissue? (Note labelling of sides).*

measure the total renal function by measuring the GFR with ^{51}Cr-EDTA and, at the same time, to perform a DMSA renal scan to assess distribution of renal function. Alternatively, divided renal function may be obtained from the ^{99}Tc^m-DTPA dynamic renal study but this takes more time on the gamma camera and computer. The author's practice is to use the static study in preference, unless there is some other indication for dynamic imaging, or there is a question of severe obstruction because of the ^{99}Tc^m-DMSA which is excreted into the collecting system. In the obstructed system, this will still be present at three hours after injection, giving rise to an over-estimate of the function of that kidney. Alternatively, the divided renal function may be estimated from the dynamic study at two minutes after injection, when there has been no excretion.

Indications for Static and Dynamic Renal Imaging

Investigation of Renal Masses

Occasional problems arise with patients whose IVU's

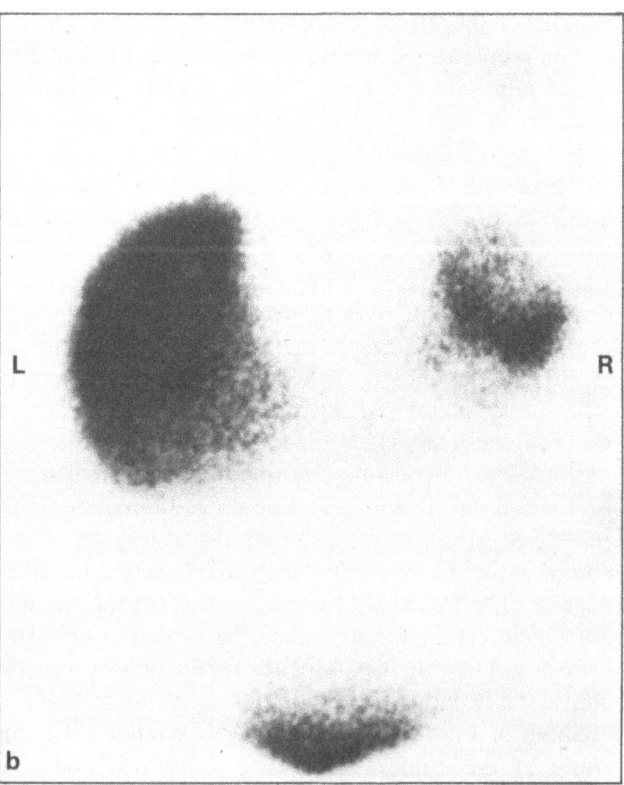

Figure 7.4 *Static renal scan in a patient with a horse-shoe kidney* (a—*anterior view and* b—*posterior view). Computer analysis shows that the hydronephrotic right portion contributes 20 per cent of the total renal function.*

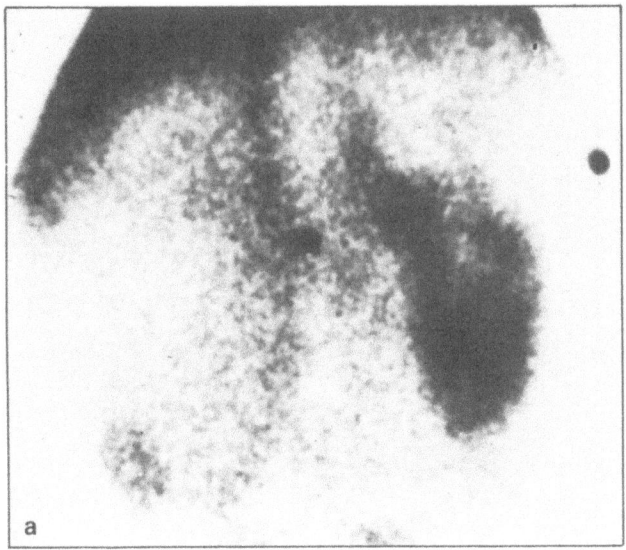

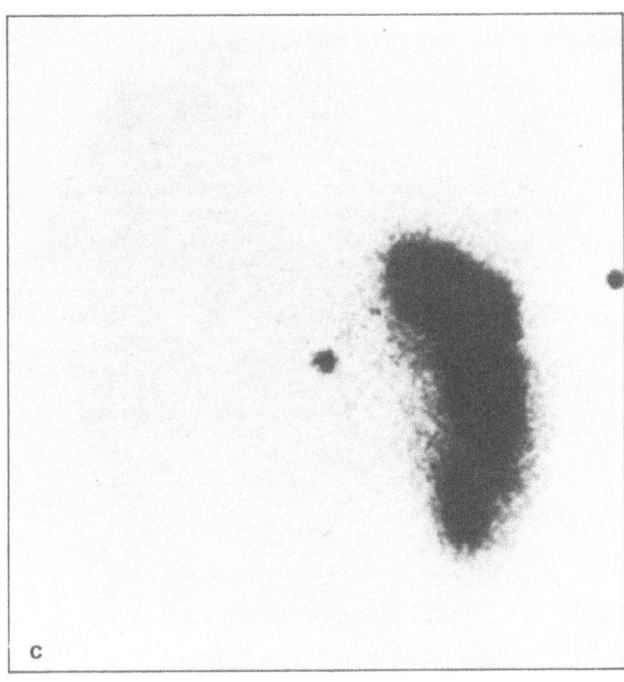

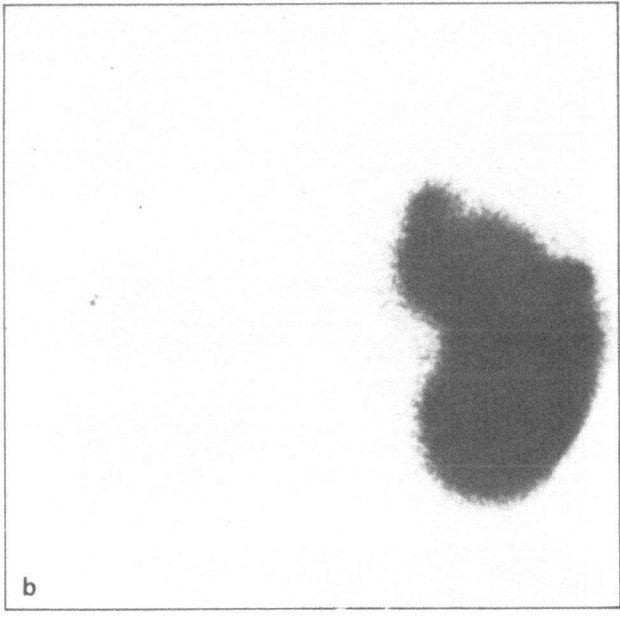

Figure 7.5 *Note ease with which distribution of parenchyma is seen (on same patient as Figure 7.3) in both* **(a)** *0-30 seconds* $^{99}Tc^m$-DTPA *and* **(b)** *3 hour* $^{99}Tc^m$-DMSA *static image, in spite of hydronephrosis shown by* **(c)** *2 hour* $^{99}Tc^m$-DTPA *images.*

Obstruction

A problem which arises regularly in urology is the patient with apparent obstruction, which has been detected on the IVU. It may be difficult to distinguish the partially obstructed PUJ from the renal pelvis which is merely dilated, especially when the patient has had previous surgery. As has been noted already, one approach is to see whether there is any progressive impairment of function. An alternative approach is to use the dynamic renal study. As described above, our current approach is to use frusemide-induced diuresis. In a dilated renal pelvis there appears to be good clearance by 15 minutes, whereas in the obstructed kidney there is increasing activity. Intermediate degrees may also be recognized. Quantitative analysis improves the accuracy of the method.

Other centres are working on mathematical approaches to assess obstruction which may appear on the dynamic renal study, and this is a field of great interest.

Assessment of Renal Perfusion

The dynamic study with $^{99}Tc^m$-DTPA allows major changes in renal perfusion to be seen, and is of value especially where the question is one of presence or absence of renal perfusion. An example of this is the patient with dissecting aortic aneurysm.

Renal artery stenosis is more difficult to assess, as the

show parenchymal distortion and it is not clear whether this represents a renal tumour, a cyst, or a 'pseudotumour' (i.e. phantom tumour). This is becoming less of a problem, but still arises, especially as it may not be possible, when using ultrasound, to distinguish a tumour from a 'pseudotumour', as they are both solid. On these occasions a DMSA scan will show whether the apparent mass represents functioning renal tissue (implying pseudotumour) or is non-functioning (cyst or tumour—Figures 7.7 and 7.8). Dynamic imaging or imaging after injection of $^{99}Tc^m$-labelled red blood cells will then show the vascularity of the lesion. Additionally, the information available about the distribution of renal function is again of value to the surgeon planning his approach.

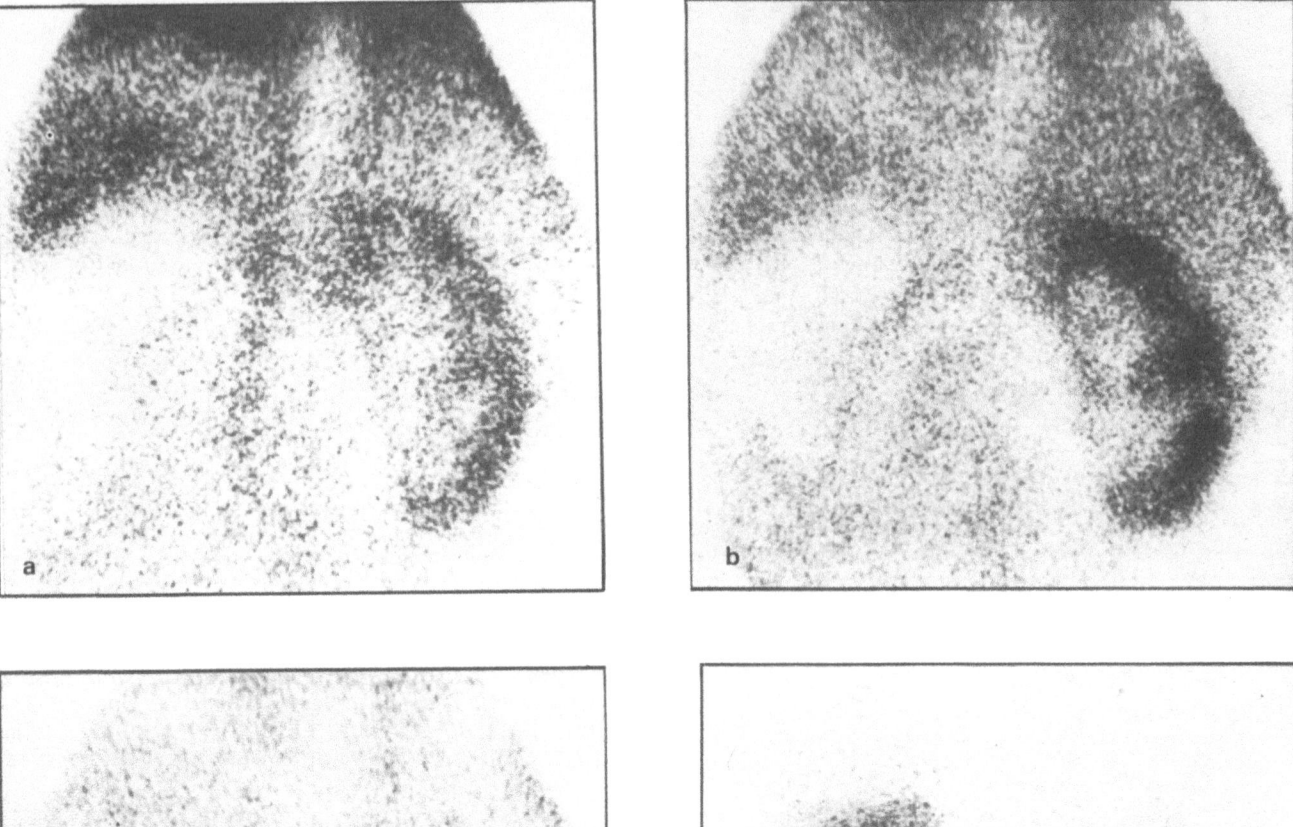

Figure 7.6 *Patient with hydronephrosis and reflux from neurogenic bladder. The distribution of functioning renal tissue is clearly seen. Note the slow passage of $^{99}Tc^m$-DTPA into the collecting systems.* (**a**) *0-30 seconds,* (**b**) *two minutes,* (**c**) *five minutes and* (**d**) *two hours.*

two kidneys have different vascular backgrounds (the liver receiving the bulk of its blood supply from the portal circulation shows a vascular perfusion peak some nine seconds later than the spleen, which forms the background to the left kidney). Because of this, unilateral renal artery stenosis is best detected using CABBS renography, when a delayed, higher peak is seen on the affected side.

Renal Failure

In the patient with apparent acute renal failure, the dynamic renal study with $^{99}Tc^m$-DTPA is the method of choice. It takes only 30 minutes and is atraumatic, and is, therefore, a suitable study for the ill patient. In this study, the size of the kidneys is readily assessed, as is their vascularity. In acute-on-chronic renal failure, the

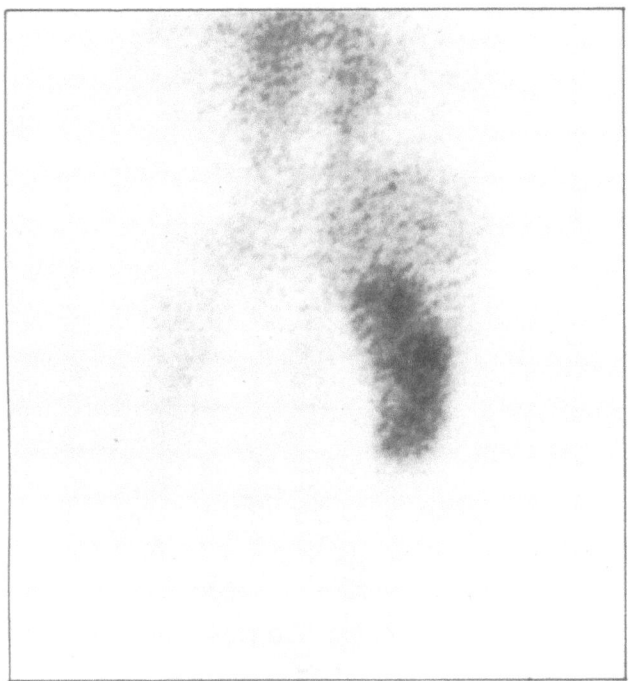

Figure 7.6 (e) *Shows the same patient (compare Figure 7.6 b) after surgery, at two minutes. The improvement in function of the kidneys, especially the right, is obvious.*

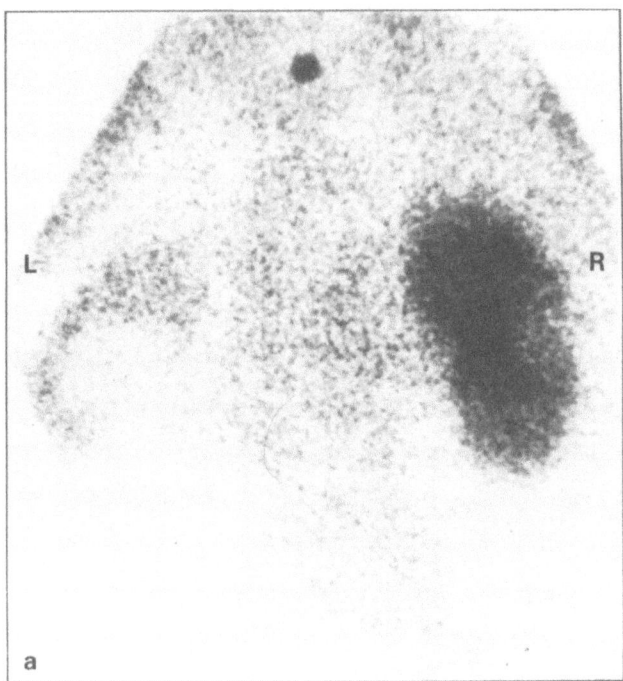

small kidneys may be only poorly seen, and a follow-up scan with ⁹⁹Tcᵐ-DMSA may be helpful in confirming this. In acute nephritis, the kidneys are usually of normal size, or larger, with some impairment of perfusion. In acute tubular necrosis (ATN) the kidneys

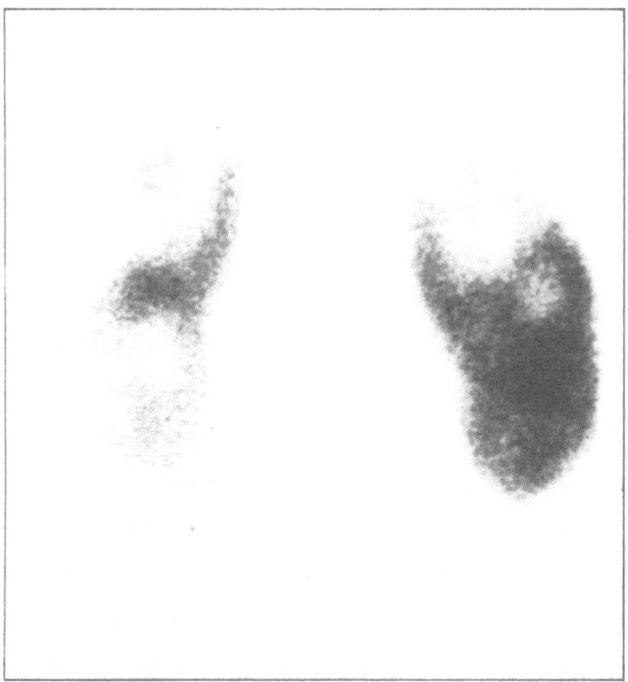

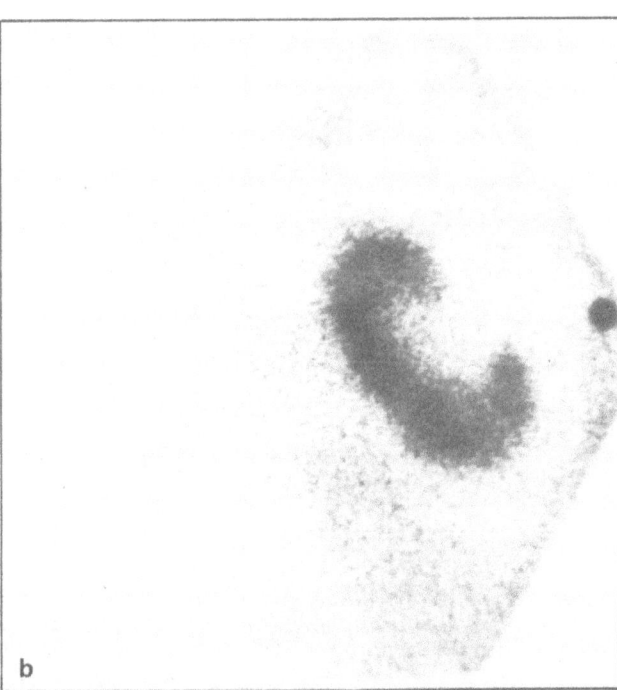

Figure 7.8 *Static renal scan in a patient whose IVU suggested a left renal tumour. The scan shows this clearly in both the posterior (a) and left posterior oblique (b) views, and also shows the (previously unnoticed) tumour in the right kidney!*

Figure 7.7 *Static renal scan in patient with polycystic kidneys.*

show a typical appearance, being well perfused and well seen at two minutes, but from then on are seen progressively less well (Figure 7.9). In obstruction, perfusion is normal in the early stages, but with prolonged obstruction impaired perfusion may be seen.

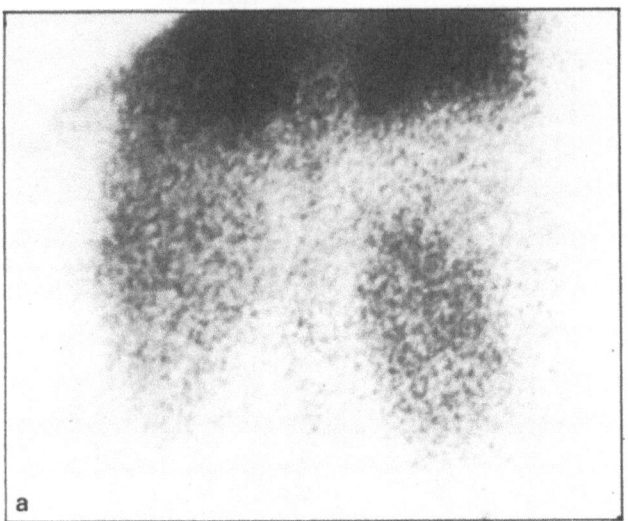

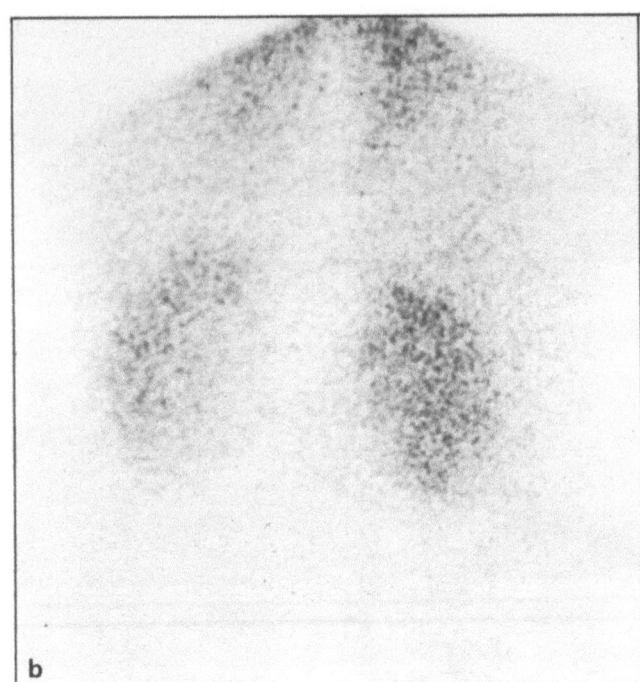

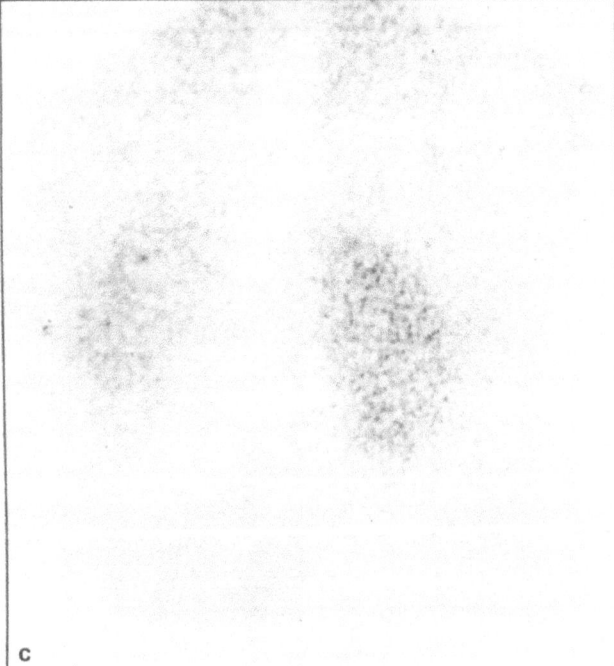

Figure 7.9 *In ATN the kidneys are well perfused and seen well at two minutes, but progressively less well thereafter. The figures show:* (**a**) *0-30 seconds,* (**b**) *two minutes,* (**c**) *five minutes and* (**d**) *30 minutes.*

Renal Transplantation

This is a specialized field where nuclear medicine has a great deal to offer. Serial studies with $^{99}Tc^m$-DTPA allow measurement of changes in the perfusion of the transplanted kidney, which is known to be one of the earliest indicators of rejection. This can be detected in the anuric patient, and rejection can be diagnosed even in the anuric patient with ATN. In addition, other complications, such as obstruction and lymphocele formation, may be detected (Figure 7.10).

Conclusion

Nuclear medicine has much to offer the urologist and nephrologist. It does not offer the structural resolution of radiology or ultrasound, or the histological accuracy of renal biopsy, but the speed and ease with which it can be performed, together with its unique ability to measure and display function, assures it of a place in the diagnostic armamentarium.

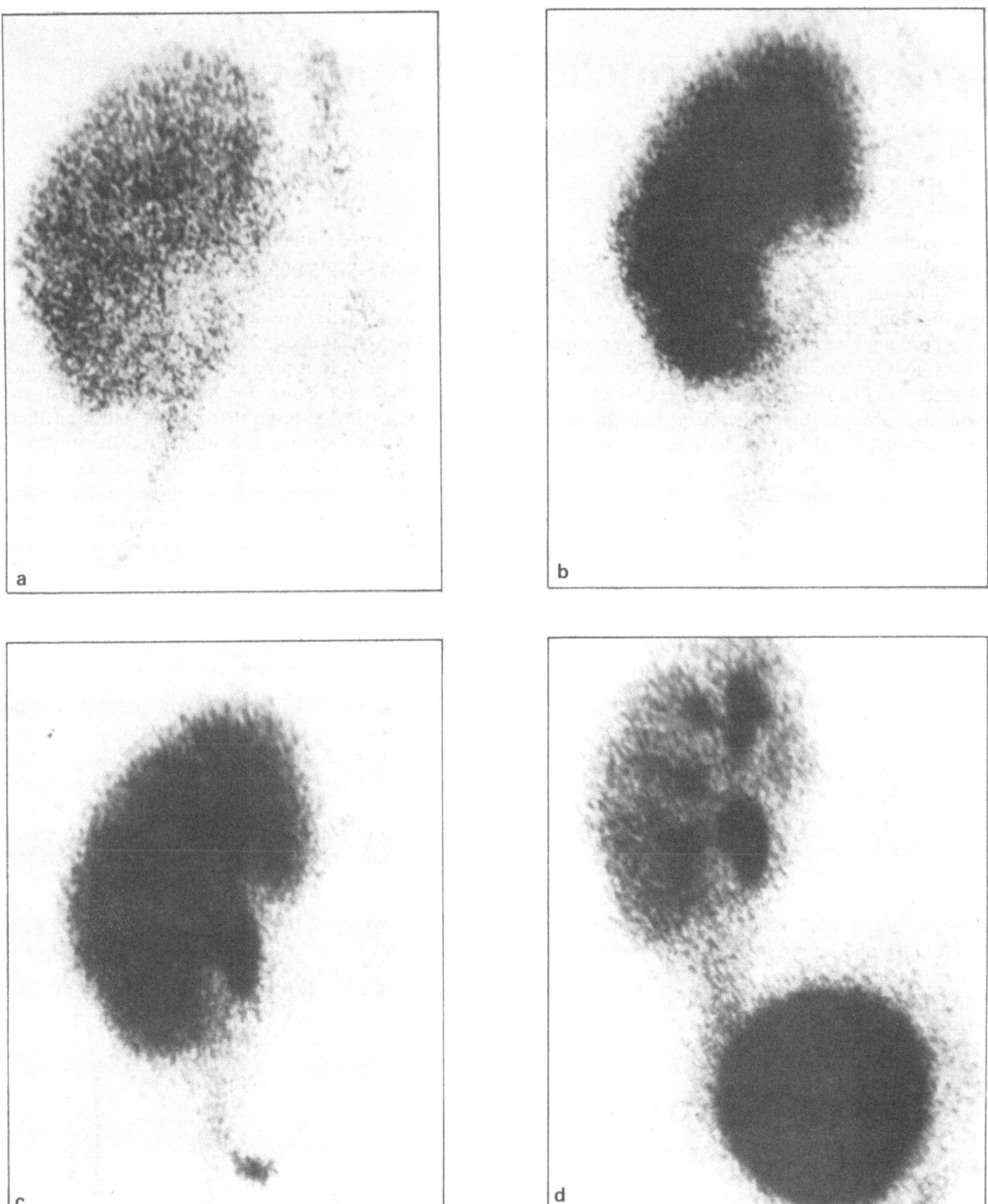

Figure 7.10 *Renal transplantation. Note visualization of artery, kidney, ureter and bladder,* (**a**) *0-30 seconds,* (**b**) *two minutes,* (**c**) *five minutes and* (**d**) *30 minutes.*

Further Reading

Britton, K. E. and Brown, N. J. G., *Clinical Renography,* Lloyd Luke, London, 1971.

Bingham, J. B. and Maisey, M. N., *Br. J. Radiol.,* 1978, **51**, 599.

Hilson, A. J. W., Maisey, M. N., Brown, C. B., Ogg, C. S. and

Bewick, M. S., *J. Nucl. Med.,* 1978, **19**, 944.

Smith, H. W., *The structure and function of the kidney in health and disease,* Oxford University Press, 1951.

Wagner, H. N., *Am. Rev. Respir. Dis.,* 1976, **113**, 203.

8. Radionuclide Thyroid Scanning

The thyroid was the first organ to be studied in vivo with radionuclide tracers. The unique property of the thyroid to concentrate and organify inorganic iodine, store the iodinated compounds and release them as active hormones into the circulation made it possible to investigate the function of the gland by means of radioactive iodine tracers, especially ^{131}I which became readily available as a by-product from nuclear reactors. More recently, the element technetium was also shown to be concentrated by the thyroid cells, but, unlike iodine, it is not organified into the thyroid hormones. The use of the radionuclide technetium-99m as pertechnetate in the investigation of thyroid function therefore provides information only on the trapping mechanism of the gland, but because of its advantageous physical properties over radioiodine (^{131}I), including a shorter physical and biological half-life (hence low radiation dose to the patient) and optimal gamma ray energy emission for scanning, technetium-99m is now widely used as an alternative to radioiodine for routine thyroid scanning.

The earliest method of investigating the thyroid with radionuclides was the 'iodine uptake test', which measured the maximum percentage uptake by the thyroid of an administered tracer dose of [131]I. This was a quantitative measure of the function of the thyroid as a whole but provided no images of the gland. Subsequently, the development of the rectilinear scanner (Figure 8.1) and, more recently, the Anger gamma camera (Figure 8.2) made it possible to measure the regional distribution of the radioactive tracer within the gland in order to build up a functional map or image of the thyroid, commonly known as a thyroid scan.

While techniques other than those involving the use of radionuclides are also available to image many organs of the body, including various radiological methods and ultrasound examinations, the radionuclide thyroid scan remains the primary and most useful method of imaging the thyroid. It is stressed that, in common with radionuclide studies of other organs, the thyroid scan provides information on the functional anatomy of the organ and for correct interpretation it should be related to the structural anatomy as readily assessed by palpation (and ultrasound examination if necessary).

Methods

The Iodine Uptake Test

This was the earliest in vivo method of using radioisotopes for the diagnosis of thyroid disease. A measured tracer dose of ^{131}I is given orally to the patient, and the percentage uptake after 4 and 24 hours is measured by means of a simple gamma counter placed in front of the neck, correction being made for background radiation and decay. In hyperthyroidism,

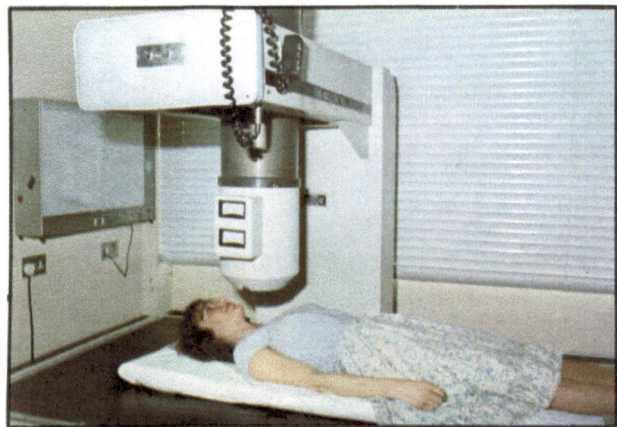

Figure 8.1 *Scanning the thyroid with the rectilinear scanner.*

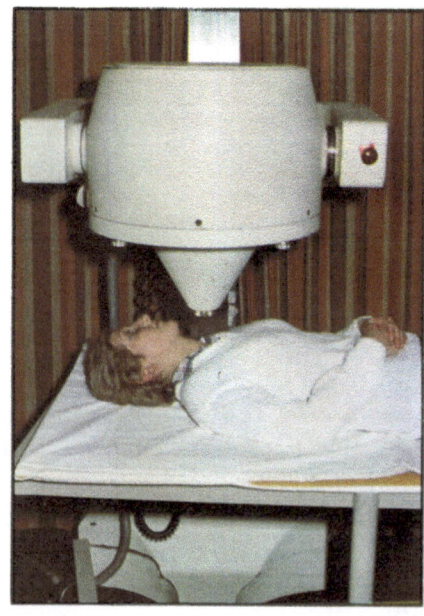

Figure 8.2 *Scanning the thyroid with the Anger gamma camera which is fitted with a pinhole collimator.*

there is an increased rate of iodine trapping and thyroid hormone production which is reflected by a raised ^{131}I uptake. Conversely, in hypothyroidism, the iodine turnover rate is low and a low ^{131}I uptake is observed.

The test, however, is invalid in the presence of excess circulating iodide, for example in patients who have received iodine-containing medication or radiological contrast media within a few weeks of the test and in patients who are taking thyroid hormone supplements. As a diagnostic investigation for hyperthyroidism or hypothyroidism, the ^{131}I uptake test has been superseded by direct measurement of serum thyroid hormone levels by radioimmunoassay. The test is now chiefly used as a guide to radioiodine dosimetry in the treatment of hyperthyroidism, as part of a T_3 suppression test to predict response to antithyroid drugs for hyper-thyroidism and for the investigation of enzyme deficiency goitres.

The Thyroid-Scan

The thyroid scan is a simple investigation which involves little discomfort to the patient. No special preparation is required, but the patient should not have received iodine compounds or thyroid supplements for at least four to six weeks prior to scanning, as uptake of tracer by the thyroid is otherwise suppressed. Scanning is carried out in the supine position 20 to 30 minutes after an in-travenous dose of 1 to 5 mCi of ^{99}Tc^m or 24 hours after an oral dose of 50 to 100 mCi of ^{131}I. With ^{99}Tc^m, a rectilinear scanner (Figure 8.1) or a gamma camera fitted with a pinhole collimator (Figure 8.2) may be used. With ^{131}I, the rectilinear scanner is probably superior. Immediately before the scan, the patient is given a drink of water to flush down any radionuclide in the pharynx or oesophagus which has originated from salivary gland secretion. Anatomical landmarks, such as the suprasternal notch, may be defined on the scan image by means of a radioactive marker placed on the patient or by triggering a point light source. This is important in patients with suspected retrosternal goitre for accurate localization and for the assessment of thyroid nodules. Interpretation of the scan should be made only in the light of the patient's clinical history, thyroid function status and the results of careful

Table 8.1 Main clinical applications of thyroid scanning.

1. Investigation of solitary thyroid nodules.
2. Assessment of the thyroid in hyperthyroidism before or after therapy.
3. Investigation of possible ectopic thyroid tissue.
4. Management of differentiated (functioning) thyroid cancer.

palpation of the neck. Thus, a non-functioning left lobe on the thyroid scan may be due to previous surgery, replacement by a non-functioning mass, agenesis of that lobe or suppression by an autonomously functioning nodule in the right lobe. When the scan is performed with the gamma camera, a percentage uptake measurement can also be carried out simultaneously.

Clinical Applications

The most important clinical applications of thyroid scanning are listed in Table 8.1.

The Normal Thyroid Scan

Typically, the normal thyroid is seen, on scanning, to consist of two lobes of nearly equal size and shape with uniformly distributed function, connected by a narrow central isthmus (Figure 8.3). However, many normal variations exist, such as absence of a functioning isthmus, asymmetry in size and function of the two lobes or presence of a small pyramidal lobe, which is often more evident in patients with Graves' disease.

Investigation of Solitary Thyroid Nodules

The Solitary Non-Toxic Thyroid Nodule

One of the commonest problems in thyroid disease is the finding of a solitary thyroid nodule in a euthyroid patient. Although the majority of such nodules are benign, a small but significant proportion are malignant but cannot usually be distinguished from the benign

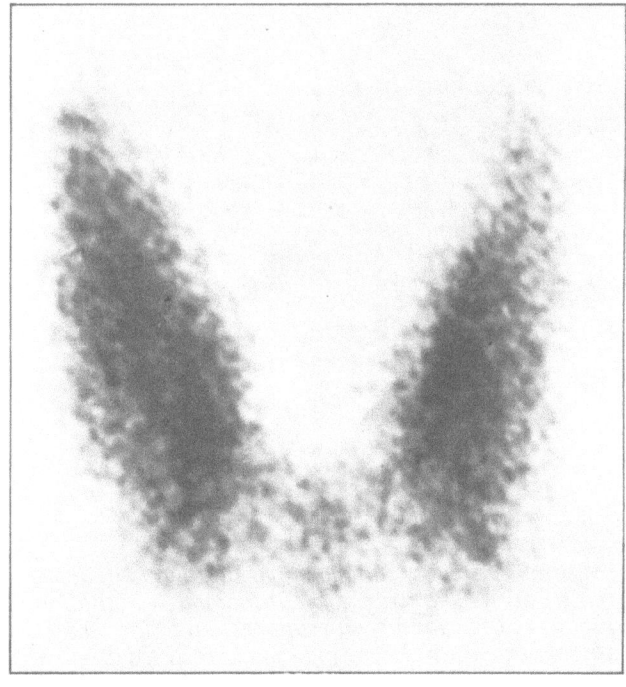

Figure 8.3 *Normal thyroid scan.*

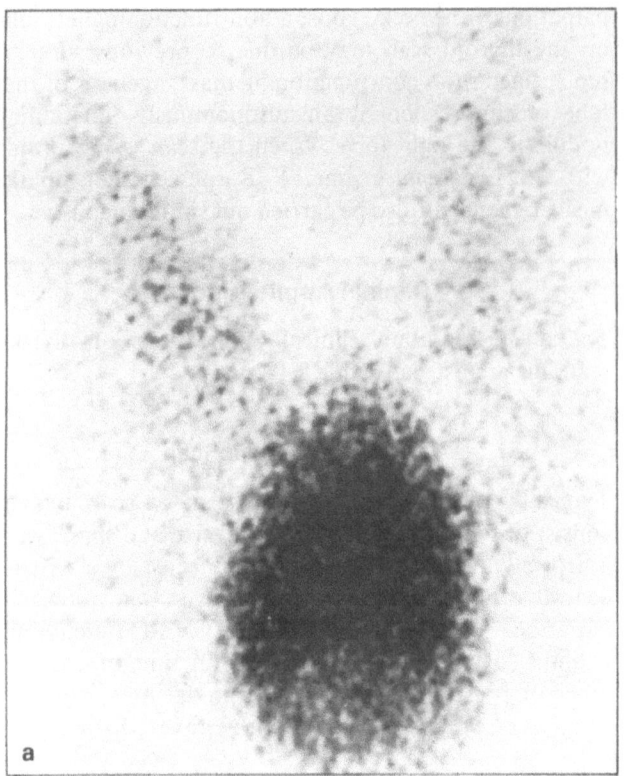

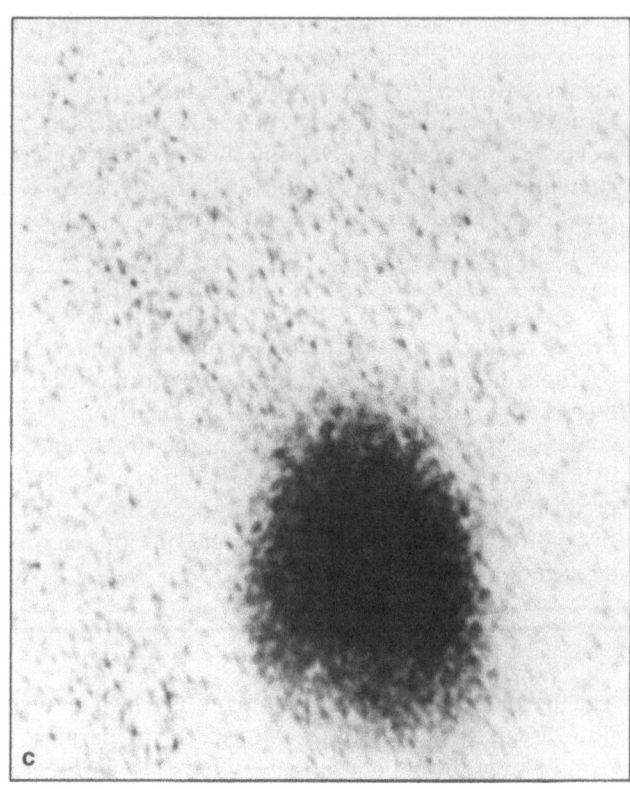

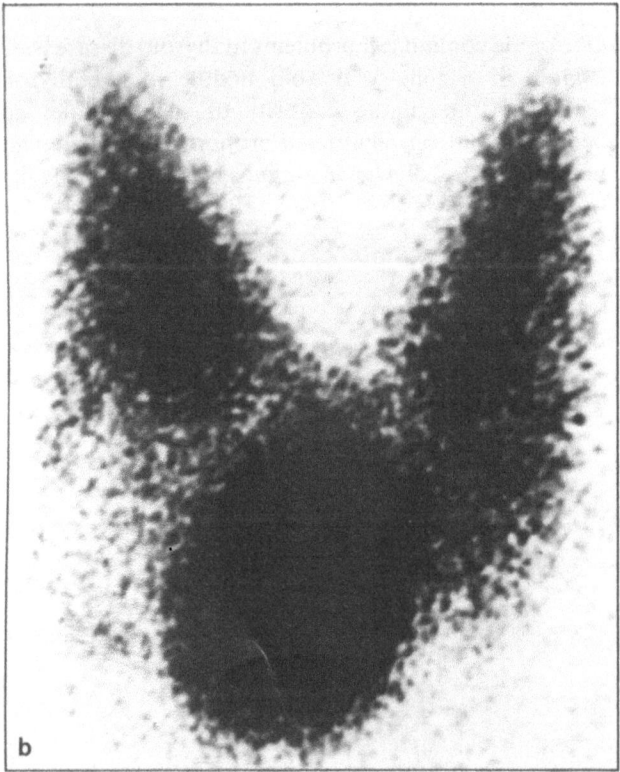

Figure 8.4 *Solitary functioning (hot) thyroid nodule.* **(a)** *Initial scan showing an autonomously functioning nodule in the isthmus with suppression of the remaining thyroid tissue.* **(b)** *Following i.m. TSH, the extranodular tissue is stimulated to function.* **(c)** *Following T₃ administration, the functioning nodule is unsuppressed.*

lesion on clinical examination. A thyroid scan will establish whether the nodule is functioning (hot) or non-functioning (cold) and whether it is associated with other nonpalpable nodules.

Solitary hot nodule. A functioning nodule (Figure 8.4a) is, as a rule, a benign lesion, although it has rarely been reported to be associated with malignancy. There have also been reports of exceptional cases of malignant nodules which appear hot on the technetium scan but cold on the iodine scan. Functioning thyroid nodules are often autonomous (i.e. they function independently of pituitary TSH control). They often secrete sufficient thyroid hormones to inhibit pituitary TSH secretion and thus cause suppression of the extranodular thyroid tissue (Figure 8.4a). This suppressed tissue can be demonstrated by repeating the scan after TSH injection (10 i.u. daily intramuscularly for 3 days), which stimulates the extranodular tissue (Figure 8.4b). On the other hand, T_3 administration (80 to 120 micrograms daily for seven days) causes no suppression of the autonomous nodule (Figure 8.4c). The autonomous nodule is associated with an absent pituitary TSH response to TRH, even though serum thyroid hormone levels are within the euthyroid range. Such nodules may eventually give rise to frank hyperthyroidism.

Solitary cold nodule. Of solitary non-functioning thyroid nodules (Figure 8.5a), 10 to 20 per cent are malignant although the majority are benign lesions, for

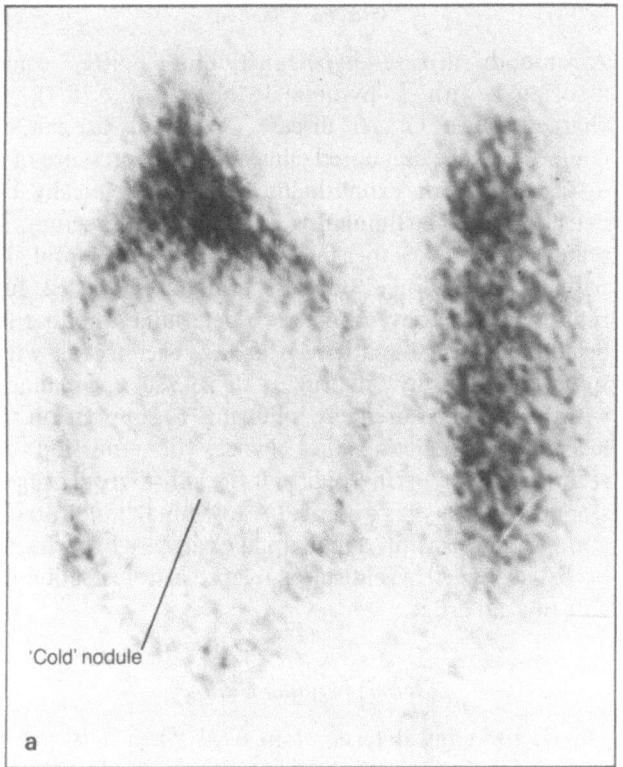

'Cold' nodule

a

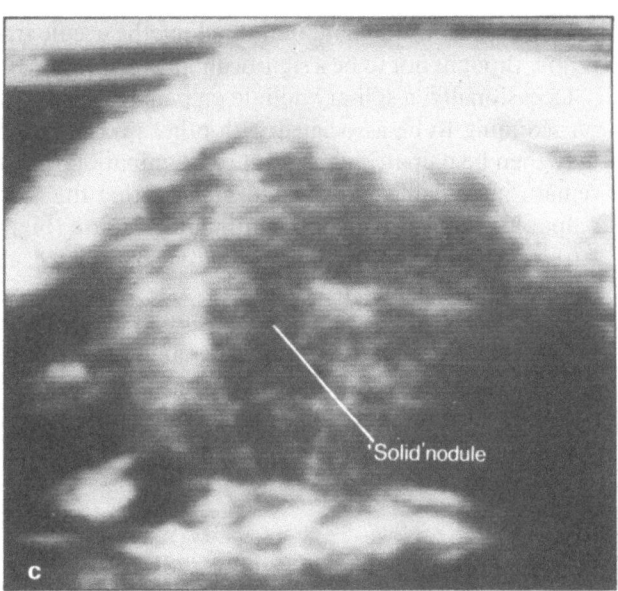

'Solid' nodule

c

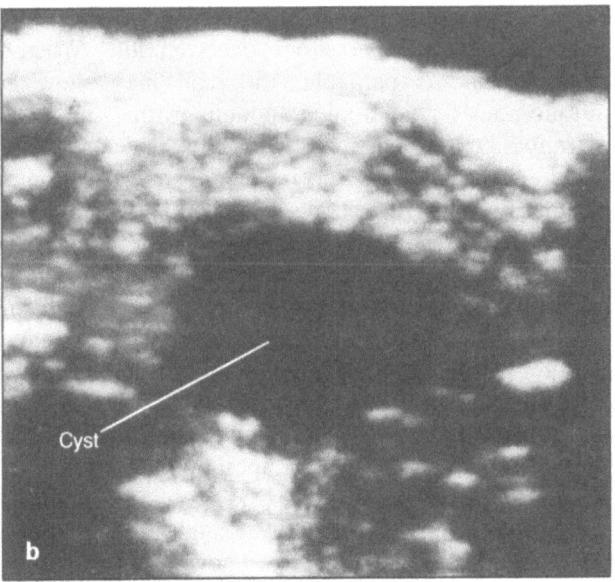

Cyst

b

Figure 8.5 (a) *Solitary non-functioning (cold) thyroid nodule in the right lobe. Ultrasound investigation of such a nodule showing (b) a transonic lesion, i.e. a cyst, and (c) a solid lesion producing echoes, which can be benign or malignant.*

percutaneously and cytological examination of the aspirate for malignant cells can be performed. Continued observation is necessary after cyst aspiration, and persistence, recurrence or enlargement of the nodule may be an indication for surgical excision. Solitary cold nodules that appear solid on ultrasound should be removed for a histological diagnosis. Percutaneous needle biopsy of solid cold nodules, although not routinely practised in this country, is commonly performed elsewhere and provides useful information.

example benign cysts, adenomas or localized thyroiditis, but the distinction cannot be made on the scan. Ultrasound examination has proved to be valuable to distinguish cystic from solid nodules (Figure 8.5b, c). Cysts are usually, although not always, benign and, following ultrasound diagnosis, can be aspirated

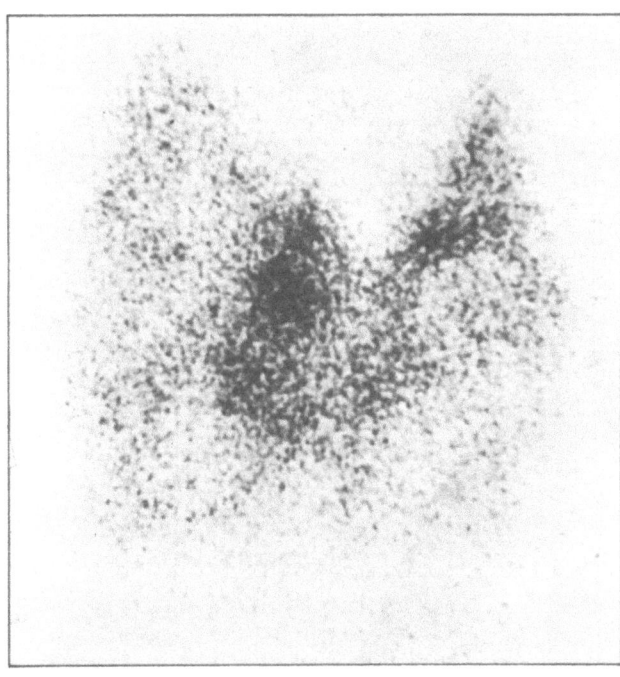

Figure 8.6 *Simple non-toxic multinodular goitre. The scan shows enlarged lobes with irregularly distributed function and multiple areas of reduced or absent function corresponding to degenerative nodules.*

The spread of a malignant tumour along the needle tract is now thought not to be a significant problem.

Occasionally, a solitary nodule on palpation is shown on scanning to be associated with other nodules which may then be palpated on careful re-examination or may remain impalpable. This would indicate that the easily palpable nodule is part of a multinodular goitre (Figure 8.6) and the scan findings would thus reduce the probability of malignancy.

Using the above techniques, it should therefore be possible to assess the risk of malignancy in a solitary palpable nodule and select the cases that definitely require surgery. Large nodules which cause local symptoms should, of course, be removed, irrespective of investigation findings.

Management of Hyperthyroidism

The diagnosis of hyperthyroidism is confirmed by elevated serum thyroid hormones and not by thyroid scan. However, a scan is essential for the assessment and appropriate management of some patients with confirmed hyperthyroidism. On clinical palpation, the majority of hyperthyroid patients have a smooth diffuse goitre or a nodule goitre which may be either uninodular or multinodular. Occasionally a goitre is not palpable or is not well defined. A thyroid scan demonstrates accurately the nature of the thyroid causing hyperthyroidism.

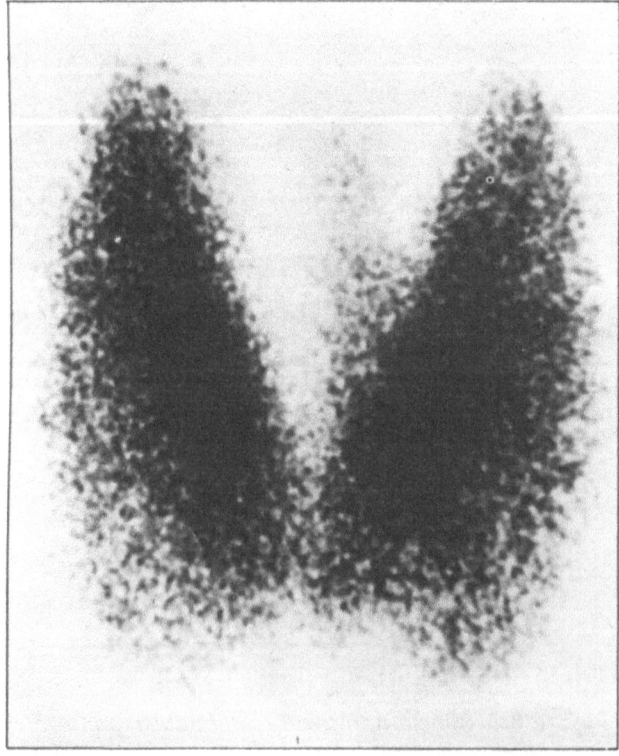

Figure 8.7 *Graves' disease. Smooth diffuse hyperplasia and hyperfunction of both lobes with a pyramidal lobe.*

Graves' Disease

A smooth diffuse hyperfunctioning goitre, often associated with a pyramidal lobe (Figure 8.7), is characteristic of Graves' disease. Graves' disease can, of course, often be diagnosed clinically in the presence of a diffuse goitre or exophthalmos, or biochemically by detecting thyroid stimulating antibodies in the serum. A scan and uptake measurement may be helpful in patients with Graves' disease, who are selected for radioiodine therapy, in order to determine the dose to be administered. In patients who have been treated with a course of anti-thyroid drugs, a thyroid scan, combined with uptake measurement following T_3 suppression, is helpful in predicting the chances of remission or recurrence of hyperthyroidism if the anti-thyroid drug is stopped after a year's course. A low uptake indicates a good prognosis while a high uptake carries a high risk of persistent hyperthyroidism or relapse after cessation of anti-thyroid drugs.

Toxic Nodular Goitre

This is the clinical term often used when a palpable uninodular or multinodular goitre is found in association with hyperthyroidism, but a scan is necessary to define the exact nature of the nodules in relation to thyroid hormone oversecretion. When a single nodule is palpable, the scan may show an autonomously functioning nodule with suppressed extranodular tissue, i.e. a solitary toxic adenoma (Figure 8.8a, b), or an incidental non-functioning nodule in a diffuse toxic goitre (Figure 8.8c), or asymmetrical enlargement of a diffuse toxic goitre (Figure 8.8d). Similarly, when hyperthyroidism is associated with a multinodular goitre, a scan is indicated to distinguish autonomously functioning nodules with suppressed extranodular tissue (Figure 8.9a, b) from incidental non-functioning nodules in the presence of diffuse hyperfunction of the extranodular tissue, i.e. Graves' disease superimposed on a longstanding multinodular goitre (Figure 8.9c and d). Hyperthyroidism caused by single or multiple autonomous nodules is also known as Plummer's disease, and it is characteristic of this condition that intramuscular TSH causes stimulation of the suppressed extranodular tissue in contrast to variants of Graves' disease where no such change is observed.

The distinction between Plummer's disease and Graves' disease is of therapeutic and prognostic significance when treatment with radioiodine is contemplated. Hyperthyroidism due to Graves' disease can usually be treated with an average dose of 4 to 8 mCi of ^{131}I, but a high incidence of postradiation hypothyroidism is generally observed, averaging 20 per cent in the first year with a subsequent steady annual rise of about three per cent to reach 50 per cent after 10 years.

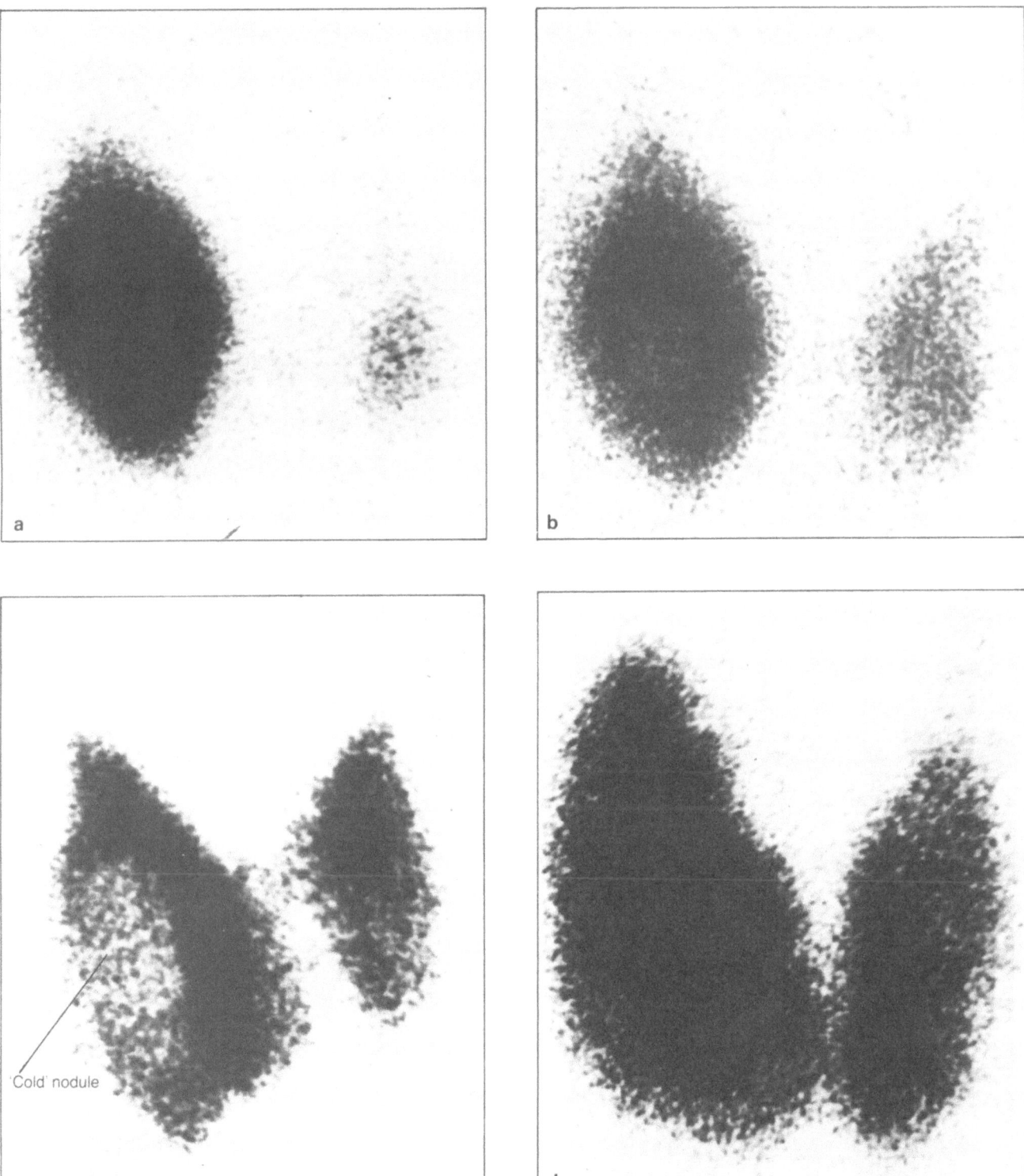

Figure 8.8 *Hyperthyroidism associated with a single nodule on palpation.* **(a)** *Solitary autonomously functioning nodule with suppressed left lobe which after TSH* **(b)** *becomes stimulated.* **(c)** *Incidental cold nodule in a diffuse toxic goitre (Graves' disease).* **(d)** *Asymmetrical enlargement of the right lower pole in Graves' disease accounting for the apparent palpable nodule.*

On the other hand, hyperthyroidism due to Plummer's disease is more resistant to radioiodine and requires larger doses of ^{131}I, but, despite this, postradiation hypothyroidism is rarely observed. This is explained by the fact that in Plummer's disease, the radioiodine administered therapeutically concentrates mainly in the

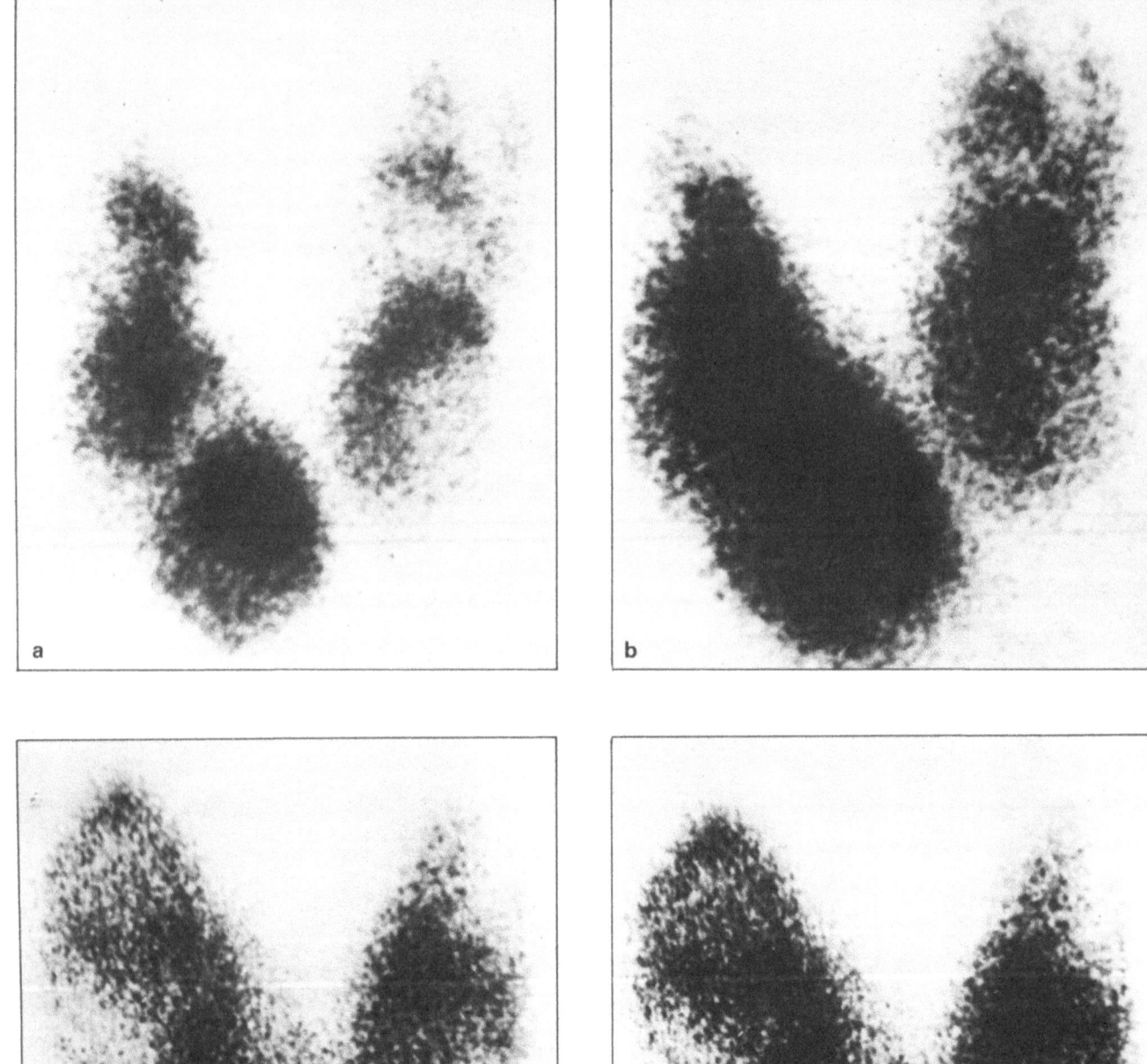

Figure 8.9 *Toxic multinodular goitre. On scanning, this may be due to either (i) multiple autonomously functioning nodules (**a**) with suppressed extranodular tissue which after TSH (**b**) becomes stimulated or (ii) Graves' disease superimposed on a long-standing multinodular goitre (**c**). After TSH (**d**) the distribution of function remains unchanged.*

autonomous nodules which are destroyed, while the extranodular tissue being suppressed does not take up any significant amount of radioiodine and subsequently

is able to function and maintain the euthyroid state (Figure 8.10). We have found a standard dose of 15 mCi of ^{131}I to be a simple way of treating hyperthyroidism

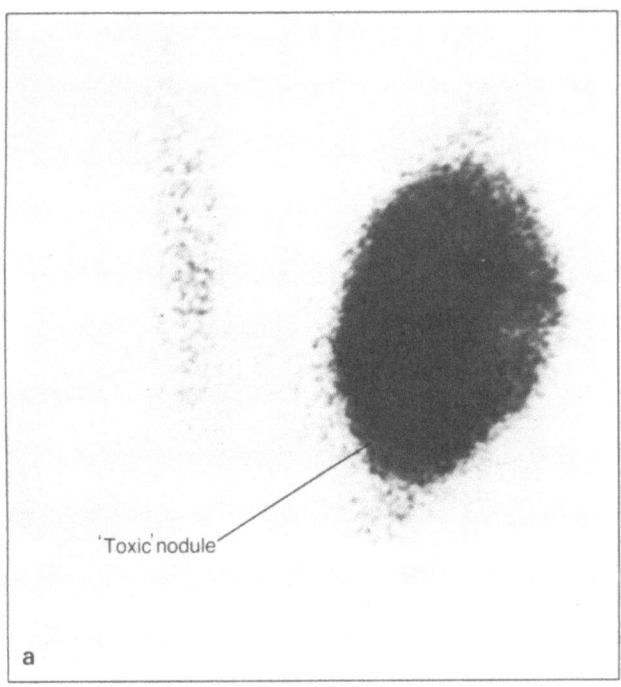

'Toxic' nodule

a

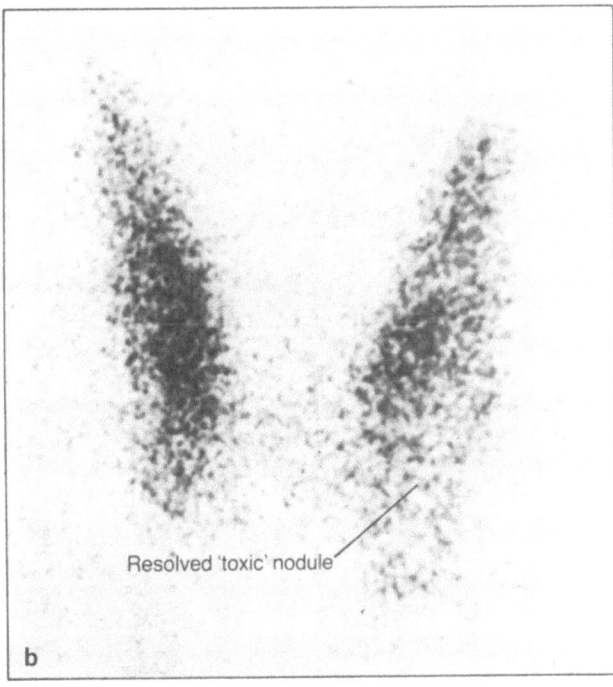

Resolved 'toxic' nodule

b

Figure 8.10 *Radioiodine therapy of autonomous toxic nodules. The scan before therapy* (a) *shows a single functioning nodule with suppression of the remaining thyroid. Six months after* ^{131}I *therapy* (b) *the nodule has resolved, and the extranodular tissue is functioning normally.*

due to autonomous nodules confirmed on scan, resulting in a high incidence of cure and a low incidence of hypothyroidism.

Abnormally Situated Thyroid Tissue

Embryologically, the thyroid originates as a midline structure from the back of the tongue, and descends down the middle of the neck to its final position in the lower half of the neck, where it divides and enlarges into two lateral lobes and an isthmus. Failure of descent results in a lingual or sublingual thyroid which may present as a swelling at the back of the tongue or upper part of the neck, occasionally causing hypothyroidism. Such swellings may be confirmed by scanning to be functioning thyroid tissue (Figure 8.11) and should of course not be removed as they may represent the patient's only functioning thyroid. It is recommended that every patient with a midline swelling in the neck should have a thyroid scan before surgical excision to exclude ectopic thyroid tissue.

A normally situated thyroid may enlarge downwards into the upper mediastinum to produce a retrosternal goitre. This appears as an upper mediastinal opacity on the chest radiograph and may cause deviation or compression of the trachea or the oesophagus resulting in dyspnoea or dysphagia. Such retrosternal goitres can be diagnosed by scanning, using the sternal notch as a reference point (Figure 8.12). Scanning with ^{131}I is preferable to $^{99}Tc^m$ when investigating retrosternal goitres, in view of the high absorption by the chest wall of the lower gamma energy of $^{99}Tc^m$ and the poor function often associated with a retrosternal goitre which forms part of a multinodular goitre.

A goitre with retrosternal extension which is diagnosed on scan is usually an indication for surgical treatment (in view of the risk of tracheal compression from the enlarging goitre at any time).

Thyroid Cancer

Scanning with radioiodine plays an important part in the management of differentiated (i.e. papillary and follicular) thyroid cancer. The vast majority of malignant thyroid tumours, whatever their histological types, appear as solitary cold nodules when scanned at the time of presentation (Figure 8.13a), reflecting their relative lack of endocrine function compared to adjacent normal thyroid tissue. Scanning for evidence of spread at this stage is usually of no value, as any metastases which are present, like the primary tumour, do not concentrate iodine to any significant extent and cannot therefore be detected.

However, when the normal thyroid tissue associated with the tumour has been completely ablated by surgery (Figure 8.13b) and/or by an ablative dose of ^{131}I (e.g. 80 mCi), the differentiated papillary and follicular carcinomas and their metastases usually show significant iodine uptake after about four weeks, due to stimulation by the high TSH levels. Scanning with tracer

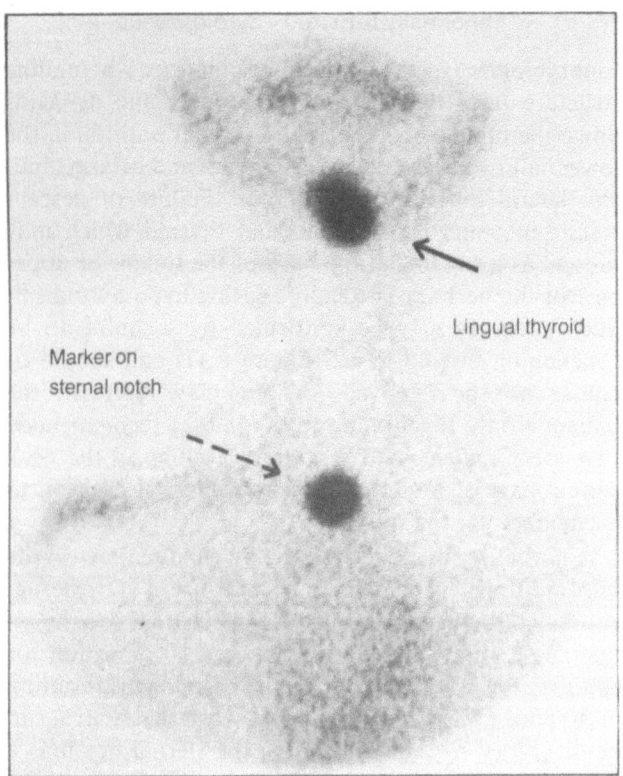

Figure 8.11 *Lingual thyroid (↖) in a child and absent functioning thyroid tissue in the normal position. Note the radioactive marker on the suprasternal notch. (⇢)*

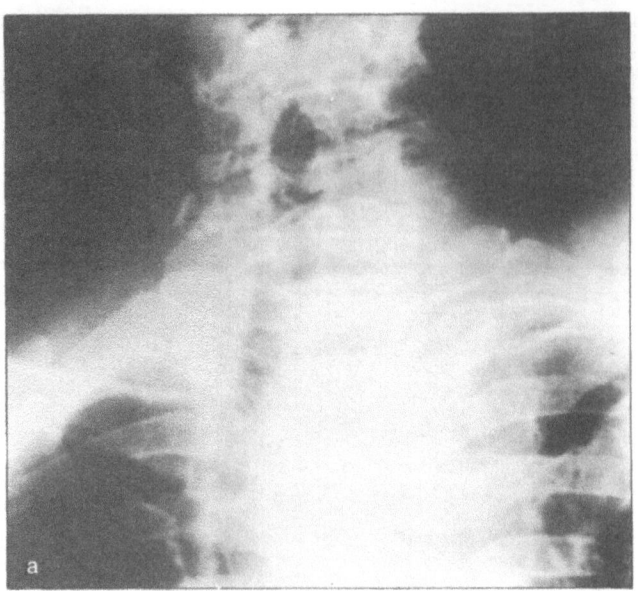

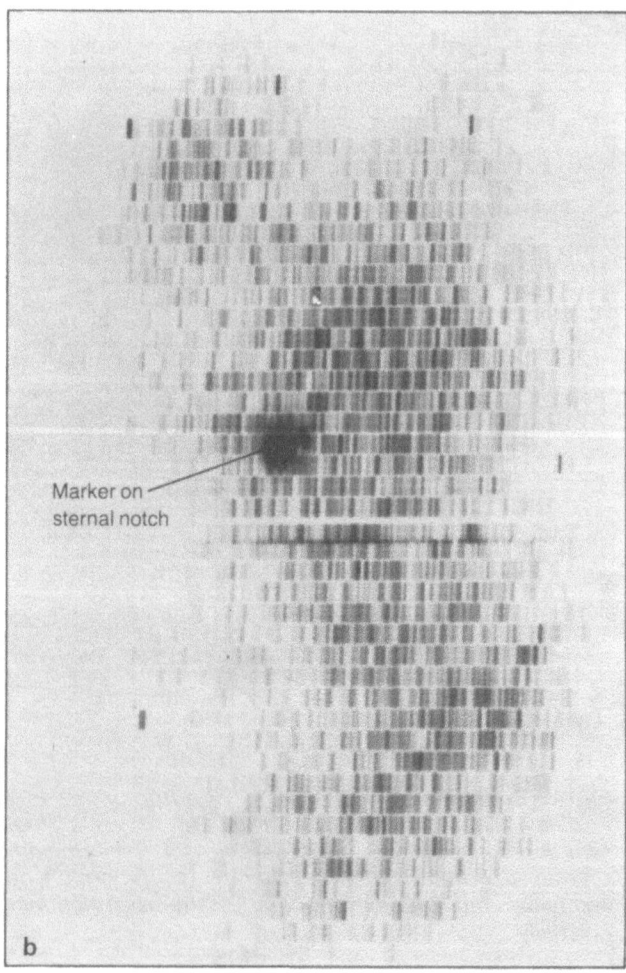

Figure 8.12 *Retrosternal goitre. (a) Radiographic examination showing deviation of the trachea caused by a left upper mediastinal mass. (b) ¹³¹I thyroid scan showing a corresponding left-sided retrosternal goitre. The middle dot is a marker on the suprasternal notch.*

doses of ¹³¹I will then detect and localize any residual or recurrent functioning tumour (Figure 8.13c) and its metastases (Figure 8.14) as hot areas, usually in the neck, lungs or bones. In many cases, these functioning tumours can then be destroyed by the administration of large doses of ¹³¹I orally (for example 150 mCi) to allow radiotherapeutic levels of isotope to concentrate in the tumour cells. Response to therapy can be assessed by repeating the scan after three to six months and, if necessary, the high dose of ¹³¹I therapy and a follow-up iodine whole body scan can be repeated until evidence of tumour uptake is no longer present. After each therapeutic ¹³¹I administration, the patient is given full suppressive doses of thyroid hormone (T_4 or T_3 which is stopped before the next scan, for one month in the case of T_4 or two weeks with T_3, to allow the rise in endogenous serum TSH level necessary to stimulate iodine uptake by the tumour). Up to five or six treatment doses of ¹³¹I may be required in advanced or resistant cases before the whole body scan shows absence of iodine uptake by a tumour.

Complications from repeated high dose ¹³¹I therapy are rare but include bone marrow hypoplasia or aplasia, leukaemia and, rarely, acute radiation pneumonitis or chronic fibrosis in cases of widespread pulmonary metastases. Routine blood counts, as well as respiratory function tests in patients with pulmonary metastases,

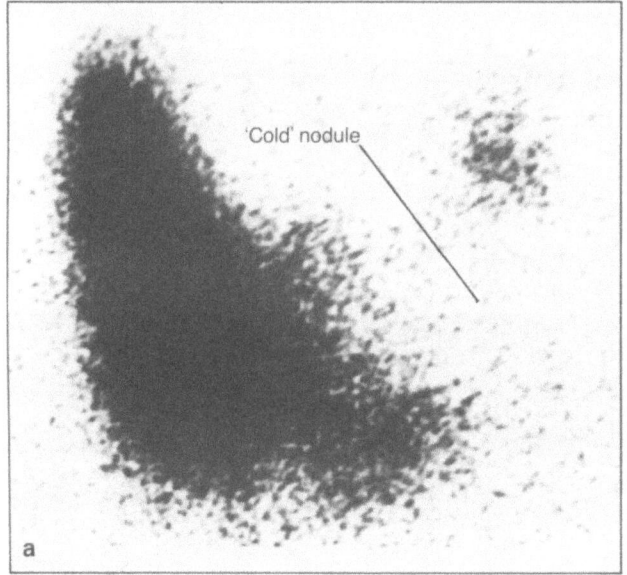

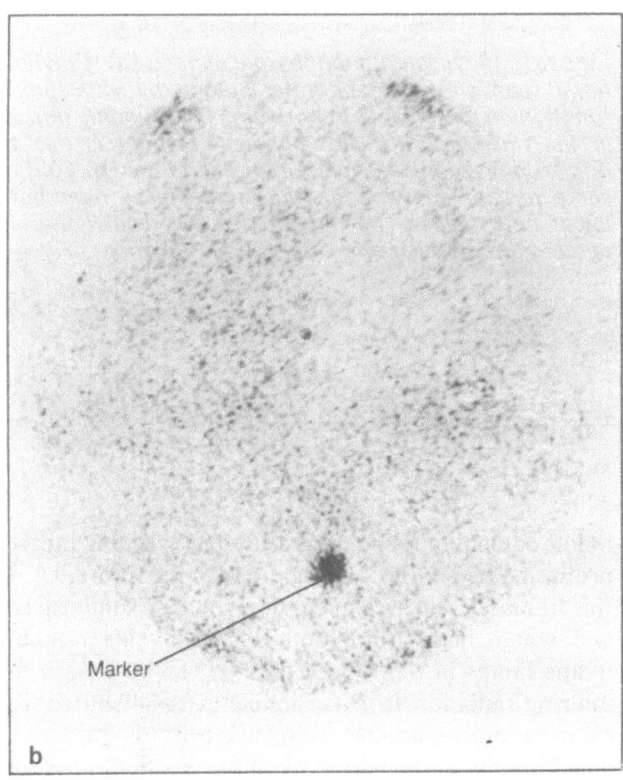

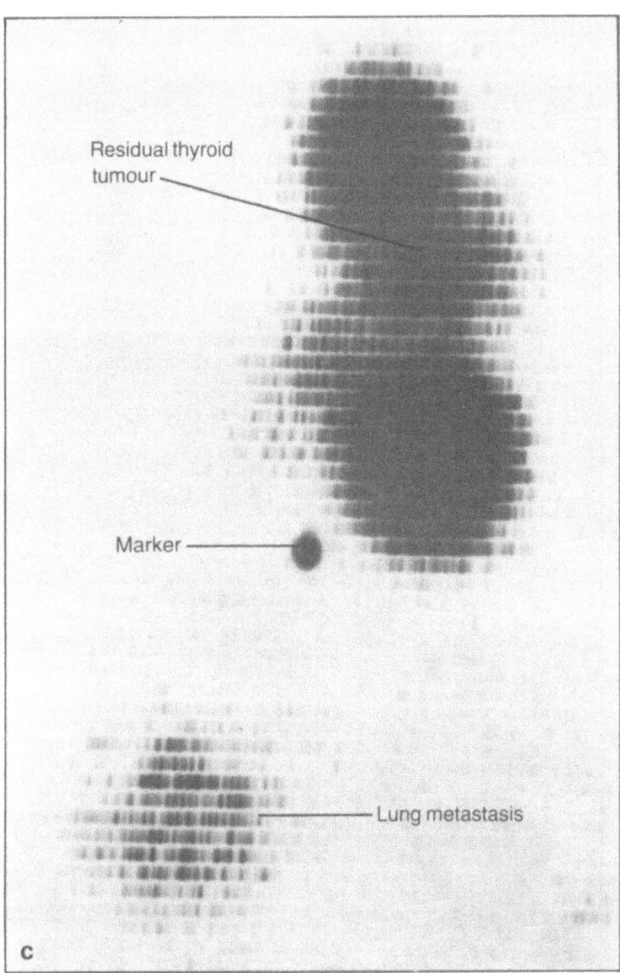

Figure 8.13 *Differentiated thyroid cancer.* **(a)** *Solitary cold nodule in the left lobe due to a follicular thyroid carcinoma.* **(b)** *Scan following total thyroidectomy showing absent uptake throughout.* **(c)** *131I scan on same patient a month later showing now functioning residual tumour in the left thyroid bed and metastatic spread in the right side of the chest.*

tumours, e.g. anaplastic or medullary carcinomas, with little or no iodine uptake may have extensive metastases that are evident clinically or radiologically but are either poorly or not visualized on the iodine scan (Figure 8.15). Radioiodine therapy is of no value in treating such tumours.

Conclusion and Future Development

In conclusion, the radionuclide scan is a simple, useful and cheap investigation in the diagnosis or management of thyroid disease. Although it is useful in the investigation of solitary thyroid nodules and in the selection of those nodules that definitely require surgery owing to the risk of malignancy, it has not entirely solved the problem of accurate presurgical diagnosis of thyroid cancer. It is hoped that the future development

are therefore advisable before each therapeutic dose of 131I.

It is stressed that thyroid cancer detection by the radioiodine scan is based on the degree of iodine uptake by the tumour cells. Well differentiated tumours with good iodine uptake are thus readily detected, and pulmonary or bony metastases from such tumours can be detected with greater sensitivity by the radioiodine scan than by radiography (Figure 8.14). On the other hand, non-differentiated or poorly differentiated

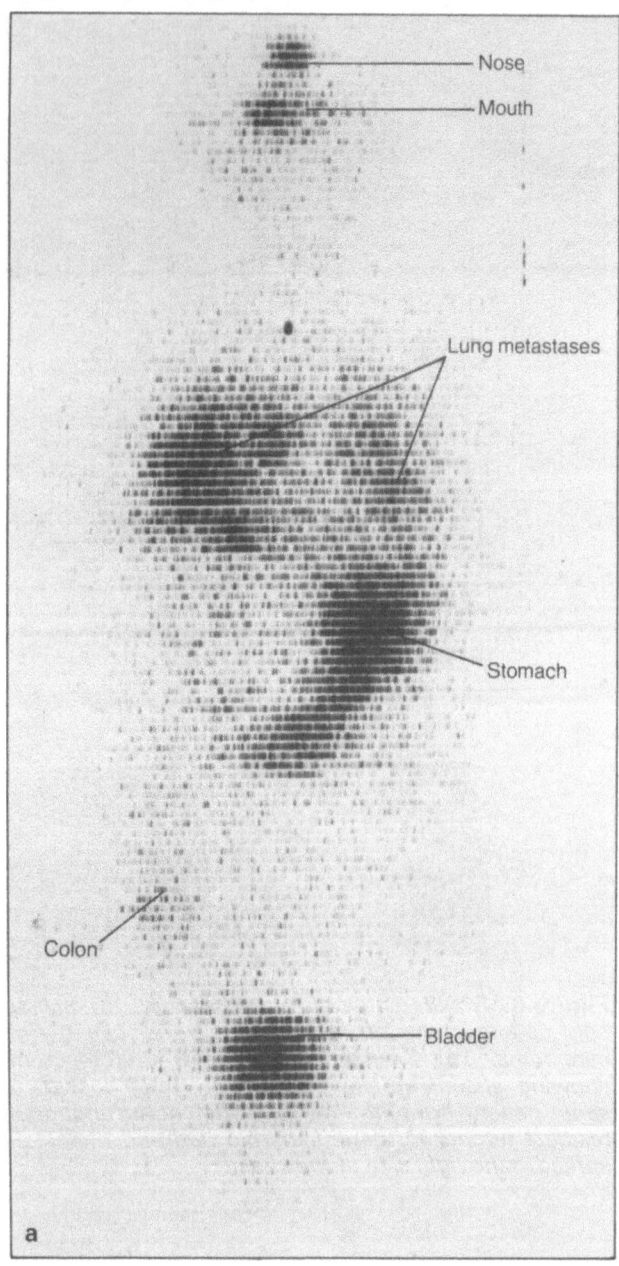

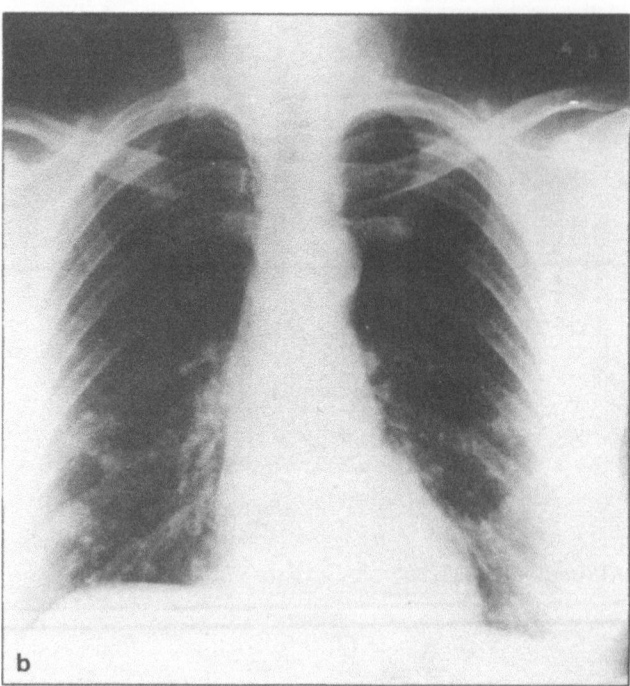

Figure 8.14 *Differentiated thyroid cancer. (a) ^{131}I whole body scan showing abnormal uptake by widespread functioning metastases in both lungs. The iodine uptake in the nose, mouth, stomach and bladder is due to normal physiological secretion or excretion. (b) CXR of same patient showing multiple metastases over both lower lung fields. The patient had a follicular thyroid carcinoma removed and total thyroid ablation six years previously.*

of radiopharmaceuticals that act as specific tumour markers will contribute a great deal to an accurate and easier diagnosis of malignant thyroid cancers and their metastases. Radioimmunoassay of serum thyroglobulin as a simple and specific marker for thyroid cancers, following ablation of the associated normal thyroid tissue, is currently being assessed, and early comparative studies with the iodine whole body scan described above appear promising.

The recent development of the radiographic fluorescence technique for the measurement of total iodine content of regional areas of the thyroid is another promising diagnostic investigation for the future. Using this technique, no systemic radionuclide is administered and whole body irradiation is thus avoided. Stable iodine atoms in the thyroid are excited by a beam of ionizing radiation from a suitable external source, for example americium-241, directed towards the neck, which results in the release of characteristic fluorescent x-rays from the excited iodine atoms. Quantitative analysis of the characteristic iodine x-rays by a semiconductor detector provides a measure of the total iodine concentration inside a particular region of the thyroid towards which the radiation beam is directed. In vitro measurement and early in vivo studies have indicated that this technique is most likely to be useful in the diagnosis of thyroid cancers as these have an undetectable total iodine content compared to normal thyroid tissue or most benign adenomas which have measurable levels. Further development and evaluation of this technique is in progress.

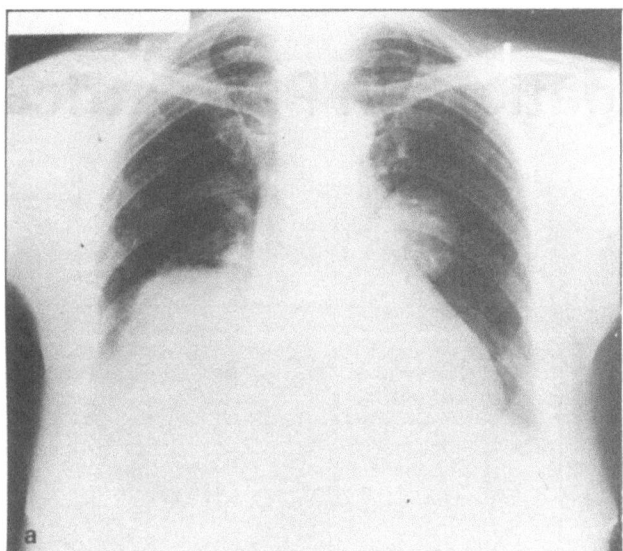

Figure 8.15 *Undifferentiated thyroid cancer.* **(a)** *CXR showing massive pulmonary metastases.* **(b)** *[131]I whole body scan showing relatively little iodine uptake by the right lower lobe metastatic mass, and negligible uptake by the left lung metastasis. Physiological uptake in the abdomen, pelvis and face are again noted.*

Further Reading

Charkes, N. D., *Semin. Nucl. Med.,* 1971, **1**, 316.

Hoffer, P. B., Gottschalk, A. and Quinn, J. (Chapter 28), *Diagnostic Nuclear Medicine,* Gottschalk, A. and Potchen, E. J. (Eds), Williams and Wilkins, USA, 1976.

Ng Tang Fui, S. C. and Maisey, M. N., *Clinical Endocrinology,* 1979, **10**, 69.

Pochin, E. E., *Semin. Nucl. Med.,* 1971, **1**, 503.

Acknowledgement

I wish to thank Dr Barbara King, Ultrasound Department, Guy's Hospital for Figs 8.5(b) and (c).

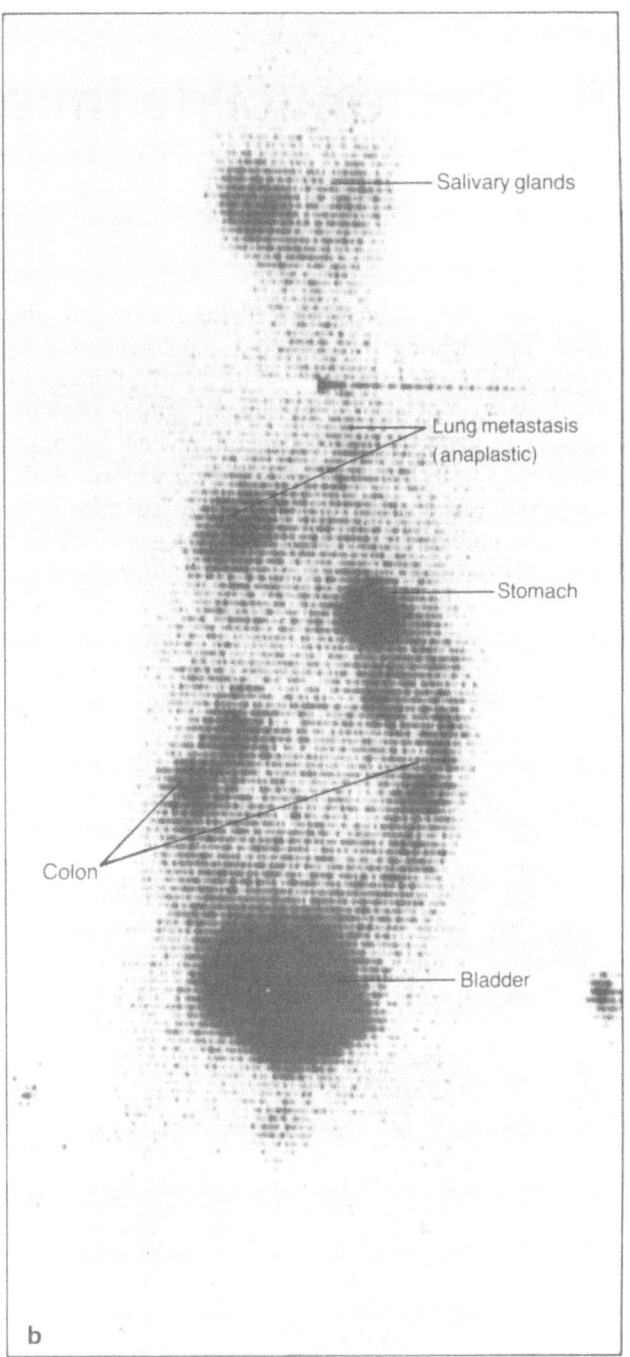

Salivary glands

Lung metastasis (anaplastic)

Stomach

Colon

Bladder

9. Radionuclide Investigations in Paediatrics

The primary difference between the method of diagnostic investigation of adult and child patients is the result of the different range and incidence of diseases in the respective groups. There are, of course, technical differences related to instrumentation and radiopharmaceutical doses but these will not be discussed. Radionuclide tracer procedures have many advantages (as discussed previously), which are suitable for application in paediatric medicine, i.e. they are non-invasive and atraumatic, have essentially no morbidity and mortality, and, consequently, are easily repeatable. They are functional investigations which display abnormalities of pathophysiology, and they may be used to complement conventional radiology, computerized tomography and ultrasonography, in revealing structural changes. The radiation doses, whilst they are important and must be considered when the decisions about the need for investigation are being made, are small and often far less than those received from conventional radiological procedures for similar studies. In order to maximize the information obtained it is essential that there is a full understanding of the clinical problem and careful tailor-

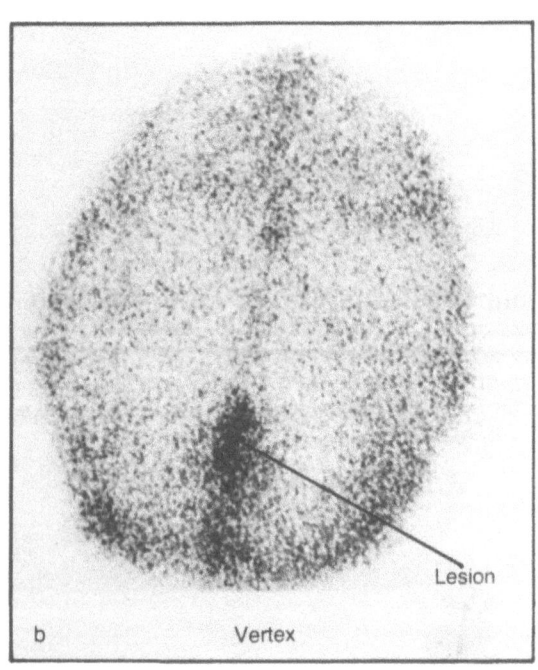

b   Vertex

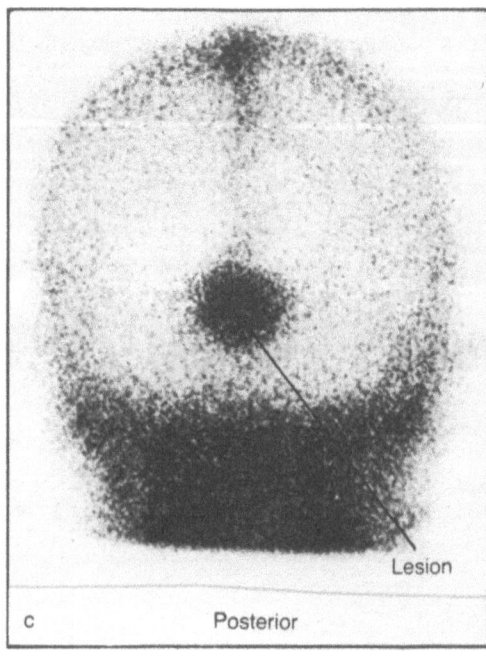

c   Posterior

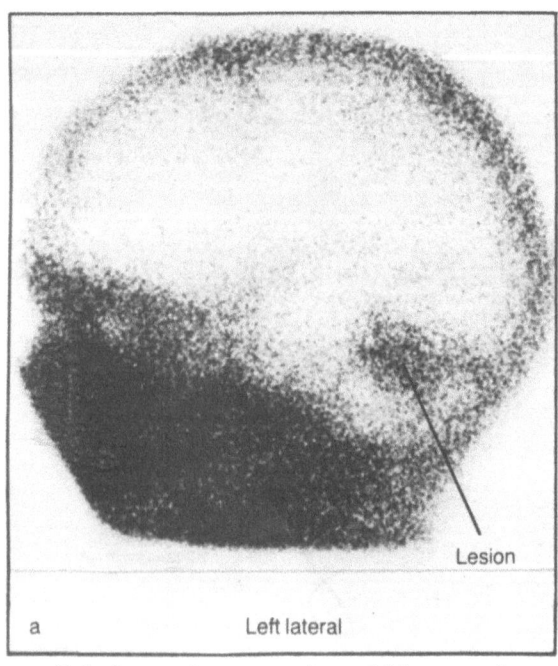

a   Left lateral

Figure 9.1 *A vermis tumour in a child presenting with gait disturbances.* **(a)** *Left lateral,* **(b)** *vertex and* **(c)** *posterior.*

ing of the investigation to try to provide the answers. In the remainder of this chapter, some of the ways in which nuclear medicine techniques can be employed to solve

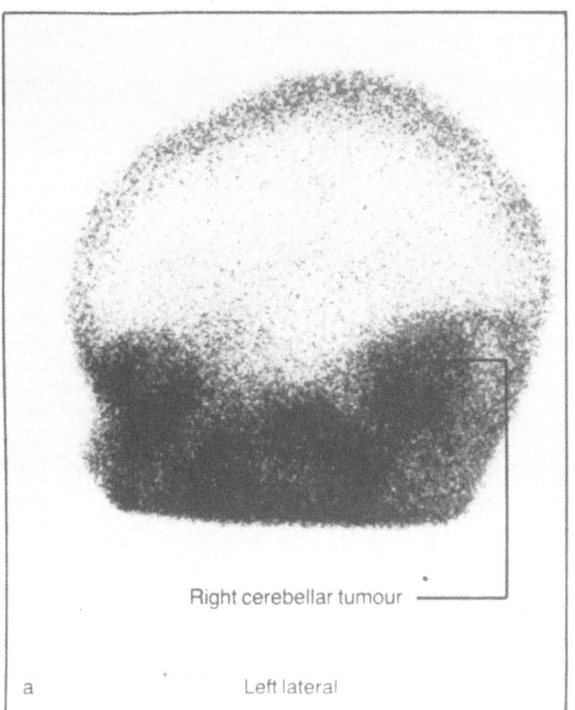

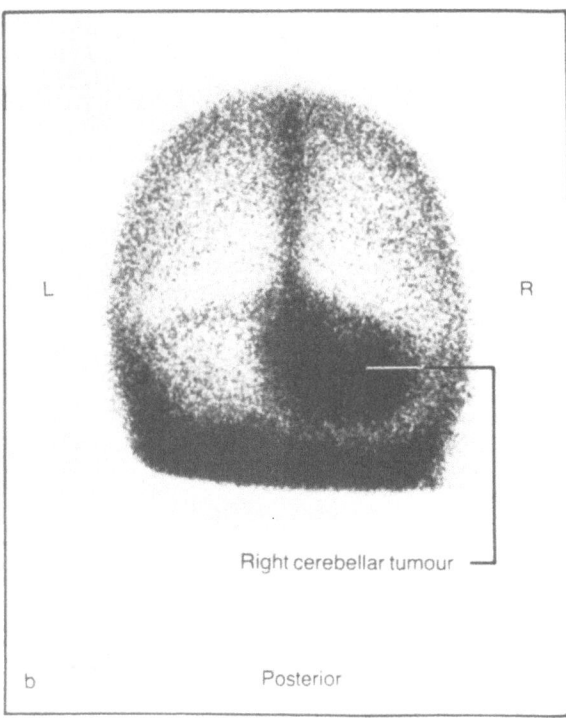

Figure 9.2 *The brain scan of a child with a medulloblastoma.* (a) *Left lateral view and* (b) *posterior view.*

clinical problems in children will be discussed and illustrated.

The Brain and CSF

There is an increased incidence, in paediatrics, both of primary tumours (rather than secondary tumours) and posterior fossa lesions (rather than cerebral lesions) with gait disturbances. It is in this area that the investigation of brain disease in children and in adults has more obvious differences.

Figures 9.1 and 9.2 show brain scans of children in whom the gait disturbance was dominant, and there was

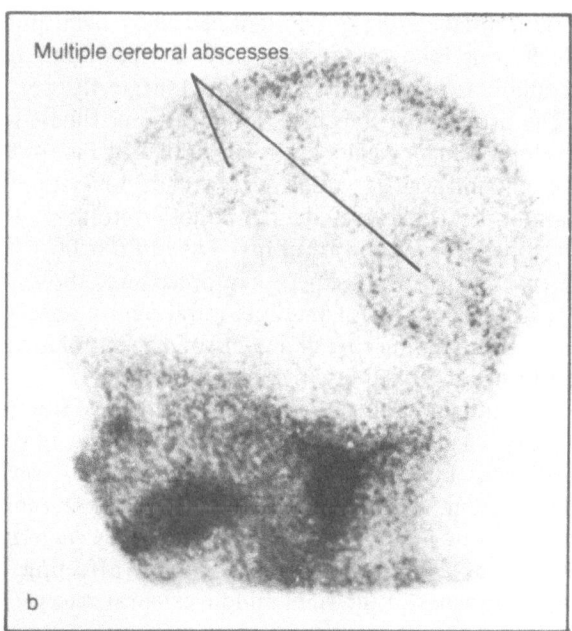

Figure 9.3 *The scan of a child with multiple cerebral abscesses which were associated with cyanotic congenital heart disease.* (a) *Posterior view and* (b) *Left lateral view.*

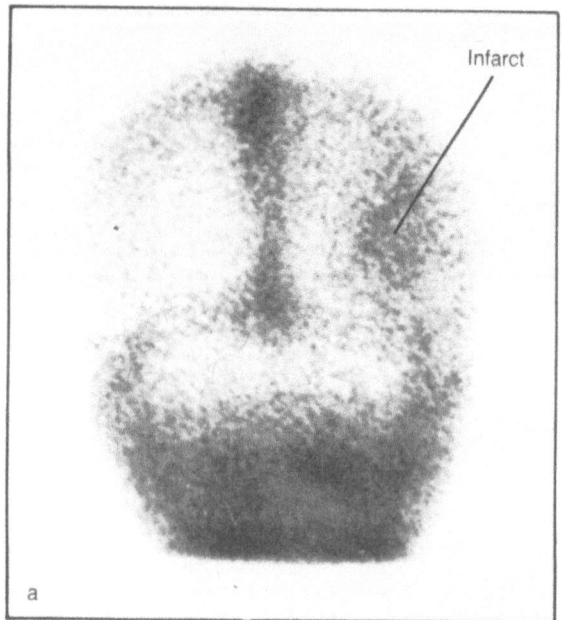
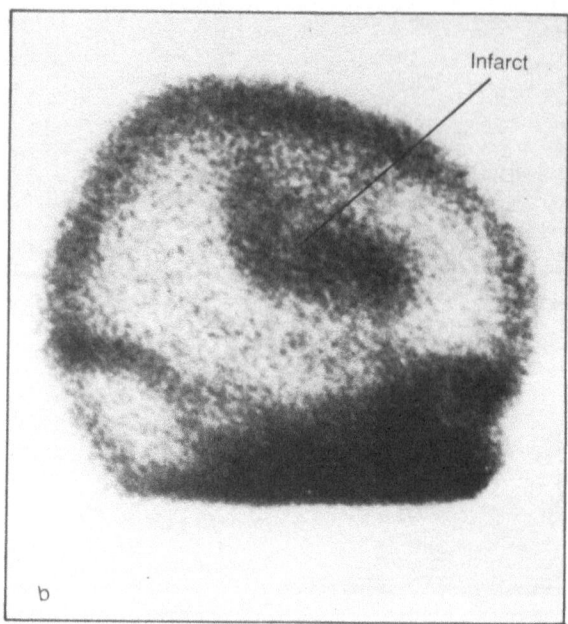

Figure 9.4 *Scan of a child with hypertension, who developed left-sided hemiparesis. This was due to infarction in the distribution of the right middle cerebral artery.* **(a)** *Posterior view and* **(b)** *right lateral view.*

strong reason to suspect an organic lesion. The first patient had a slow onset of an unstable gait, together with more recent headache and vomiting. The brain scan shows a very well-defined midline lesion lying adjacent to the confluence of the sinuses, but the lesion is seen to be anterior to this on the left lateral view. This is the typical appearance of a midline vermis lesion. Figure 9.2 shows a child with a gait disturbance but whose principal problem was the associated ataxia. In this case, the brain scan shows a massive area of abnormal uptake lying in the right cerebellar hemisphere, which was shown subsequently to be due to a medulloblastoma which was removed surgically.

The problem of the child with a systemic illness who develops neurological signs is illustrated in Figure 9.3. The patient was a young girl with a long-standing cyanotic heart disease, due to Fallot's tetralogy, who developed a fever and focal fits. The brain scan, which was performed as an emergency procedure, shows the typical appearances of multiple intracerebral abscesses with a surrounding ring of activity and a central area of diminished radioactivity (the 'donut' sign).

The sudden onset of hemiparesis, which is so frequent in adult neurological practice, is relatively rare in paediatrics but may occur in association with severe hypertension, as shown in the child whose brain scan is illustrated in Figure 9.4. This shows the characteristic features of a large intracerebral infarct affecting the major branches of the right middle cerebral artery. The demonstration of subsequent resolution of these lesions (e.g. abscesses, primary tumours and infarcts) after treatment, is another important application of the brain scan.

The importance of knowing the physiological sites of tracer excretion and common artefacts is shown in Figure 9.5, where the possibility of multiple lesions on the brain scan was raised. Later, however, it was recalled that the mother had been assisting the child to lie still, resulting in some salivary contamination of the mother's hand. Afterwards, this was confirmed by a gamma camera picture.

The investigation of a hydrocephalus in childhood, although characteristic (Figure 9.6), is unrewarding with radionuclide brain scanning, in view of the low incidence of normal pressure hydrocephalus and tumour as a cause. This is an area where the CT brain scan has revolutionized the investigation. After treatment of hydrocephalus, however, tracers may be valuable in assessing the patency of a ventriculo-atrial or ventriculo-peritoneal shunt as the clinical problem—frequently, it is necessary to discover whether the shunt is blocked. Figure 9.7 shows the normal result of injecting a small amount of tracer into the shunt; if this is patent the flow of cerebrospinal fluid (CSF) down the shunt allows a rapid wash-out of the tracer which can be visualized with the gamma camera and displayed graphically, using the area of interest facility from the computer. Figure 9.8, on the other hand, shows a similar clinical situation of increasing headaches and increasing head size in a child whose shunt was, in fact, blocked and, in this case, there is practically no wash-out of tracer confirming the blockage of the shunt. This is a simple atraumatic procedure which rarely gives equivocal results.

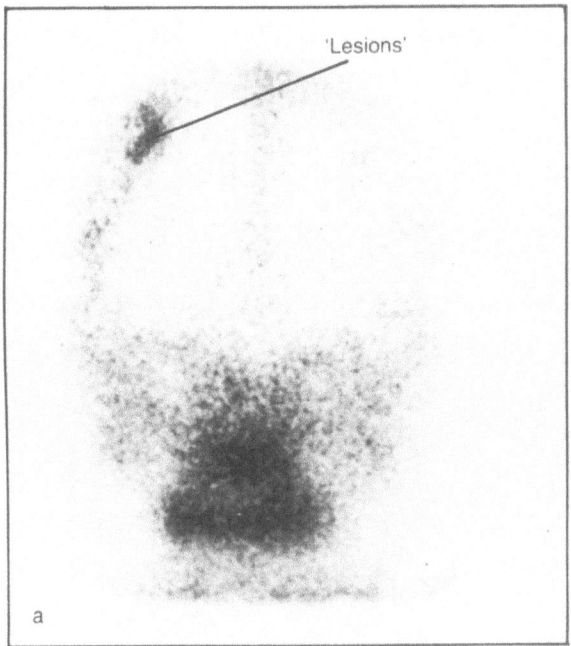

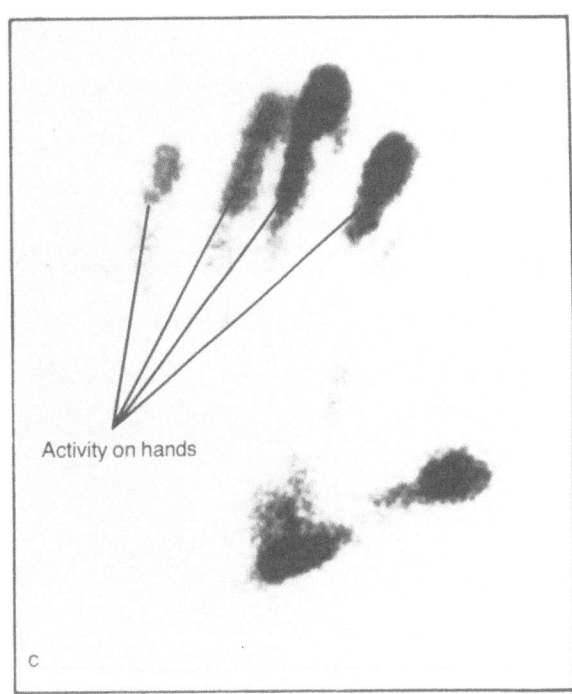

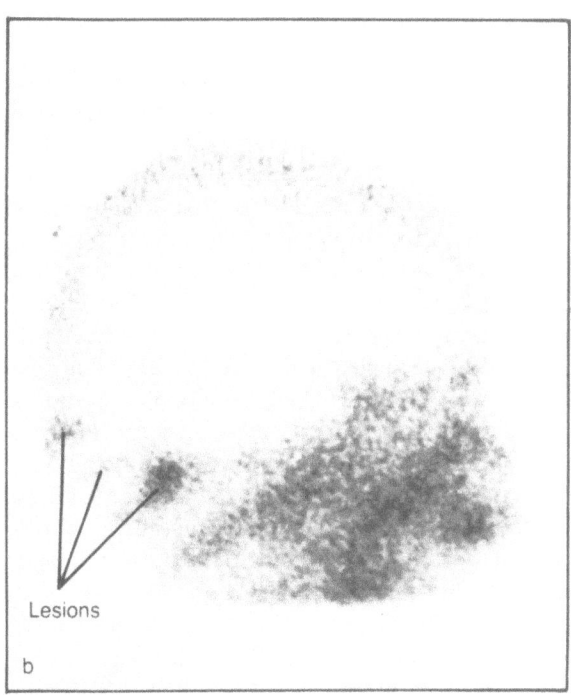

Figure 9.5 *This scan shows the possibility of artefact from salivary contamination. The mother's hands were contaminated whilst she held the child's head for imaging.* **(a)** *anterior view,* **(b)** *left lateral view and* **(c)** *the mother's hand.*

Liver, Spleen Scanning

The most frequent clinical problem which leads to a liver/spleen scan is the finding of hepatomegaly in a child who is receiving medical attention for some other reason. Figure 9.9 shows the liver/spleen scan of a child who was found to be mentally delayed in development and shows diffuse hepatosplenomegaly with some increased uptake in the bone marrow, indicating impairment of overall liver function. Biopsy demonstrated a glycogen storage disease and the liver scan was used subsequently to assess response to therapy. Figure 9.10 shows the liver/spleen scan of a newborn infant who was found, on routine examination, to have a palpable liver in addition to persistent cardiac failure. The liver/spleen scan shows an enlarged liver, which may be found in any cause of heart failure, but in addition multiple focal defects were found, which were subsequently shown to be multiple haemangiomata with a high blood flow resulting in a high output cardiac failure. The staging of paediatric patients with known carcinoma should be applied in the same way as in adults, and, again, can be a very valuable way of following response to therapy as it may be the only measurable lesion available for sequential investigation.

Bone Scanning

The bone scan has been used for a wide variety of problems in childhood. The important advantage it has over skeletal radiology is its markedly increased sensitivity, due to the ability to detect functional changes in bony metabolism before they give rise to structural abnormalities on the radiograph.

Part of the bone scan of a child with a primary bone tumour in the right humerus, subsequently shown to be a Ewing's sarcoma, is shown in Figure 9.11. The scan permitted rapid exclusion of any other lesions in the skeleton with a high degree of confidence. Incidentally, it provides an excellent demonstration of the

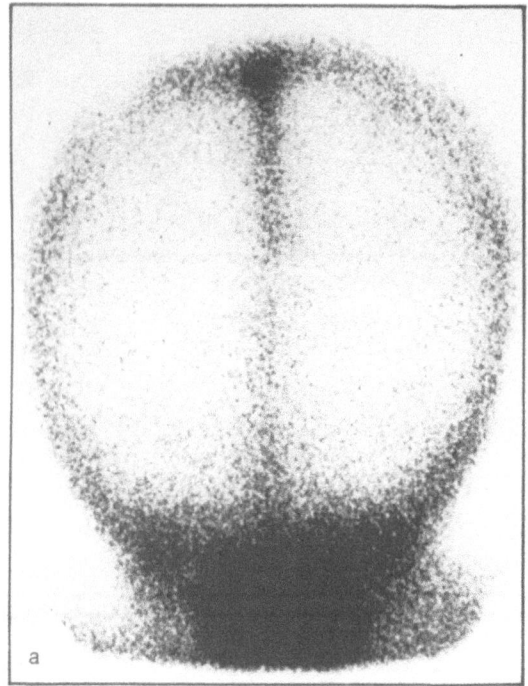

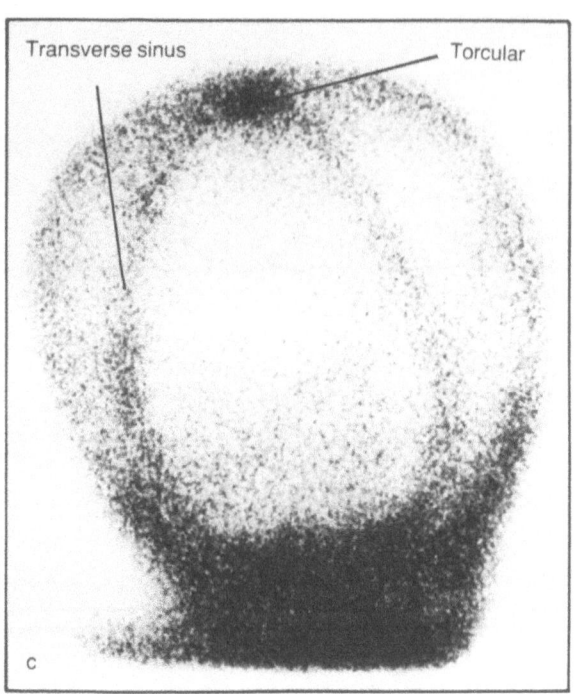

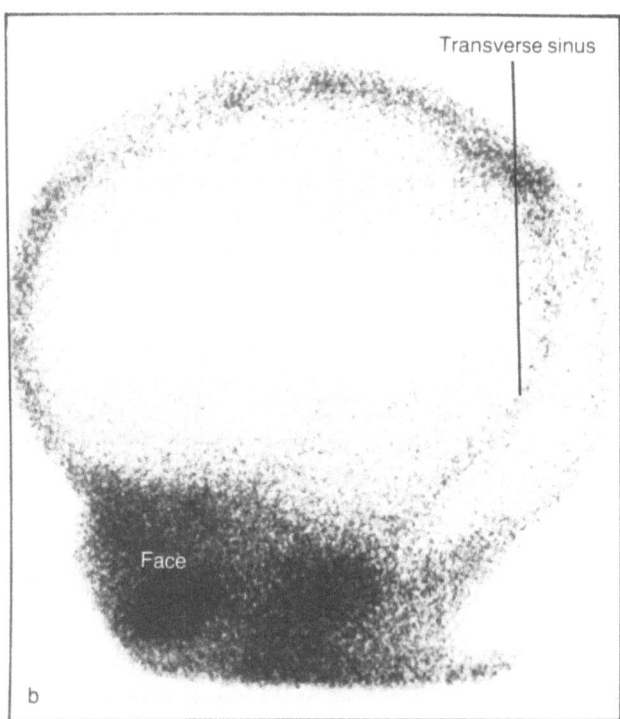

Figure 9.6 *A patient with internal hydrocephalus. The scan shows the large head and the grossly distorted venous sinuses.* (**a**) *Anterior view,* (**b**) *left lateral view and* (**c**) *posterior view.*

physiological and functional changes which are displayed by the bone scan where the actively growing bone at the epiphyses is clearly shown as areas of increased radionuclide accumulation.

Pain, experienced in the bony areas of the body, is a frequent clinical problem in childhood. Figure 9.12 shows the radionuclide scan of a child with pain in the tibia and an equivocal radiograph. The markedly increased uptake was associated with an osteoid osteoma and confirmed the suspicion on the radiograph.

Frequently, a negative bone scan is even more helpful in the management of cases which, on the radiograph, are suspected of having bone lesions. The reason for this is that with the higher sensitivity of the bone scan, a negative one, in the face of an equivocal radiograph, makes an active lesion extremely unlikely. Figure 9.13 shows three patients in whom associated trauma with bone pain was the clinical problem. Figure 9.13a is the scan of a young boy who was an enthusiastic athlete, who developed tibial pain—the radiograph was negative but the bone scan was clearly positive, both of these were used in the diagnosis of a stress fracture caused by excessive training. Subsequently, this was shown to become positive on the radiograph. Figure 9.13b is of a child who fell on an outstretched hand and had clinical features suggestive of a scaphoid fracture, but the radiograph (Figure 9.13c) was equivocal. The bone scan clearly confirmed an active lesion at the site of the scaphoid, and subsequent radiographs confirmed a scaphoid fracture. Figure 9.13d shows the bone scan of a child who fell off her skateboard, but the bone scan showed diffuse, rather than focal, uptake and there was no further evidence radiographically or clinically to suggest a fracture.

Bone scanning has been used to advantage in other important areas, such as in the identification of fractures associated with battered children, and in the

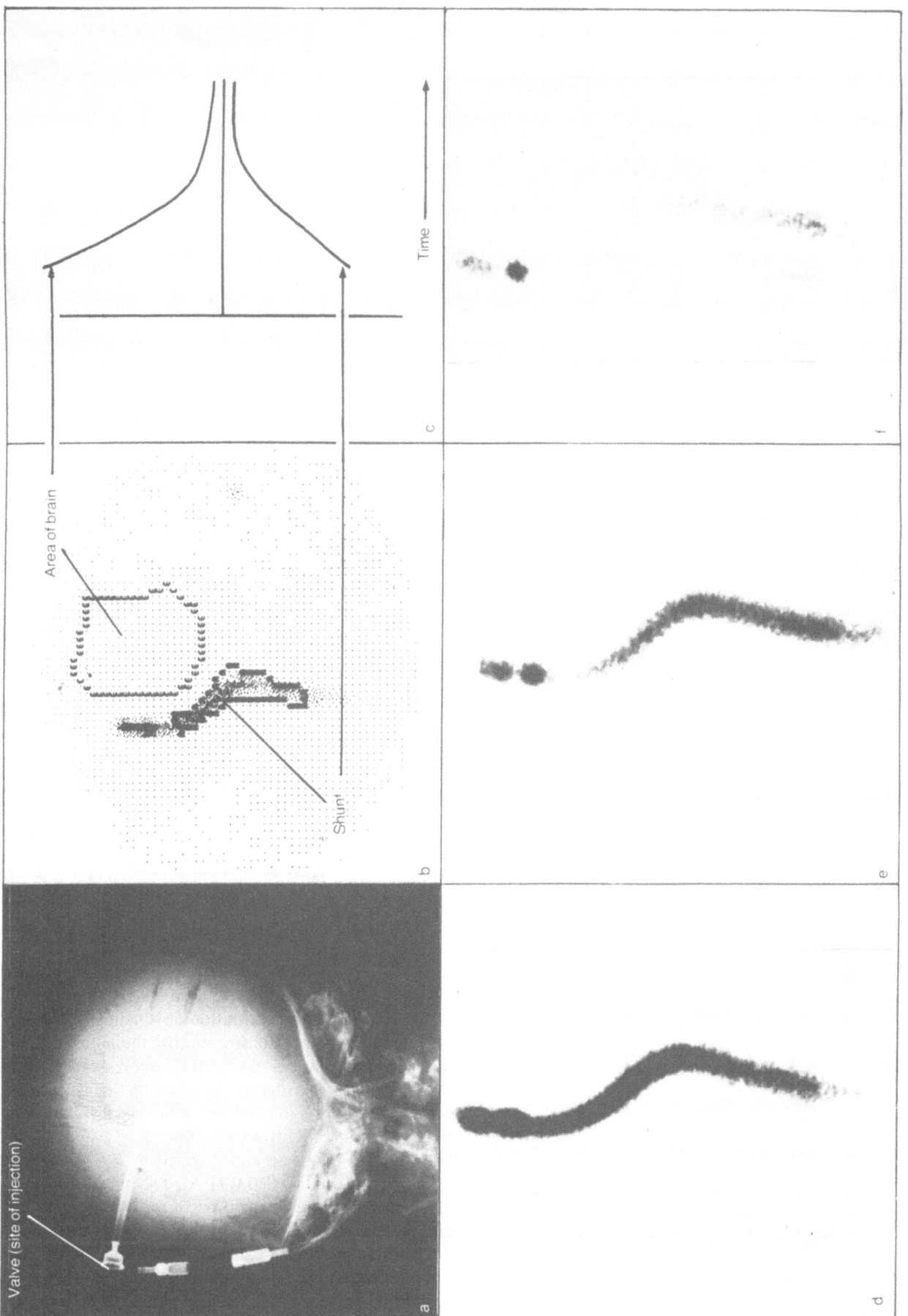

Figure 9.7a Radiograph showing the position of the shunt, (**b**) the areas of interest are marked on the computer oscilloscope from which time activity curves (shown in Figure **9.7c**) are generated. (**d**, **e** and **f**) Activity in the shunt is 'washing-out' rapidly.

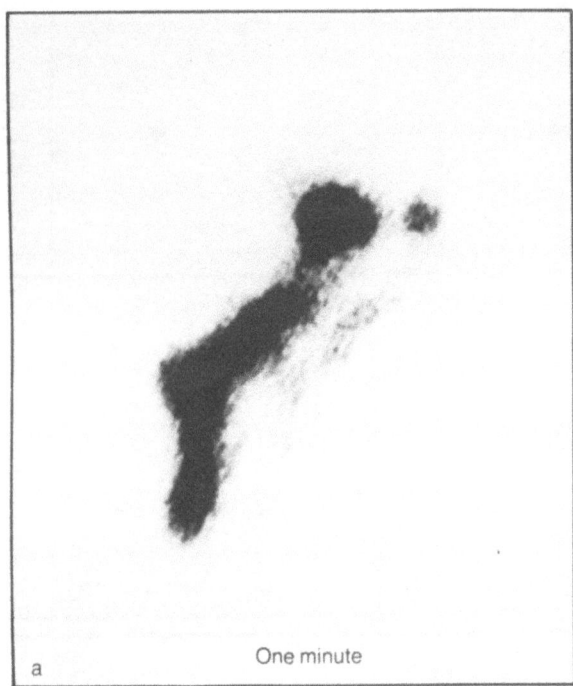

a   One minute

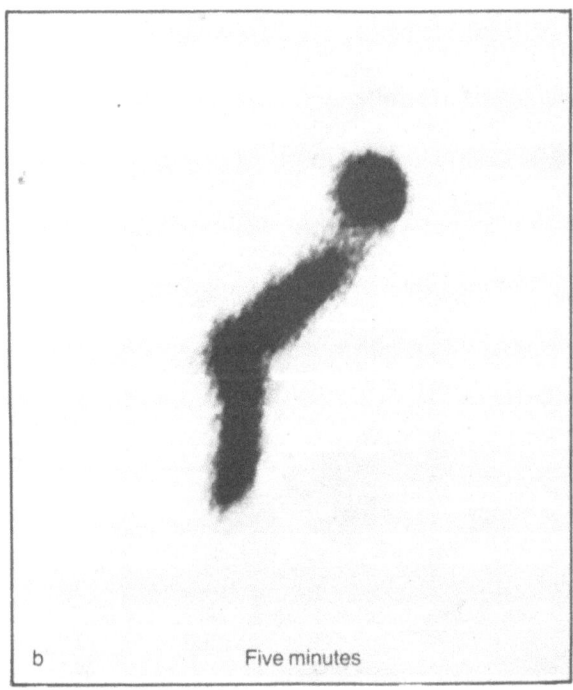

b   Five minutes

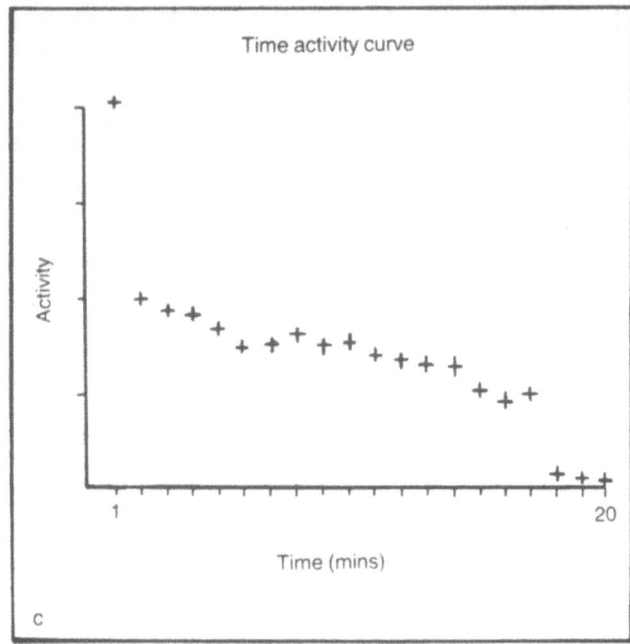

c

Figure 9.8 *Scan showing a blocked VA shunt for hydrocephalus, with no significant 'wash-out' of tracer with time* **(a)** *after one minute and* **(b)** *after five minutes.* **(c)** *Time activity curve taken from the area of interest over the shunt.*

differential diagnosis of the irritable hip syndrome where the earlier detection of bony disease, in particular osteomyelitis, results in very important improvement in management.

The Genitourinary Tract

Where the use of radionuclide investigation of renal and renal tract disorders has been systematically applied, the results have been extremely rewarding, probably more

so than in other organ systems. The clear delineation of the clinical problem in renal disease is essential to the effective use of radionuclides. When the clinical problem is one of the measurement of divided renal function prior to surgery or as a means of follow-up then an agent, such as technetium-99m labelled DMSA, must be used. Figure 9.14 shows the DMSA scan of a baby presenting with an abdominal mass due to left-sided hydronephrosis. The contribution of the left kidney to total renal failure which was contained in the rim around the 'blown up' collecting system was measured as 30 per cent. Figure 9.14b shows the left kidney postoperatively having decreased in size to normal, and quantitatively maintaining approximately 30 per cent of the total renal function. Figure 9.15, similarly, shows the distribution of function in a horse-shoe kidney, and demonstrates how the anterior view, without interference from the spine can clearly demonstrate the bridge of functioning tissue between the two moieties. The child in acute renal failure may benefit considerably from a radionuclide scan, using an agent that is taken up and excreted by the glomerulus (technetium-99m labelled DTPA). The main advantages are that a measure of renal perfusion can be obtained and that characteristic patterns of causes of renal failure have been identified, e.g. acute glomerulonephritis, pre-renal failure and acute tubular necrosis. However, perhaps of greatest importance, is that the large and potentially toxic load of osmotic material that has to be

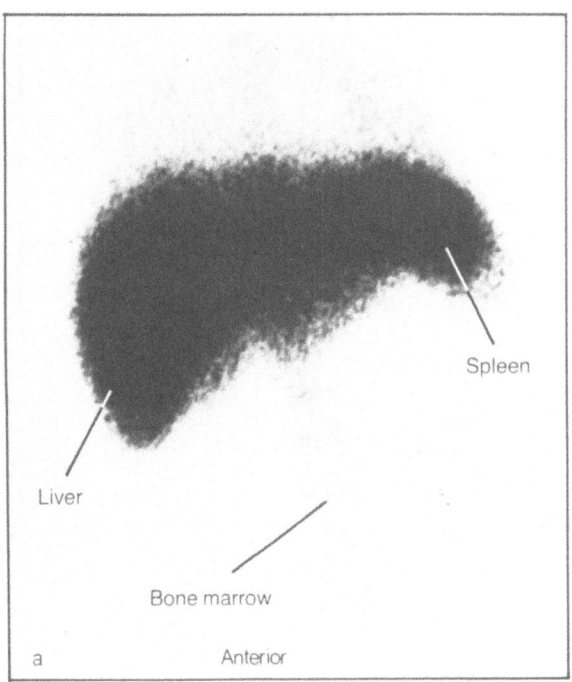

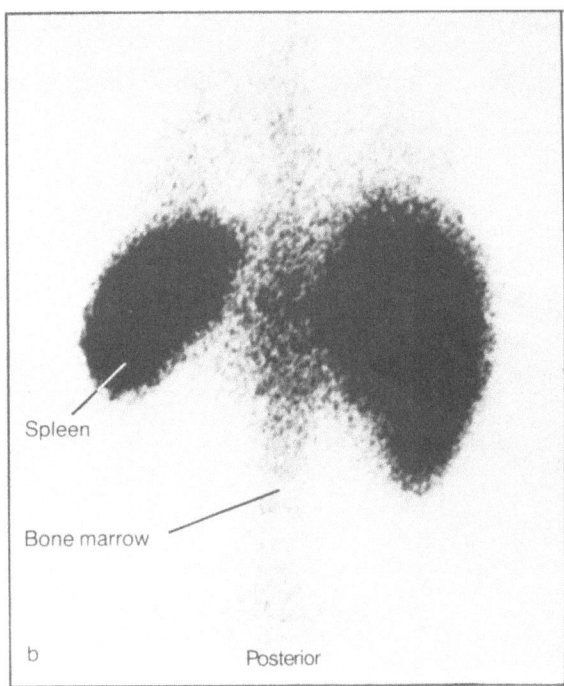

Figure 9.9a and b *The liver/spleen scan of a child of two years who was suffering from hepatosplenomegaly. The scan shows the larger liver and spleen without focal lesion—this was shown later to be due to glycogen storage disease.*

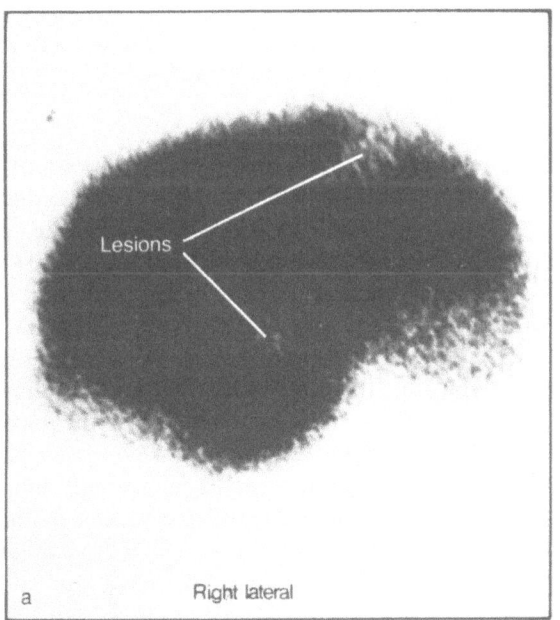

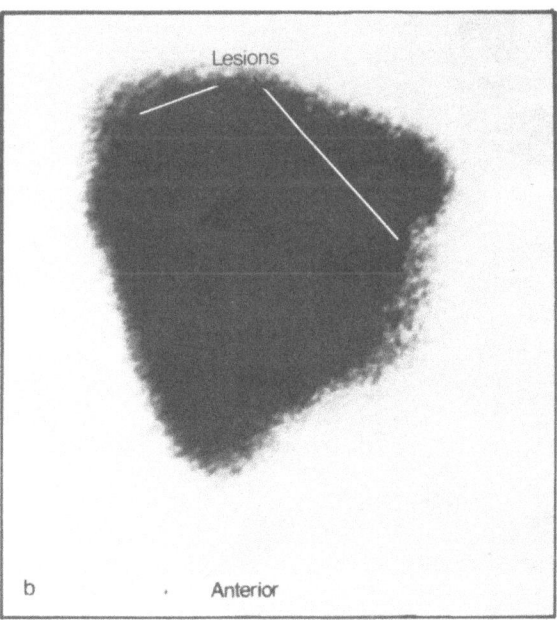

Figure 9.10a and b *The liver/spleen scan of a baby who presented with hepatomegaly, due to multiple haemangiomata.*

given for a high dose intravenous urogram (IVU) is not necessary. Consequently, the information can be obtained with no risk to the infant.

Figure 9.16 is the scan of a one-week-old baby with acute oliguria following diarrhoea. Both kidneys are seen to be well perfused, they are well visualized at five minutes, and there has been some excretion of tracer. This is the appearance seen in pre-renal failure due to

dehydration, and rapid rehydration allowed a return to normal renal function.

The child with a possible pelviureteric junction (PUJ) obstruction is a not infrequent problem and there are two aspects of this which can be evaluated. The first is a measure of divided function; serial measurements allow one to assess any affect on renal function in the equivocal case. Second, it is possible to assess the degree

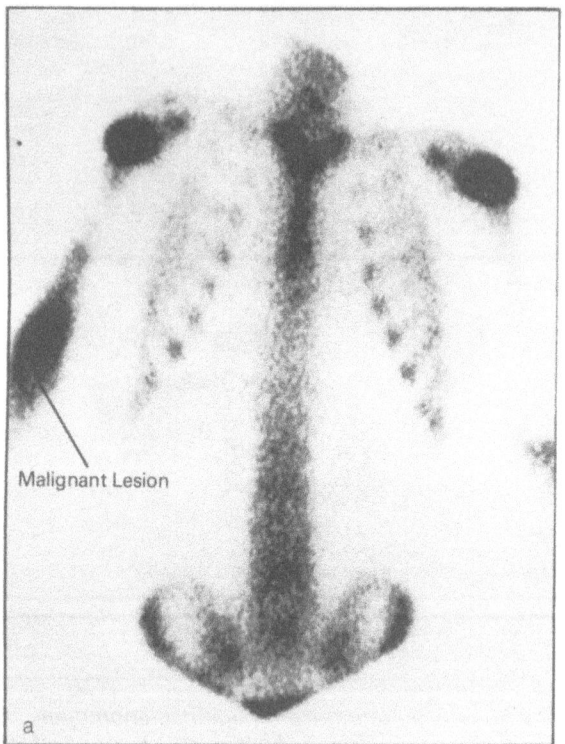

Malignant Lesion

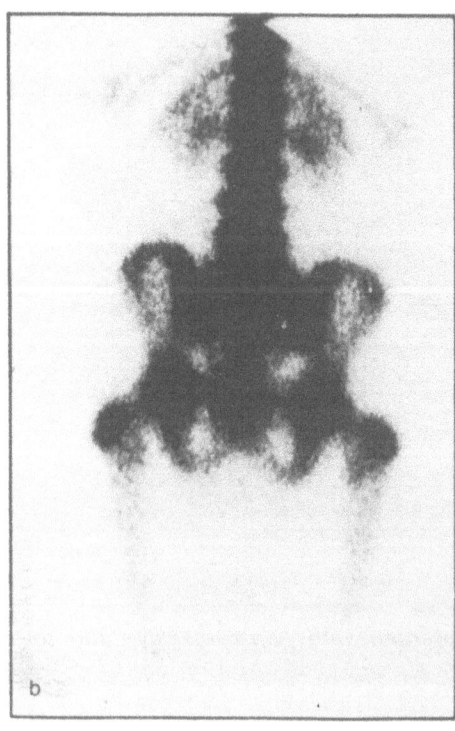

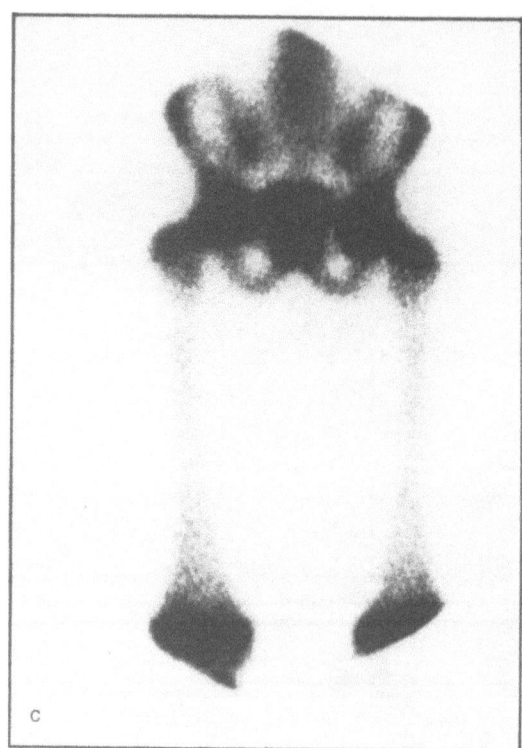

Figure 9.11a, b and c *The body scan of a child with a malignant bone lesion. The whole body scan was taken so that any other bone lesions could be detected. The scan shows the epiphyseal activity at the growing ends of bones, in addition to the malignant lesion.*

diuresis with Frusemide show rapid wash-out of the tracer on the left side, which was not obstructed, but no significant change in activity on the right side, confirming PUJ obstruction on this side. In Figure 9.18, the initial IVU on this child was reported as showing a non-functioning right kidney, and the two minute DTPA scan appears to confirm lack of function of the right kidney. However, the delayed 30 minute image shows a large collecting system lying just above the bladder which, on the anterior view, is clearly seen to be a pelvic kidney with PUJ obstruction. Renal imaging may be valuable in the location of the site of ectopic renal tissue in other congenital abnormalities, which are similar to that described above.

Respiratory Disease

Lung scanning is much less frequently used in childhood, the reason for this is mainly because the major value and indication for lung scanning—that of pulmonary embolism—is much less common in this age group. However, it is becoming apparent that the use of perfusion ventilation lung scanning in combination provides easily obtained and valuable information about the pathophysiology of lung disease in children. Figure 9.19 shows such an example of a child with

of obstruction, again, when there is doubt from the intravenous urogram (IVU). Figure 9.17 shows the scan of a child who had an equivocal IVU, suggesting right-sided PUJ obstruction. The scan, using DTPA, showed two well perfused kidneys with equal divided function with dilated pelves, more marked on the right than the left side. The images before and after an induced

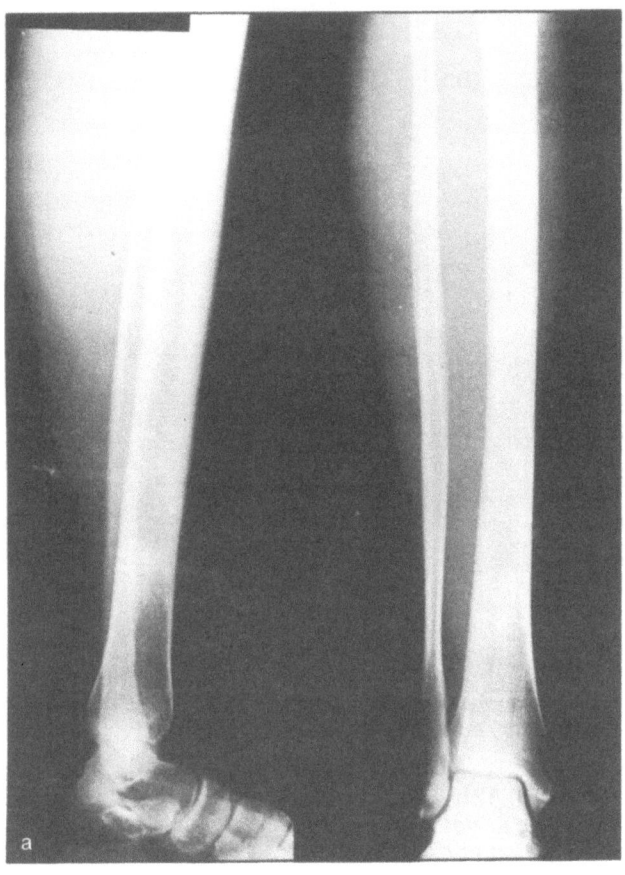

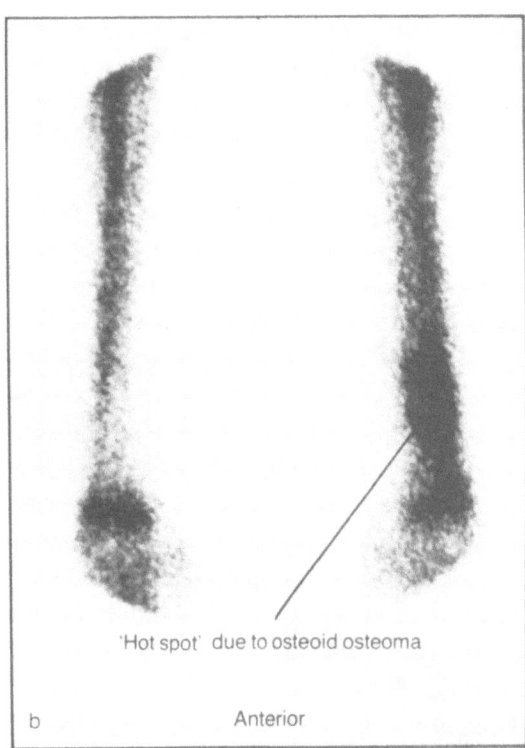

'Hot spot' due to osteoid osteoma

b   Anterior

Figure 9.12a *The equivocal radiograph and* **(b)** *the radionuclide scan of a young girl who had developed pain in her lower limb due to osteoid osteoma.*

partial atresia of subsegmental arteries to the right upper lobe. The chest radiograph showed only a suggestion of decreased vascularity to the right upper lobe, but the perfusion lung scan demonstrates very clearly that there is almost absent perfusion to the right upper lobe. However, ventilation, as imaged using krypton-81m, is entirely normal. This, of course, is the pattern which is normally seen in acute pulmonary embolus, but it may occasionally occur in abnormalities of the pulmonary arteries. Other situations in which perfusion ventilation lung scanning may be helpful in childhood include investigation of McCleod's syndrome (unilateral pulmonary hypoplasia), the investigation of patients with suspected foreign body inhalation, and in the functional assessment of patients with parenchymal lung disease such as bronchiectasis and cystic fibrosis.

The other use of lung scanning in children lies in the assessment of the size of a right-to-left shunt (cardiac shunts) and quantification of the right lung blood flow versus the left lung blood flow. The lung scan can be used in this situation because the technetium-99m labelled microspheres or macroaggregates are normally entirely trapped symmetrically by the pulmonary capillaries. However, if there is an intracardiac right-to-left shunt a proportion of the particles, depending on the size of the shunt, will by-pass the pulmonary capillary sieve and find their way into the systemic

circulation. By quantification of the ratio trapped in the pulmonary capillary bed versus the amount in the systemic circulation, the size of the right-to-left shunt can be calculated. Likewise, following by-pass operations, such as a Blalock anastomosis, where a subclavian artery has been anastomosed to the right pulmonary artery for severe pulmonary stenosis, if this is patent the proportion of microspheres which are found in the right lung field will greatly exceed those found in the left lung field and if the shunt becomes blocked this difference will disappear. Figure 9.20 shows almost the entire body of a one-year-old child with Fallot's tetralogy who had a Blalock anastomosis. The increasing cyanosis suggested strongly that the anastomosis was not working, and the scan clearly showed two factors. First, there was a large amount of activity in the kidneys and brain due to the appearance of the particles in the systemic circulation via the right-to-left shunt. Second, the uptake in the two lungs is approximately equal, clearly indicating that the shunt is obstructed.

Gallium Scanning

A frequent clinical problem in children, as well as in adults, is one of PUO (pyrexia of unknown origin)

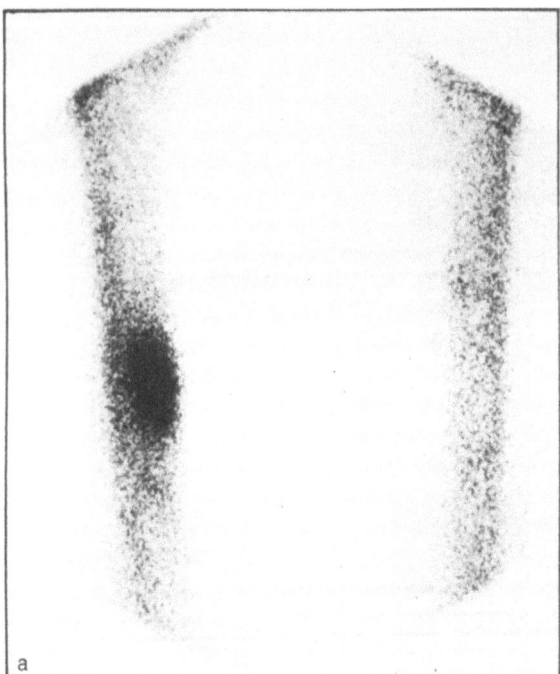

Figure 9.13a *The scan of a middle-distance athlete who developed pain in the right tibia—this was due to a stress fracture. The radiograph was negative, but the bone scan showed a 'hot' lesion due to the stress fracture.*

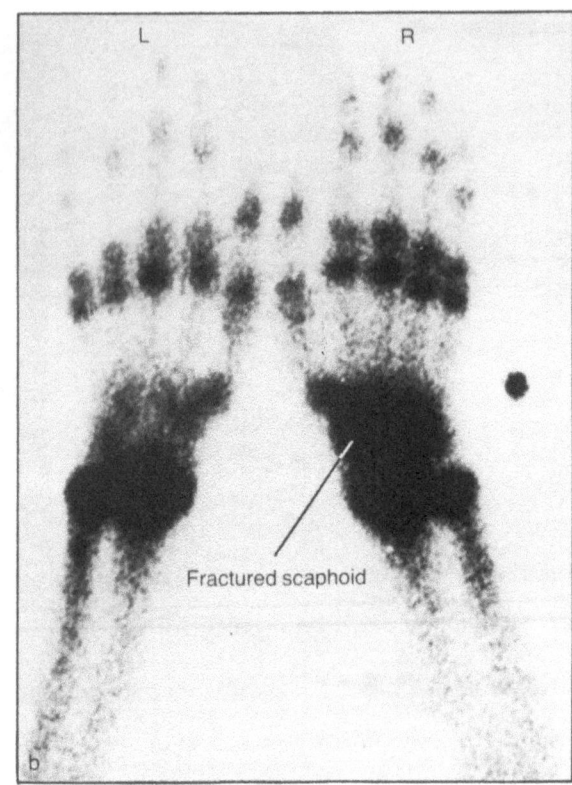

Figure 9.13b *The bone scan of a patient (after a fall) showing a 'hot' lesion in the region of the scaphoid.* **(c)** *The radiograph was equivocal.*

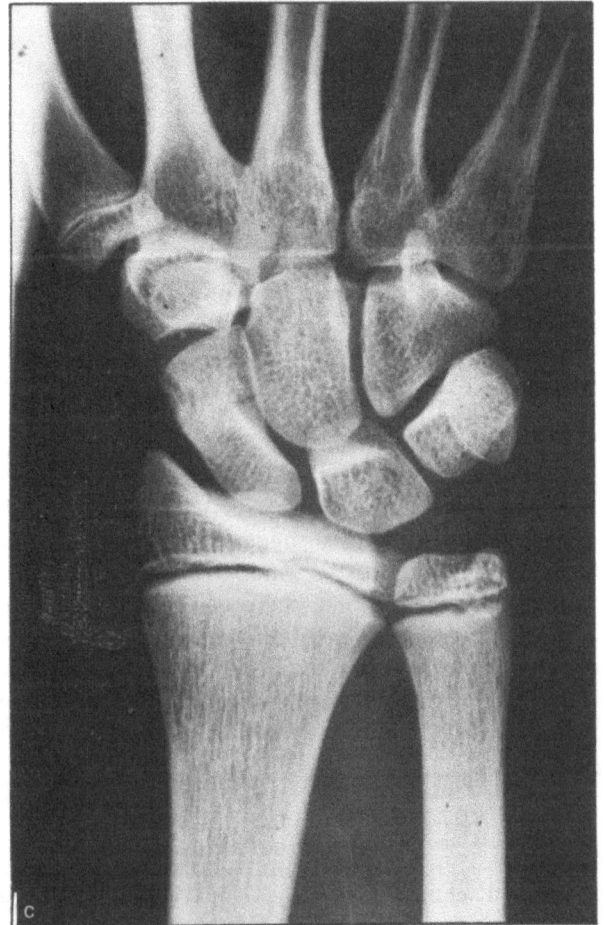

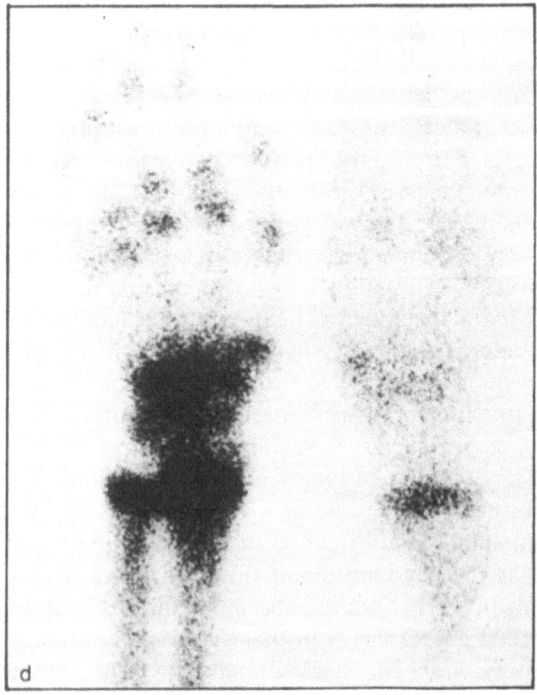

Figure 9.13d *The bone scan of a child who fell off her skateboard. There was clinical suspicion of a scaphoid fracture and the scan shows generalized non-focal uptake.*

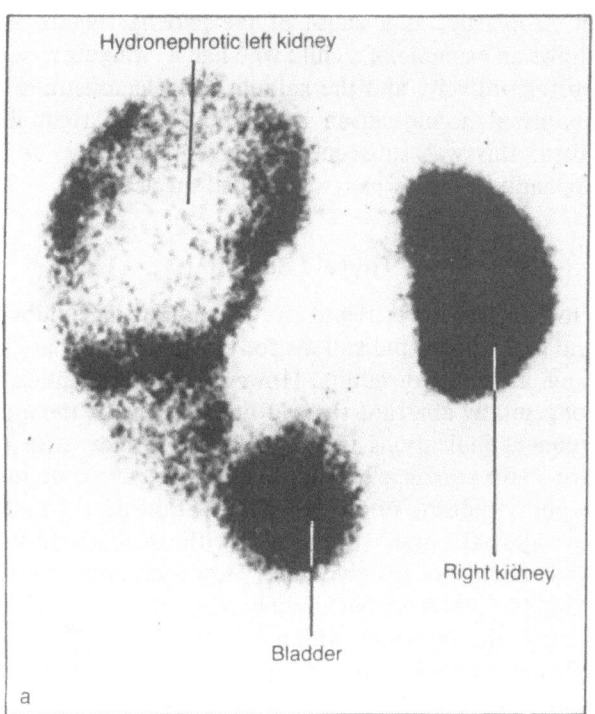

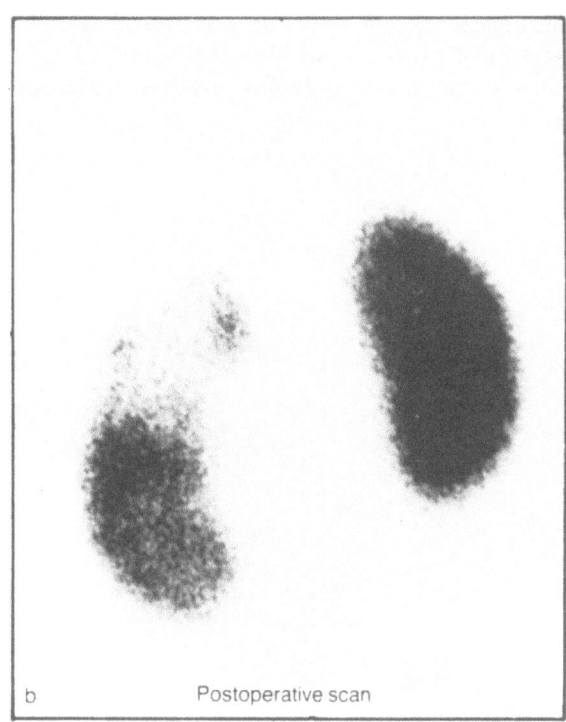

Figure 9.14a *The scan of a baby who presented with a mass in the abdomen. This was shown to be due to hydronephrosis on the DMSA scan.* **(b)** *The postoperative scan shows return to almost normal size, but with persistently decreased function.*

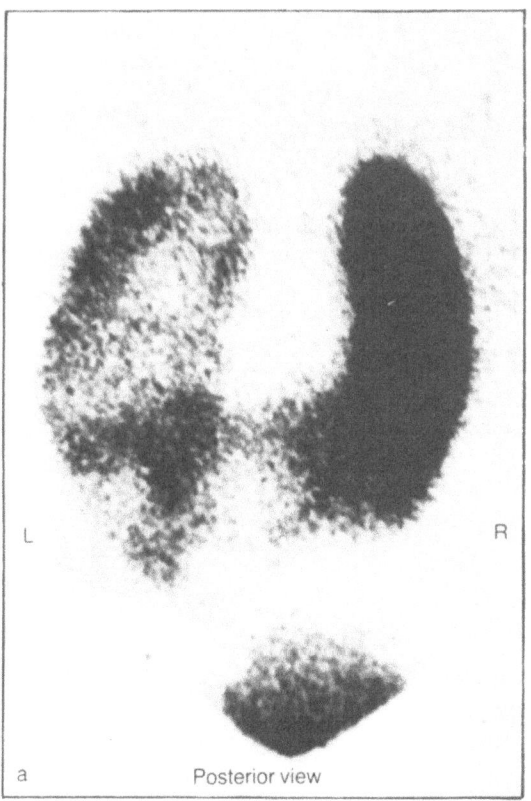

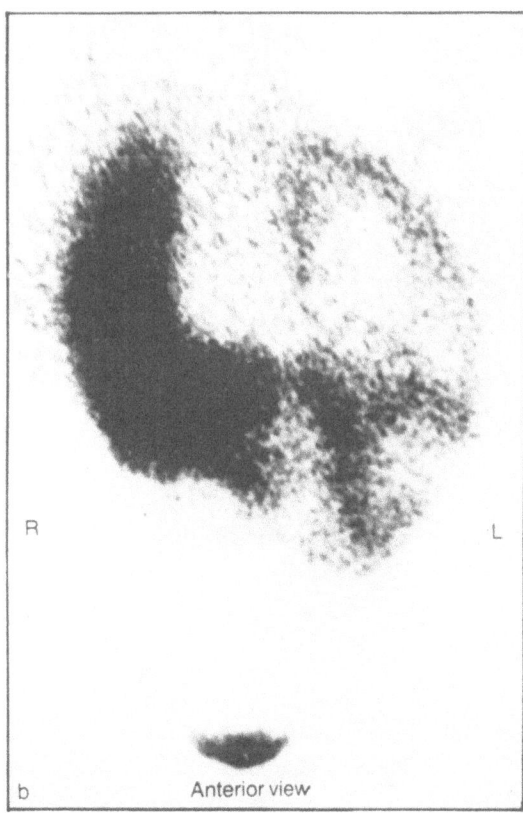

Figure 9.15a and b *The DMSA scan of a horse-shoe kidney, with left-sided hydronephrosis. The anterior view* **(b)** *shows the extent of the functioning bridge.*

either occurring de novo or postoperatively. As in adults, gallium scanning can be very valuable in localizing the site of the disease, whether inflammatory or neoplastic, as a cause of the pyrexia. Figure 9.21 shows an example of a child who had a swinging pyrexia postoperatively, and the gallium scan demonstrates an abnormal accumulation of gallium in the right iliac fossa; this was subsequently shown to be due to an appendix abscess which was treated surgically.

Thyroid Scanning

Thyroid disease is relatively uncommon in childhood and many of the indications for thyroid imaging are the same as those for adults. However, the localization of congenitally aberrant thyroid tissue is one of the more frequent indications in childhood. This may arise for two main reasons; either a child with severe or mild hypothyroidism, or in the investigation of a possible thyroglossal cyst. Scanning with technetium-99m pertechnetate or ^{123}I gives a very low radiation dose and should be performed in all such cases. Figure 9.22 shows a child who presented with a midline nodule which was thought to be due to a thyroglossal cyst. The thyroid scan shows that there is no functioning thyroid tissue in the neck and that the entire thyroid is located at the back of the tongue (a lingual thyroid).

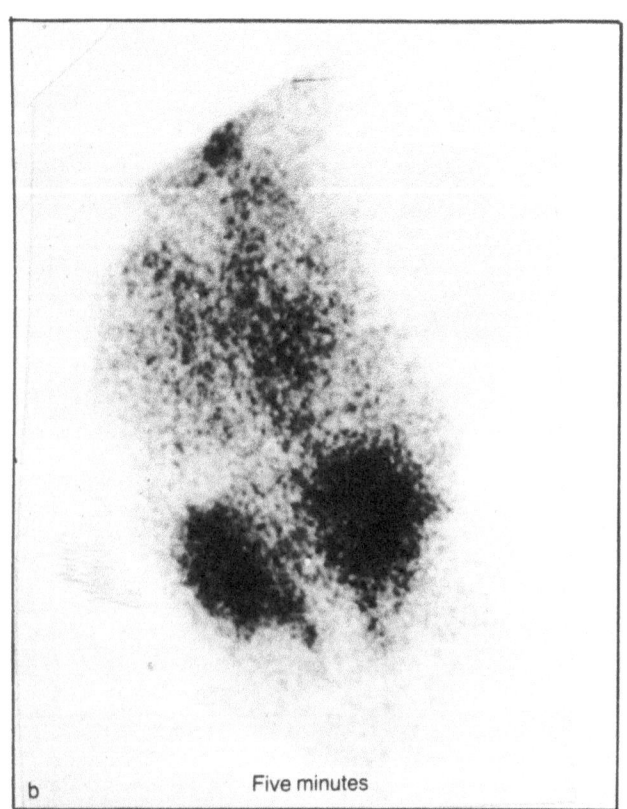

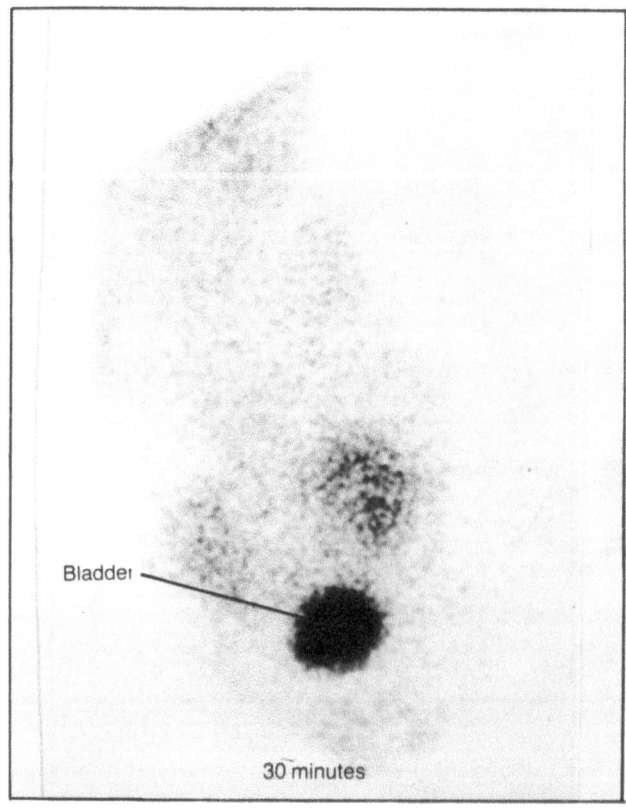

Figure 9.16 *The scan of a baby with acute oliguria—shows well perfused kidneys with some tracer excretion. Pre-renal failure responded well to rehydration. Views taken at (a) 30 seconds, (b) five minutes and (c) 30 minutes.*

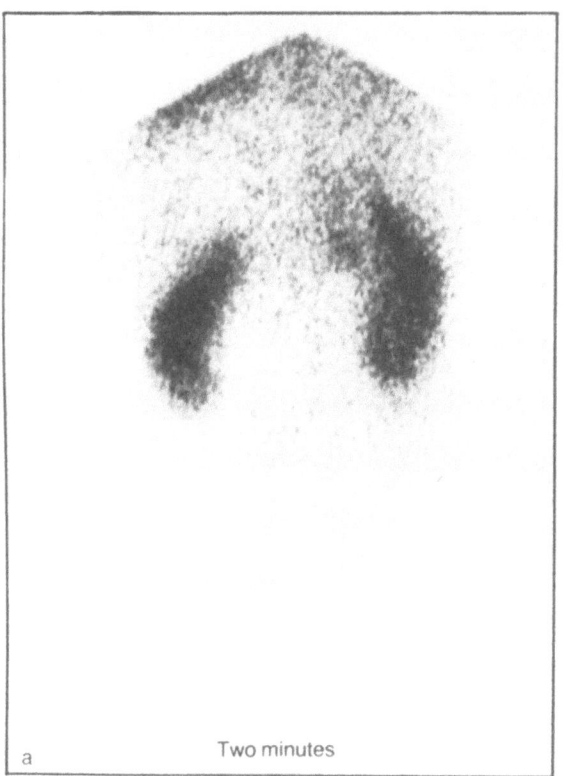

a   Two minutes

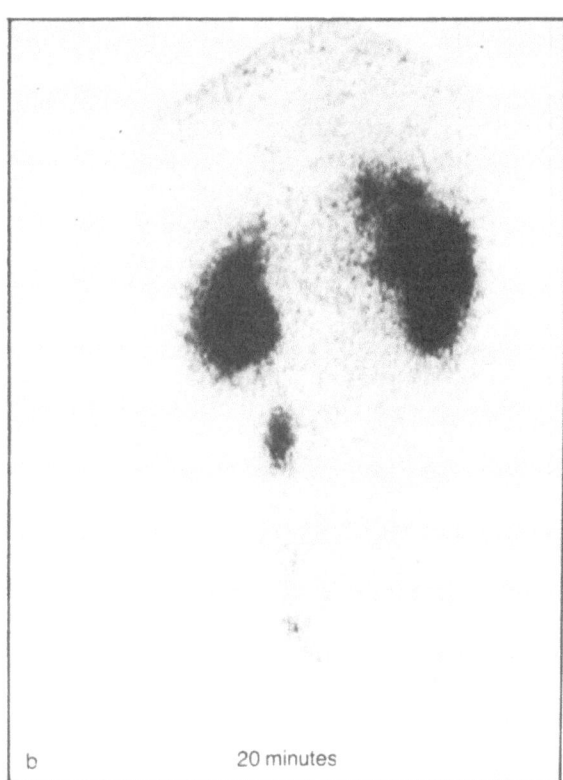

b   20 minutes

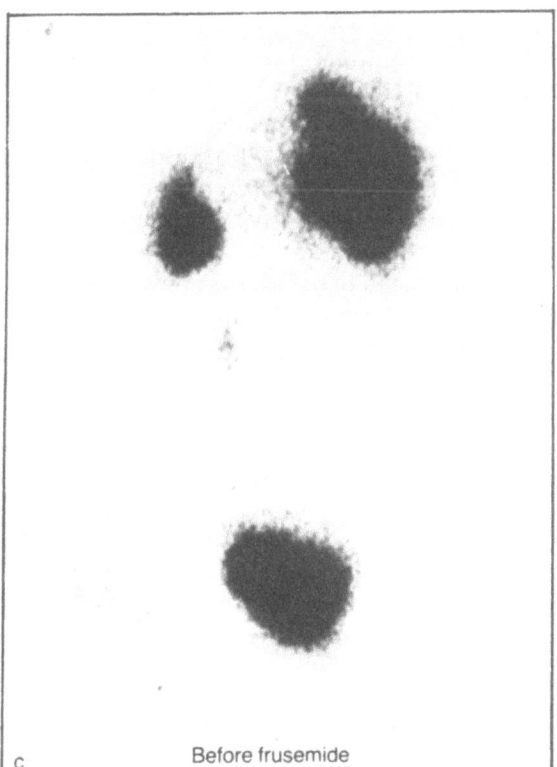

c   Before frusemide

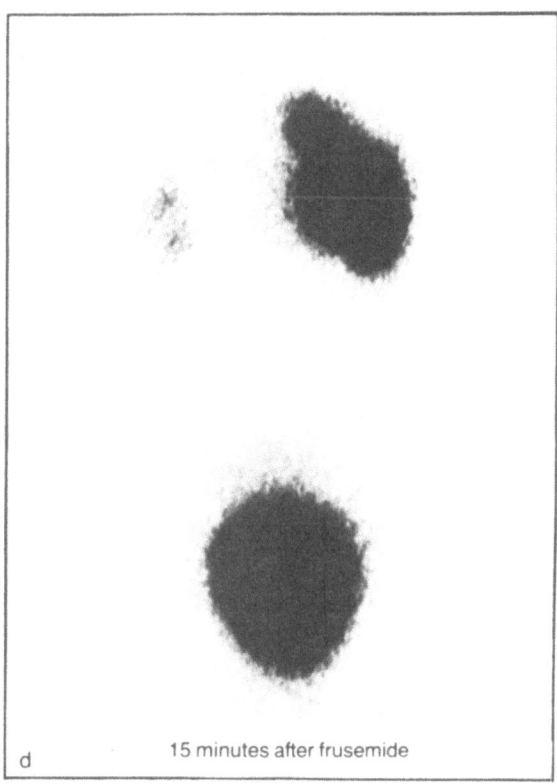

d   15 minutes after frusemide

Figure 9.17 *The scan of a child with an equivocal PUJ obstruction on IVU.* (a) *Shows good symmetrical function,* (b) *after 20 minutes both collecting systems are full of tracer and appear to be dilated.* (c) *Before and* (d) *15 minutes after diuresis, induced by frusemide, showing good 'wash-out' from the normal side, but no 'wash-out' on the right side. This result confirms PUJ obstruction.*

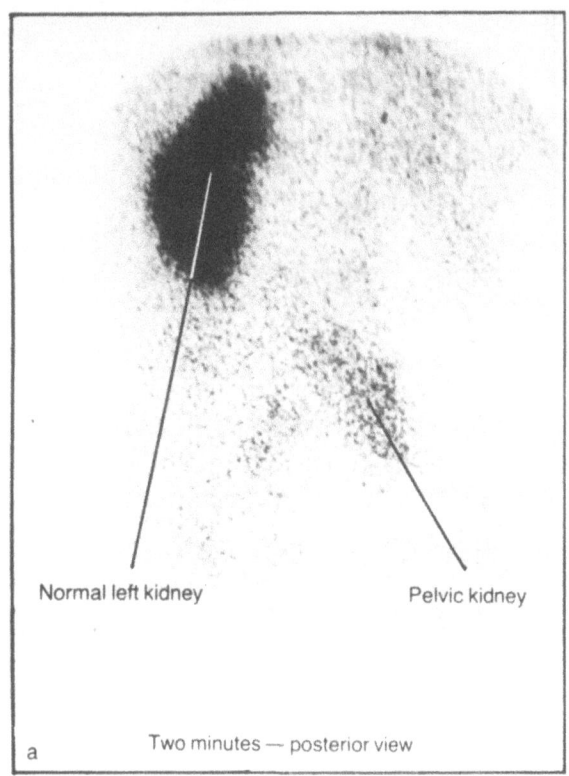

Normal left kidney

Pelvic kidney

a   Two minutes — posterior view

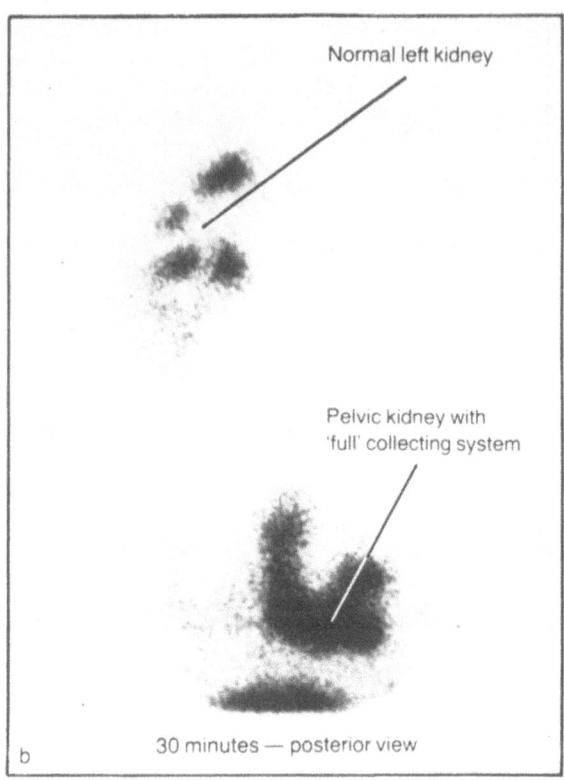

Normal left kidney

Pelvic kidney with 'full' collecting system

b   30 minutes — posterior view

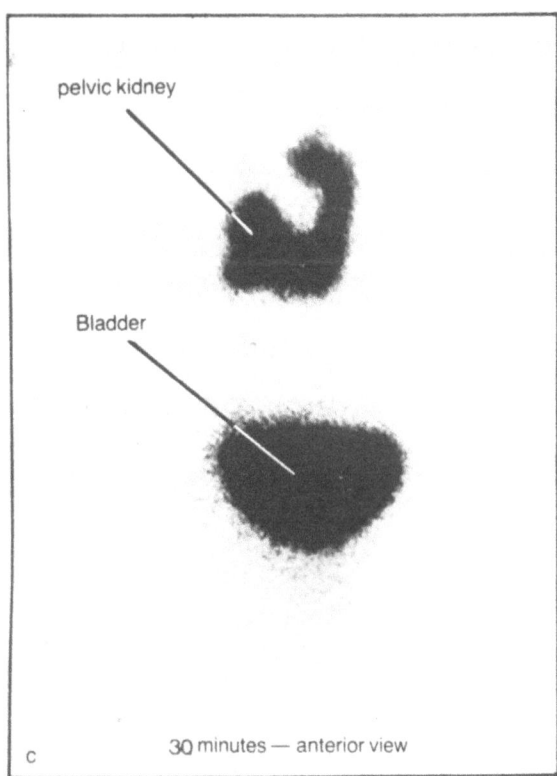

pelvic kidney

Bladder

c   30 minutes — anterior view

Figure 9.18 *The pelvic kidney on DTPA renal scan.* **(a)** *The early two minute view shows an almost non-functioning low right kidney,* **(b)** *shows a gross excess of tracer in the 'low' kidney and* **(c)** *demonstrates more clearly on the anterior view that the kidney is pelvic and obstructed.*

Meckel's Diverticulum

A clinical problem which s found, not infrequently, in childhood is recurrent or persistent gastrointestinal bleeding. A bleeding Meckel's diverticulum may be a cause of such persistent bleeding, and it is notoriously difficult to localize this when using the standard radiological techniques of barium enema, barium meal and follow-through studies. The principle of the radionuclide study lies in the fact that the bleeding Meckel's diverticulum will almost always contain gastric mucosa, and technetium, like iodine, is taken up and excreted by gastric mucosa. Figure 9.23 shows the scan of a child with a history of recurrent gastrointestinal bleeding leading to severe anaemia. The scan which was obtained 15 minutes after an intravenous injection of technetium-99m pertechnetate shows that, in addition to the stomach activity and the bladder activity, there was a small focal finger-like area of increased uptake in the right iliac fossa. The patient subsequently underwent surgical exploration, and an inflamed bleeding Meckel's diverticulum at the ileo-caecal junction was found and excised.

Cardiac Imaging

The most important use of this technique is in the identification and quantification of left-to-right shunts, and it can be an invaluable way of diagnosing or excluding a left-to-right shunt, either intracardiac or due

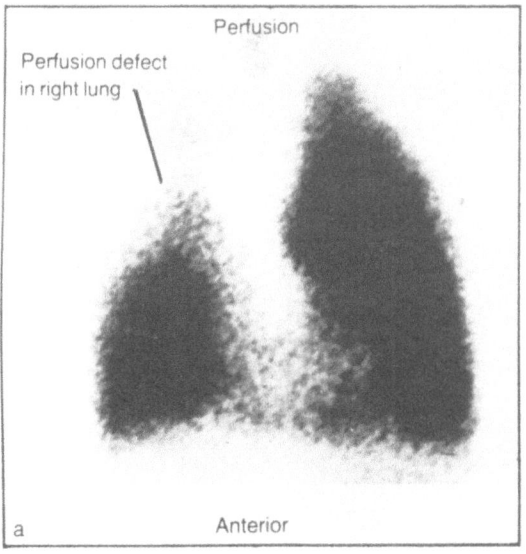

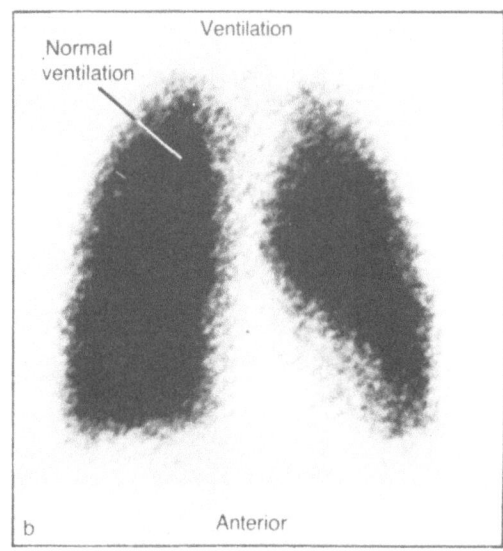

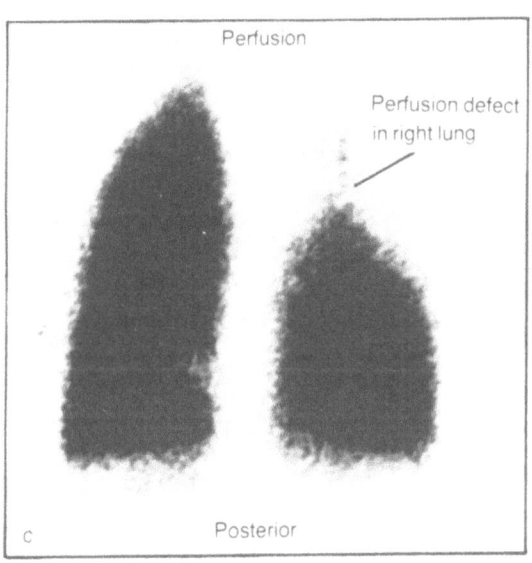

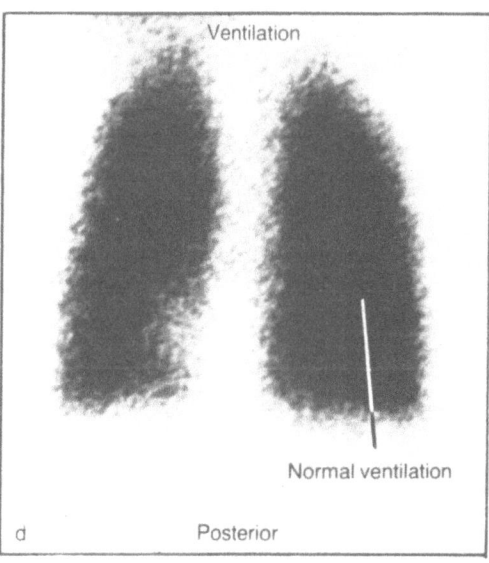

Figure 9.19a, b, c and d *Atresia of the subsegmental arteries to the right upper lobe, showing normal ventilation where there is absent perfusion.*

to a patent ductus, in a child with a suspicious cardiac murmur.

Following a rapid intravenous injection of technetium-99m pertechnetate, the normal sequence of cardiac chamber and pulmonary blood flow is seen with an unobscured left ventricular phase when there is essentially no activity in the right side of the heart or the pulmonary capillary bed. However, in the presence of a left-to-right shunt the recirculation of tracer back through the right side of the heart and the pulmonary capillary bed results in persistent activity in the lung fields and right side of the heart. By using the area of interest facility of the computer, time activity curves can be generated from over the lung fields, and the size of the left-to-right shunt can be calculated using standardized programmes. These are based on fitting a curve to

the first and second pulmonary circulation resulting from the left-to-right shunt, and then quantitating the area under these curves.

Figures 9.24 and 9.25 show the comparison between a normal study and a study of a patient with a large left-to-right shunt due to a VSD. The images from the normal patient, during the first passage of the $^{99}Tc^m$ pertechnetate bolus, show clearly delineated cardiac phases with normal sequence of chamber filling; in particular, the left ventricle is seen clearly after the pulmonary phase. In contrast, the patient with a left-to-right shunt has recirculation of tracer back through the lung fields at the same time as the left ventricle fills, thereby obscuring the left ventricle during the normal left ventricular filling phase. The time activity curves in Figure 9.25 demonstrate this more clearly. The SVC

103

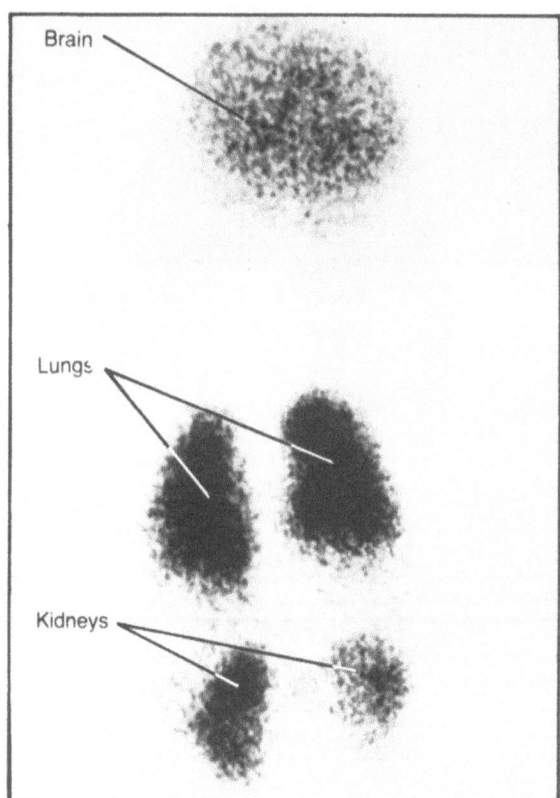

Figure 9.20 *The scan of a child with a blocked Blalock shunt, showing shunting of particles to the systemic circulation.*

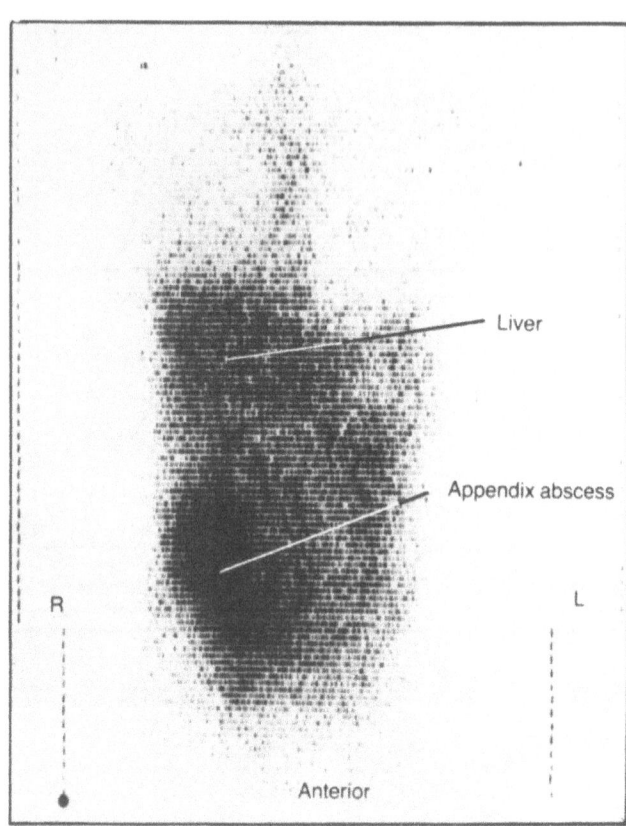

Figure 9.21 *A patient who suffered from persistent pyrexia following appendicectomy. The gallium-67 scan shows abnormal uptake in the right hypochondrium due to an appendix abscess.*

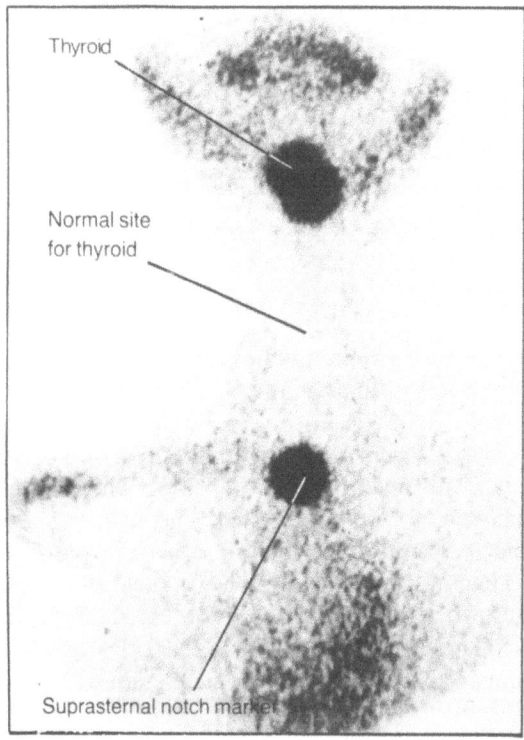

Figure 9.22 *The scan shows a child who presented with a midline 'thyroid' nodule, but was found to have a lingual thyroid. The nodule was found to be a thyroglossal cyst.*

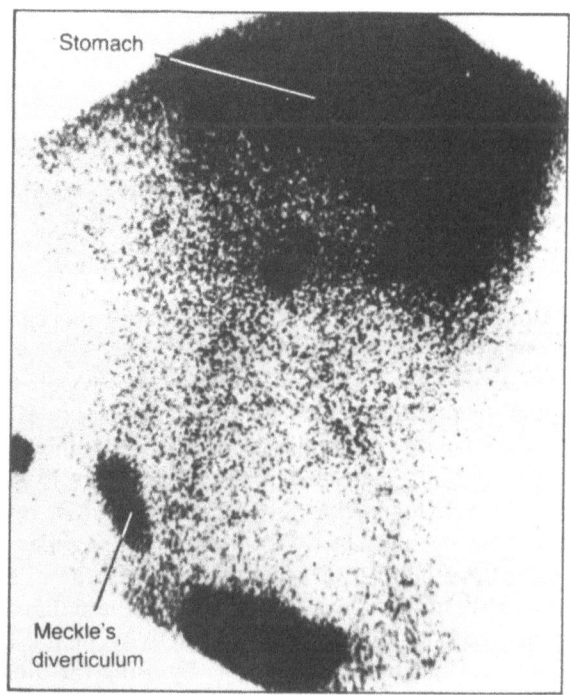

Figure 9.23 *The scan of a child with a history of recurrent gastrointestinal bleeding. The barium studies were all negative, but the scan shows clear uptake of $^{99}Tc^m$ pertechnetate in the Meckel's diverticulum.*

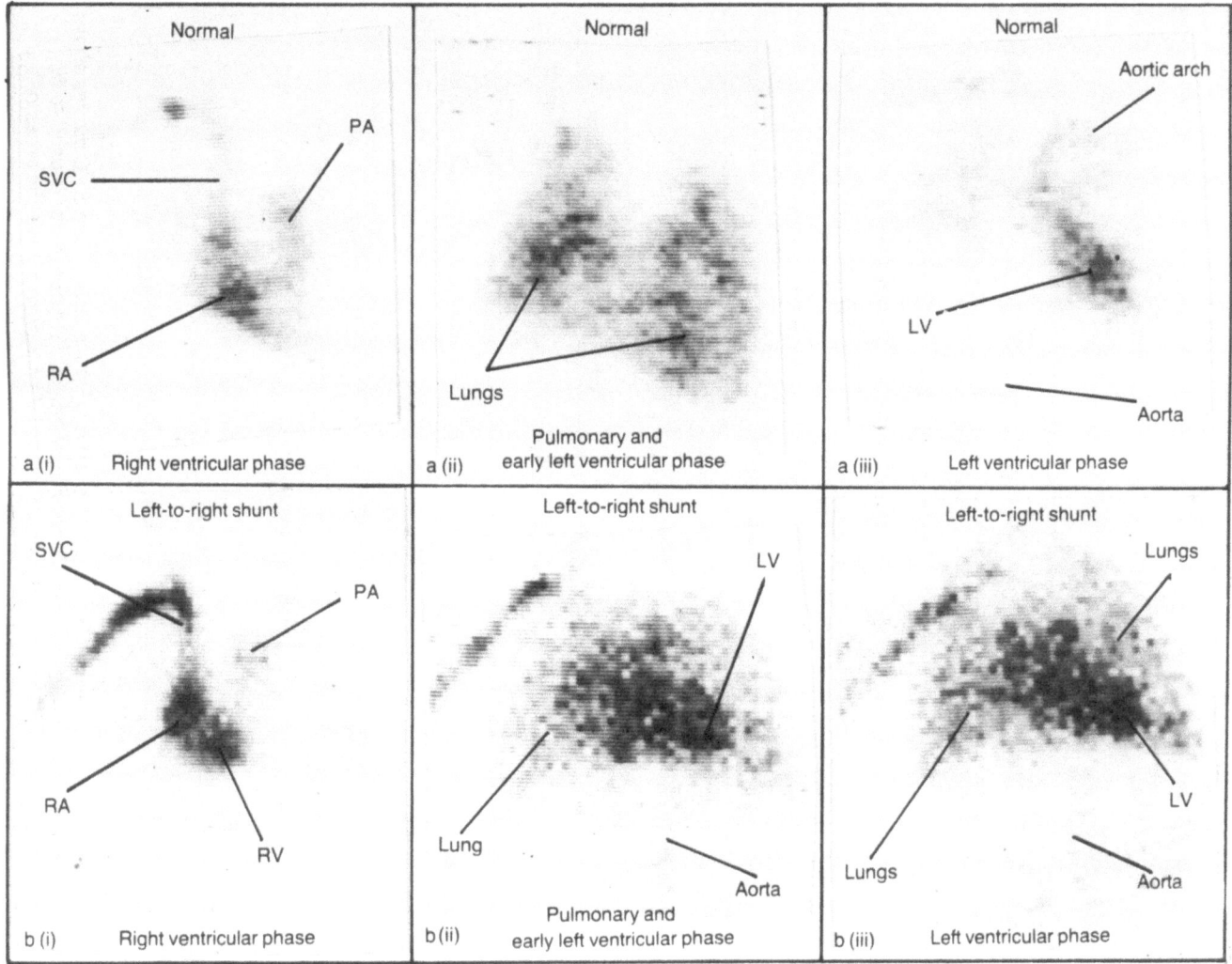

Figure 9.24 *The comparison of two first pass cardiac studies; normal and left-to-right shunt. Figure 9.24a (i, ii, iii) shows the normal sequence of chamber filling (i.e. right side, pulmonary and left ventricular). Figure 9.24b (i, ii, iii) shows the normal right side filling and pulmonary flow, but there is persistence of the lung image, which obscures the left ventricular phase due to the left-to-right recirculation.*

curve should reflect a good bolus and then, as shown in the normal case, the lung field curve should be symmetrical. However, in the case of a left-to-right shunt the downslope will be spread out by the tracer recirculating via the shunt back into the pulmonary bed. Further analysis, utilizing the computer to fit curves to the data which is obtained, enables one to calculate the contribution from the shunted blood and hence the size of the shunt.

Other areas in which cardiac imaging may be of value in children, include the initial assessment of children, particularly neonates with cyanotic disease, in order to establish, first, the presence of a cardiac rather than respiratory disease and, second, as an initial evaluation of the anatomical abnormality that is present. Thallium imaging and multiple gated isotope angiograms are becoming used more widely in paediatric cardiology but their exact role remains under evaluation.

Further Reading

Hanmaker, Hirsch, and Bowenstein, Gerald (Eds), *Nuclear medicine in clinical paediatrics.* Published by the Society of Nuclear Medicine Inc., New York, 1975.

James, A. E., Wagner, H. N., Cook, R. E., *Paediatric nuclear medicine,* W. B. Saunders, London, 1974.

▷

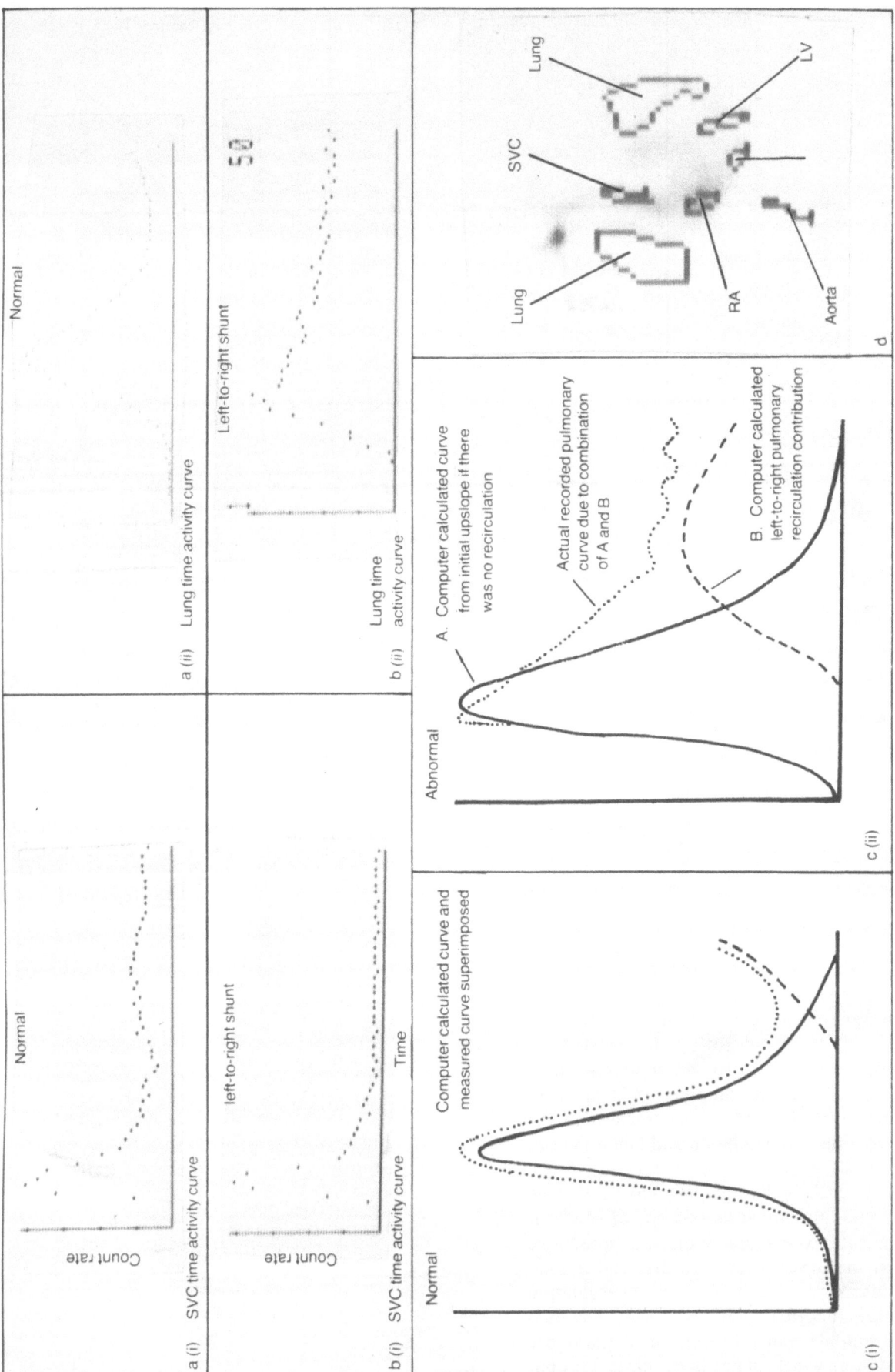

Figure 9.25a and b *Shows the time activity curves from the SVC and lung areas of interest (from the two cases shown in Figure 9.24). The SVC curves show similar sharp peaks, but the lung curve (from the left-to-right shunt case) is 'smeared', due to the left-to-right recirculation. (c) The computer is used to fit curves representing the pulmonary flow and that due to shunted blood. From this, the size of the shunt is calculated. (d) This Figure shows the areas of interest.*

10. Other Scanning Techniques

It is not intended that this book should be an exhaustive treatise on nuclear medicine. However, there are a number of imaging investigations which have not been included in the previous chapters and which may not be frequently employed in any one department, but which, nevertheless, represent important and valuable diagnostic clinical tools. In common with many situations in nuclear medicine, the scans which are described below have evolved in response to specific clinical situations. They all give answers to defined questions, and, yet again, represent largely the functional component of the organ under examination and are complementary to the structural evaluation which is made by using radiography, CT or ultrasound.

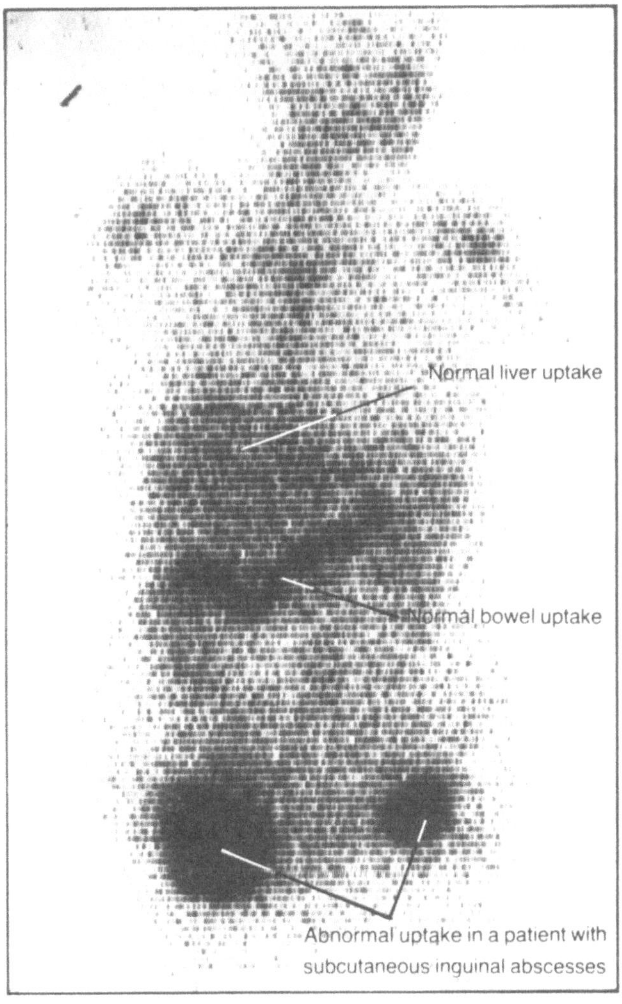

Gallium Scanning

Gallium citrate-67 (^{67}Ga) is a radioactive isotope of a trace metal and, after intravenous injection, is taken up by bone, bone marrow and, to a lesser extent, by salivary glands, lacrimal glands and the spleen. In the first 24 hours, excretion is mainly via the kidneys and subsequently via the liver in to the gastrointestinal tract.

The importance of ^{67}Ga lies in the fact that it is frequently 'taken up' by inflammatory and malignant lesions. There are many likely mechanisms for this uptake, but for the present discussion it can be regarded as a nonspecific empirical observation which has considerable clinical use.

How then is gallium-67 used? Gallium-67, as the citrate, is injected intravenously (in a dose of 50 μCi/kg body weight); an image of the distribution is obtained after 48 hours, using either a whole body rectilinear scanner, a large field of view gamma camera or a

Figure 10.1 *A gallium scan showing a couple of normal variants, together with abnormal uptake in a patient with subcutaneous inguinal abscesses.*

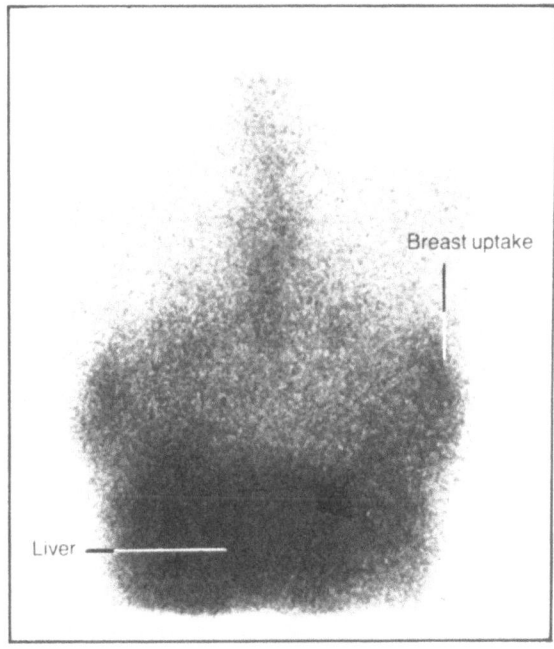

Figure 10.2 *A gallium scan showing breast uptake in a patient who was taking metoclopramide.*

scanning gamma camera. The area which is scanned is usually the anterior and posterior trunk from neck to thighs, but this will be altered depending on the particular clinical problem. Although the usual time for imaging is 48 hours, occasionally additional six hour scans and 72 hours scans may be needed, depending on the clinical situation. The normal distribution of gallium is characteristic.

A few normal variants are worth mentioning at this point (Figure 10.1 shows some of these, together with abnormal uptake in a patient with subcutaneous inguinal abscesses). First, the liver excretion into the bowel may result in clear-cut bowel visualization; bowel preparation with a laxative minimizes this effect. The kidneys are visualized in the first 24 hours, but after this time it is abnormal; the spleen, lacrimal glands and salivary glands are often faintly visualized, but after

radiotherapy salivary glands may be very 'hot'. Drugs which stimulate pituitary prolactin release may cause breast uptake (Figure 10.2). This is a frequent problem as many patients are ill and nauseated and require drugs, such as antiemetics.

Gallium scanning is a valuable diagnostic tool if there is careful attention paid to the technique, the experience of the 'normal variations' is used and there is careful tailoring of the study to answer a specific and well understood clinical problem.

Clinical Application

Gallium scanning is a non-specific localizer of disease sites. There is no difference between a focal uptake due to a tumour and that due to an abscess; if this is well

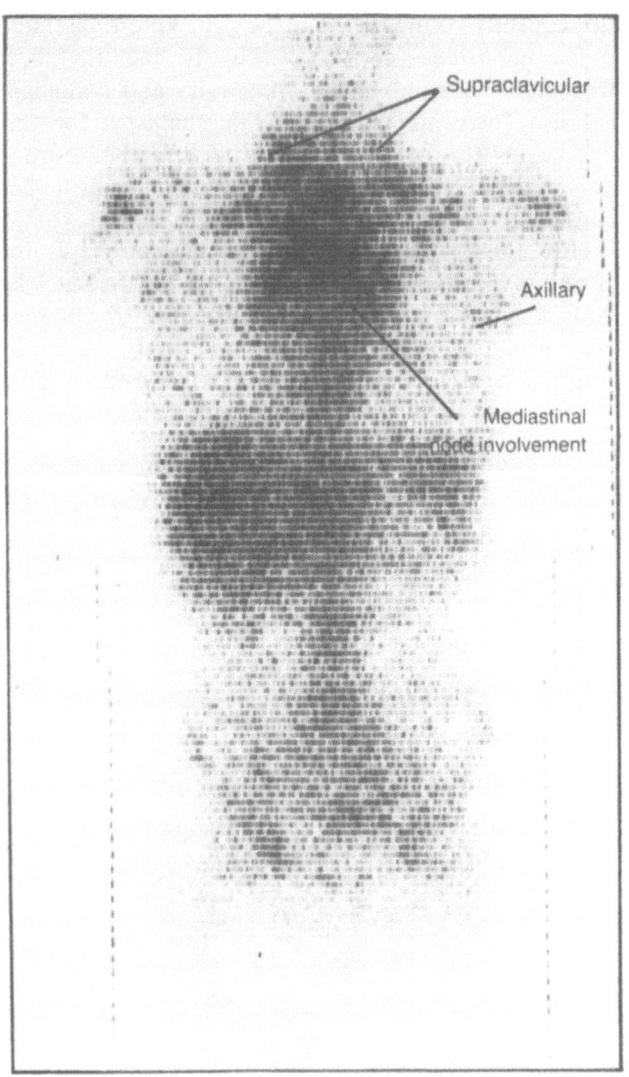

Figure 10.3 *The anterior gallium scan (day one) of a man with Hodgkin's disease—before a course of radiotherapy to the mediastinum and supraclavicular regions.*

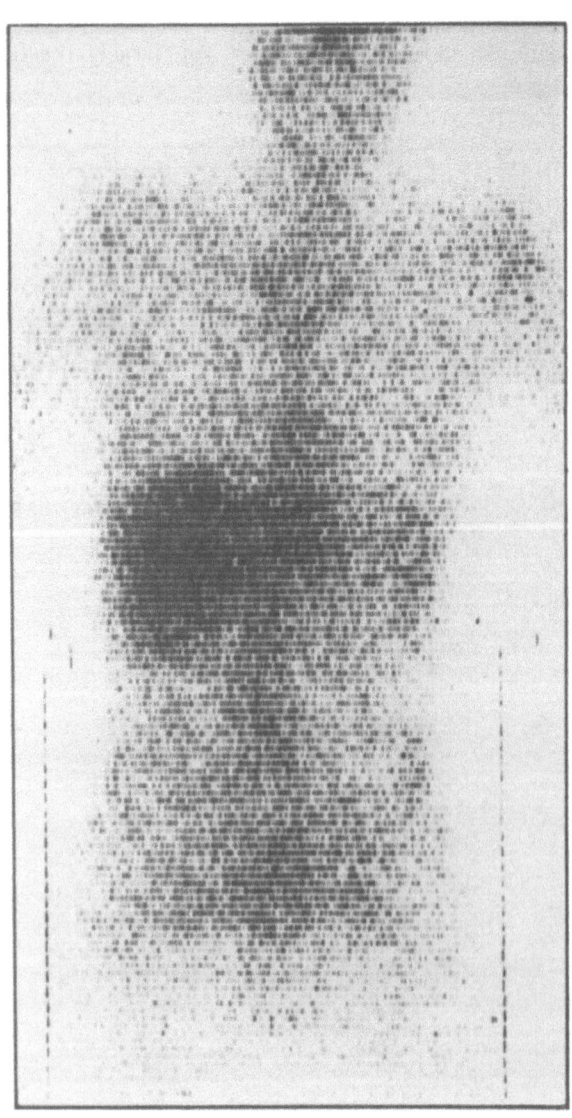

Figure 10.4 *The anterior gallium scan (day one) of a man with Hodgkin's disease (see Figure 10.3,—after a course of radiotherapy to the mediastinum and supraclavicular regions.*

108

understood, problems of interpretation are less likely. It is only by association and a priori probability that a pathological process causing abnormal gallium uptake can be inferred.

Lymphoma

Uptake of gallium by both Hodgkin's and non-Hodgkin's lymphomas has a sufficiently high positive uptake rate to be clinically useful. About 90 per cent of patients with Hodgkin's lymphoma have gallium uptake, and 80-85 per cent of those with non-Hodgkin's lymphomas. Not all sites will be positive, however, and there is a higher rate of detection above the diaphragm (>90 per cent) than below (about 70 per cent). Gallium scanning, therefore, has a small but definite place in the staging of lymphomas, although it does not replace other methods, such as lymphangiography, but is complementary to them. The reason for this is that false negative lymphangiograms, for example, are often positive on gallium scanning and vice versa. Gallium scanning probably has a much more valuable role in the follow-up of patients with 'gallium avid' lymphomas, and here the role of disease localization is well illustrated. For example, when the treated lymphoma patient develops a fever or raised ESR, gallium scanning may be the first modality to localize the site of recurrence, and also to demonstrate remission after treatment.

Figures 10.3 and 10.4 show the anterior gallium scans (day one) of a man with Hodgkin's disease, before and after a course of radiotherapy to the mediastinum and supraclavicular regions. The marked uptake in these regions at presentation has completely resolved, thus confirming the clinical impression of remission.

Other Tumours

With a few exceptions, gallium has little place in the investigation, staging and management of other malignant diseases. The exceptions are:

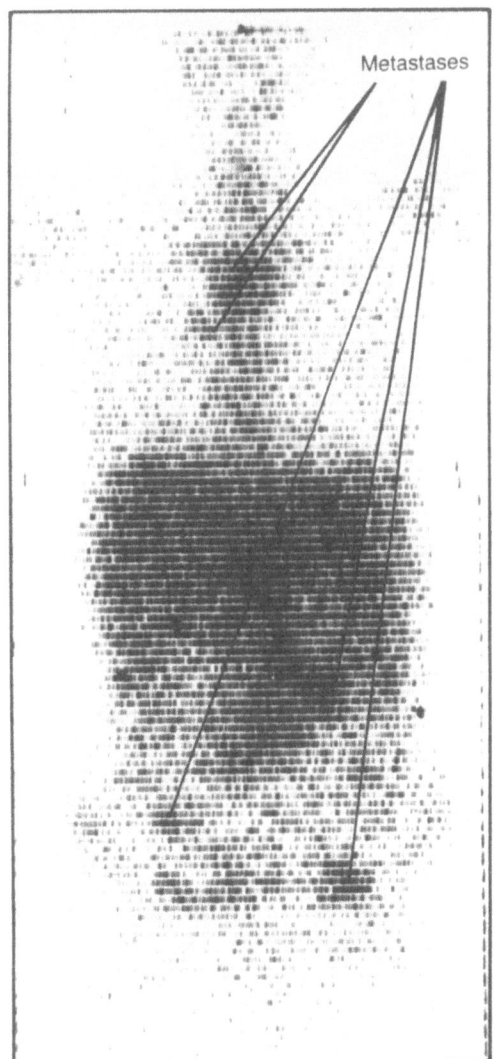

Figure 10.5 *Gallium scan of a patient with disseminated metastases from a testicular seminoma, showing good tracer uptake into the tumour.*

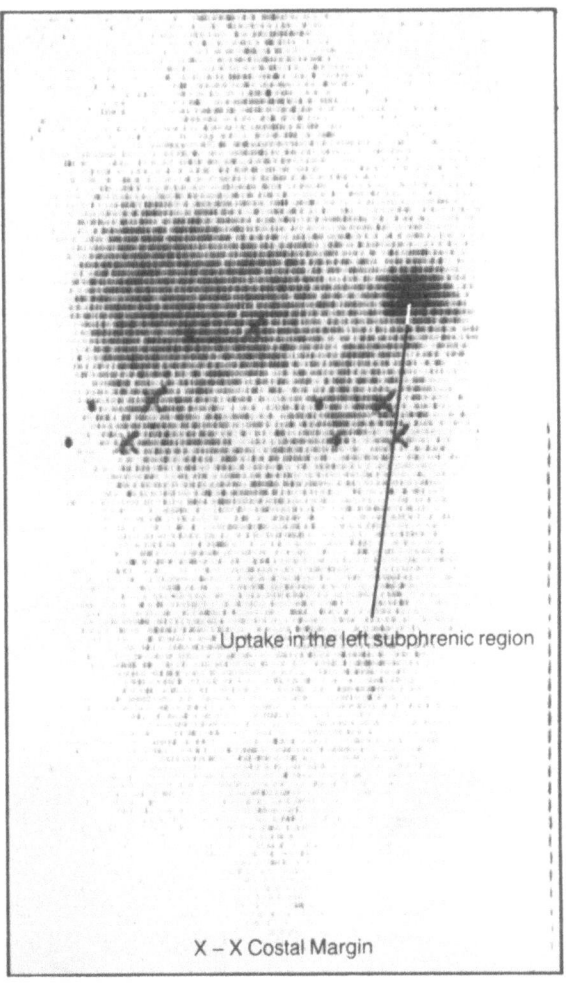

Figure 10.6 *A gallium scan showing uptake in the left subphrenic region due to a colonic carcinoma.*

1. Hepatoma, where positive gallium uptake into a 'cold' lesion on a colloid scan, in a patient with hepatic cirrhosis, has been shown to be quite specific for malignant hepatomas.

2. Testicular tumours.

3. Hypernephroma.

On the whole, the percentage of positive pick-up of gallium is too inconsistent to be of any real value. Figure 10.5 shows the appearance of an intra-abdominal testicular tumour with pelvic intra-abdominal and mediastinal metastatic spread.

Figure 10.6 shows uptake in what was interpreted as a subphrenic abscess in a man with an undulating fever. However, subsequent laparotomy showed a carcinoma of the splenic flexure.

Although gallium-67 citrate scanning is valuable at present, the future prospects must be for more specific radiopharmaceuticals which can be used non-invasively,

rapidly and accurately to stage malignant disease for the logical choice of many therapeutic possibilities.

Localization of Pus

Postoperative fever is a common and often difficult clinical problem, frequently the most worrying cause is

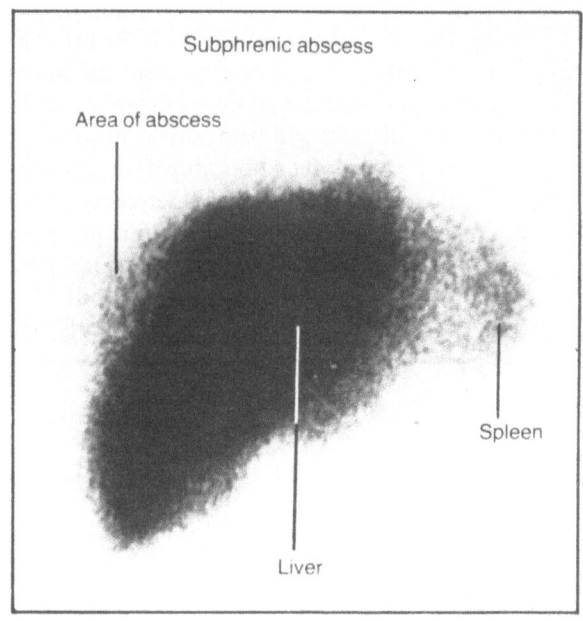

Figure 10.8 *A liver scan showing an extended right subphrenic abscess (the same patient as shown in Figure 10.9).*

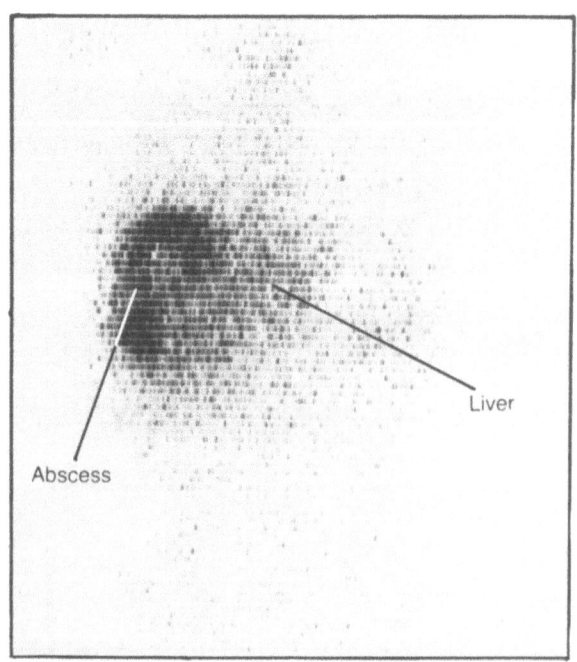

Figure 10.9 *A gallium scan performed in conjunction with a liver scan—Figure 10.8) showing an extensive right subphrenic abscess which was compressing the liver. The abscess was subsequently successfully drained.*

The maskers represent the costal margin

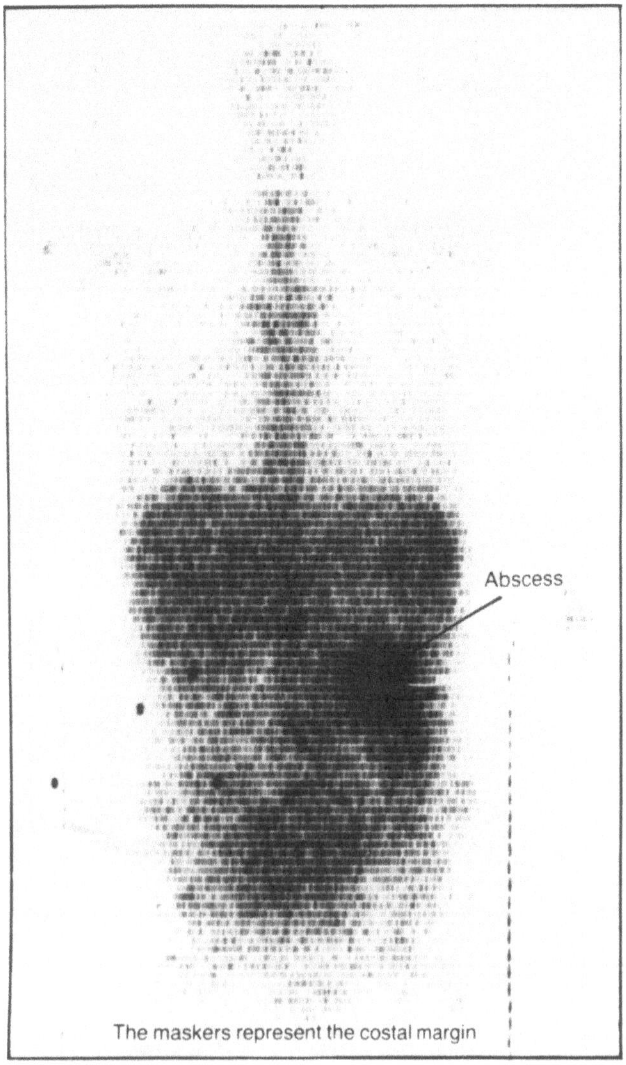

Figure 10.7 *A gallium scan showing postoperative abscess localization.*

abscess formation in an unknown site. Gallium is very effective at localizing a collection of pus, as seen in Figure 10.7. This patient had a left hemicolectomy for carcinoma and subsequently developed a swinging fever postoperatively. Abscess formation was suspected and this was confirmed by gallium scanning, the diagnosis being made on the first day's scans.

A similar problem was posed by another patient who developed a swinging pyrexia after a somewhat difficult appendicectomy (Figures 10.8 and 10.9). In this case, the clinical suspicion was of a subphrenic collection as there were changes on the chest radiograph. A gallium scan, performed in conjunction with a liver scan, showed an extensive right subphrenic abscess compressing the liver, which was subsequently successfully drained.

Investigation of Pyrexia of Unknown Origin (PUO)

A recent study from the nuclear medicine department at Guy's Hospital has shown how useful gallium scanning is in the hunt for the cause of a persistent pyrexia. In this series, 75 per cent (50) of 67 consecutive scans which were performed for PUO were found to be abnormal, and subsequent investigations confirmed a high true positive rate. Interestingly, and possibly of equal importance, there was also a high true negative rate which can be interpreted as indicating that a negative scan excludes a focal cause for the pyrexia with a high degree of probability. Since then, a few false negative cases have appeared in which the patient is being treated with what later transpired to be effective antibiotics and in immunosuppressed patients, so that care must be exercised in interpreting the results in these two situations. However, this does not mean that the investigation should not be carried out, because a positive result is as helpful as in the non-treated patient. The causes of PUO, which were discovered in this series, underlined the non specificity of the examination and ranged from subphrenic abscess to hypernephroma via stitch abscess, TB, chicken pox, lung and inflammatory intramuscular injection sites.

An example of the usefulness of gallium scanning in finding a cause for persistent pyrexia was illustrated by a young man who presented with a persistent pyrexia and gradual weight loss. Multiple investigations over a period of four months had failed to find a cause. Gallium scanning (Figure 10.10) showed an area of increased uptake in the mediastinum which was subsequently shown by mediastinoscopy and biopsy to be due to a tuberculous focus.

Adrenal Imaging

Retroperitoneal insufflation of air was for years the rather unpleasant and somewhat inaccurate Hobson's Choice for adrenal localization. Adrenal venography and arteriography were then developed, but these are invasive procedures and are not without hazard, although venography does allow adrenal vein sampling for the measurement of adrenal hormone levels.

In 1971 Beierwalters and his colleagues (Blair 1971) in Ann Arbor began imaging the adrenals using labelled cholesterol, cholesterol being the building block of adrenocortical function. The original tracer used was ^{131}I-labelled cholesterol, but recently selenium-75 labelled cholesterol has been used. The latter has the advantage of lower radiation doses, especially to the thyroid, more in vitro stability and consequently more reliability in the clinical field.

Method

A renal image (posterior view) using $^{99}Tc^m$ DMSA is obtained to localize the kidneys, the upper poles being marked on the patient by using an indelible marker pen and the scan being stored on computer. 200 μCi of ^{75}Se-cholesterol is then injected intravenously. One week later, posterior images of the adrenals are obtained by using a gamma camera and a high energy collimator, and this scan is placed on computer so that the adrenal

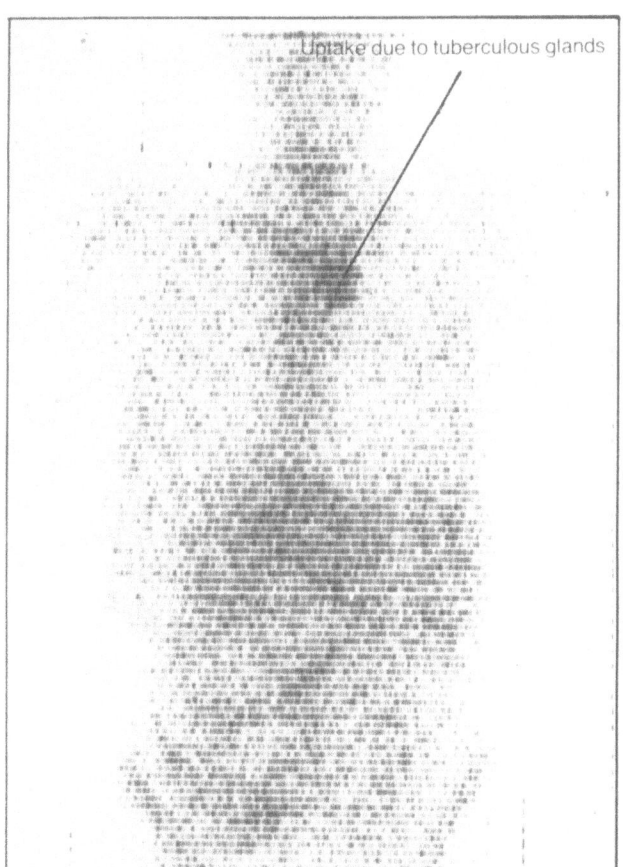

Figure 10.10 *A gallium scan of a patient with PUO.*

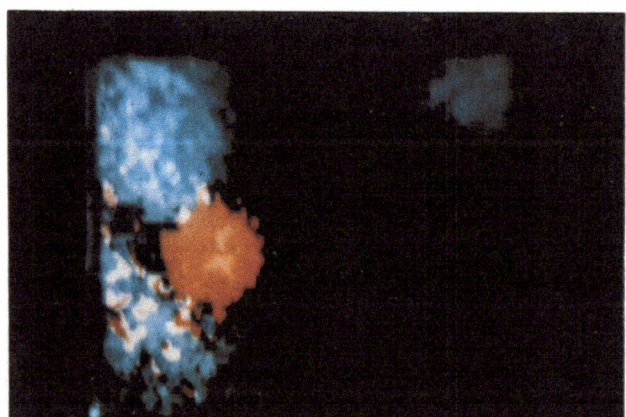

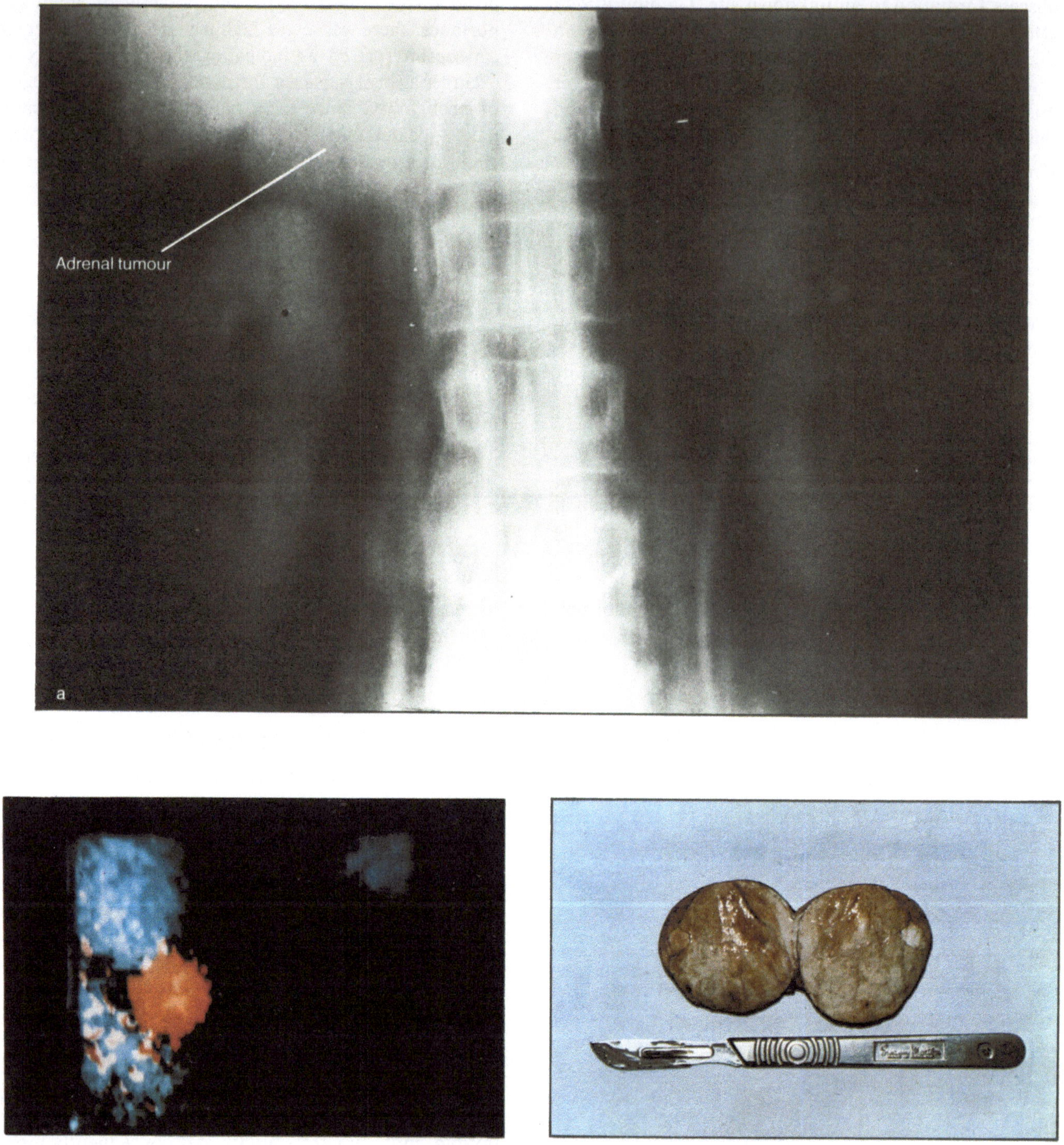

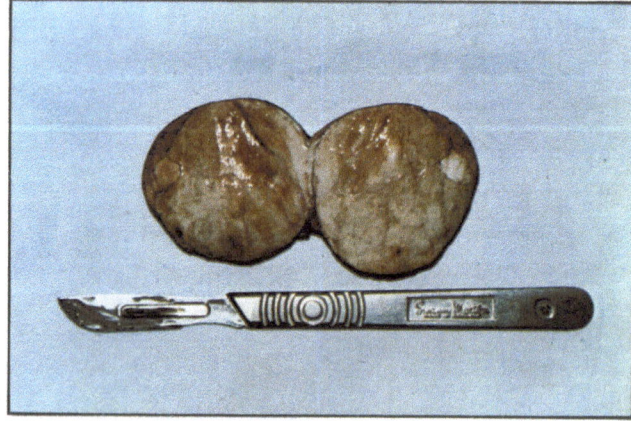

Figure 10.11 *A patient with Cushings syndrome. The IVU (a) suggested a possible mass above the kidney. The adrenal scan (b) demonstrated marked unilateral uptake of tracer, thereby confirming a solitary adrenal adenoma as the cause of the Cushings syndrome. This was successfully removed surgically (c).*

and renal images can be superimposed to localize the adrenal uptake accurately.

On the final day of scanning, a sulphur colloid liver and spleen scan may be obtained and placed on computer to enable further, more accurate localization of adrenal uptake.

Clinical Indications

The adrenal scan is *not* used to diagnose adrenal dysfunction. This is a clinical and biochemical diagnosis. The adrenal scan is used in the differential diagnosis and the localization of disease.

Cushings Syndrome

Non-iatrogenic Cushings syndrome can be caused by pituitary ACTH dependent adrenocortical hyperplasia, by an autonomous cortisone producing adrenal tumour, by ectopic ACTH production, or, rarely, by bilateral autonomous nodular hyperplasia. The problem that can be solved by adrenal imaging, in this situation, is whether the syndrome is due to bilateral or to unilateral disease (i.e. adrenal tumour), and if unilateral, which side? In this latter situation, the uptake of the contra-lateral adrenal will be diminished because of ACTH suppression.

Figure 10.11a shows the IVU of a man who presented with the classical clinical features of Cushings syndrome and it shows a left-sided adrenal mass which was

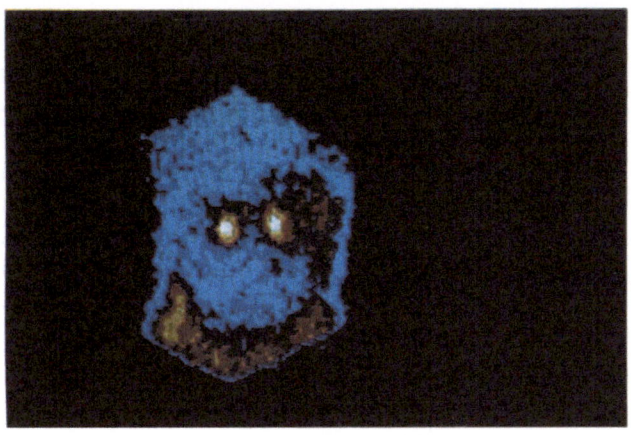

Figure 10.12 *This scan shows bilateral hyperplasia of the adrenals causing Cushings syndrome.*

Figure 10.13 *The arteriogram of a patient in whom the mass was thought to be adrenal.*

Nuclear Medicine

confirmed biochemically. The adrenal scan (Figure 10.11b) shows uptake in the tumour but none on the opposite side due to suppression of ACTH. At operation, the tumour was removed (Figure 10.11c) and found to be a single adrenocortical adenoma. In contrast, the scan seen in Figure 10.12 shows bilateral increased uptake due to classical ACTH dependent Cushings syndrome.

Taken in conjunction with the biochemical findings, the adrenal scan thus provides an accurate non-invasive part of the investigation of these patients and has an advantage over ultrasound and CT. It identifies the functional abnormality in a disease in which the disorder of function predominates.

Conns Syndrome

The place of adrenal imaging in Conns syndrome has not, as yet, been decided, but it seems highly probable that an approach similar to that taken for Cushing's syndrome will be appropriate, as the problem is essentially one of differentiating bilateral from unilateral disease. The addition of exogenous steroid, to suppress the normally functioning adrenal cortex, and quantitation of uptake are likely to be valuable adjuncts to the technique.

Upper Pole Mass

A mass which is seen on a plain radiograph or IVU that could be either adrenal or renal in origin is not an infrequent clinical problem.

The patient whose arteriogram and scan are seen in Figures 10.13 and 10.14 presented precisely this problem and from the IVU it was thought that the mass was probably adrenal. The adrenal scan showed a normal looking right adrenal but the left appeared to be 'squashed' by the mass confirmed on the arteriogram. At operation a large renal carcinoma was removed.

Phaeochromocytoma

Logically, the use of adrenal cortical scanning agents in this situation is not indicated. Occasionally, however, scanning may be useful in that a medullary tumour, if large enough, may destroy, displace or distort the surrounding shell of normal adrenal cortex and hence help in the localization of the phaeochromocytoma.

The future developments in this area are likely to include increasingly specific radiopharmaceuticals, possibly with the use of ^{123}I for lower radiation doses, and more reliable quantification.

Lacrimal Scintillography

The investigation of the common clinical problem of epiphora has been hampered by the lack of a suitable, simple non-invasive physiological method of imaging the lacrimal drainage system. Lacrimal scintillography

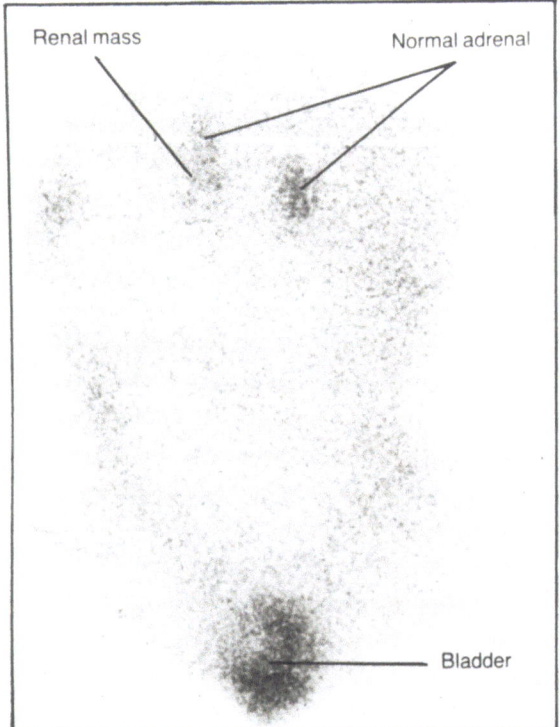

Figure 10.14 *The scan of the same patient (Figure 10.13)—the mass was found to be a renal carcinoma, which was distorting an otherwise normal adrenal.*

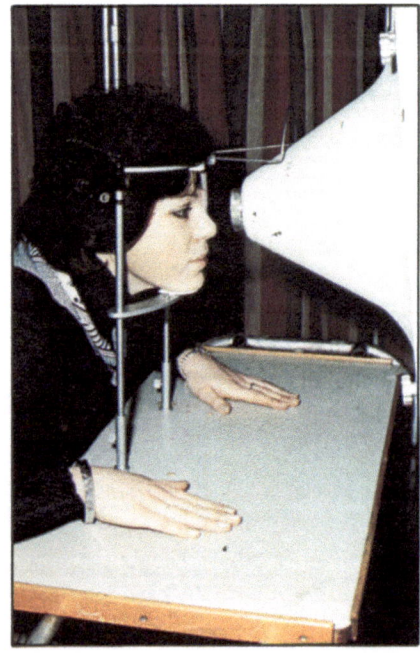

Figure 10.15 *A patient who is being assessed by lacrimal scintillography.*

114

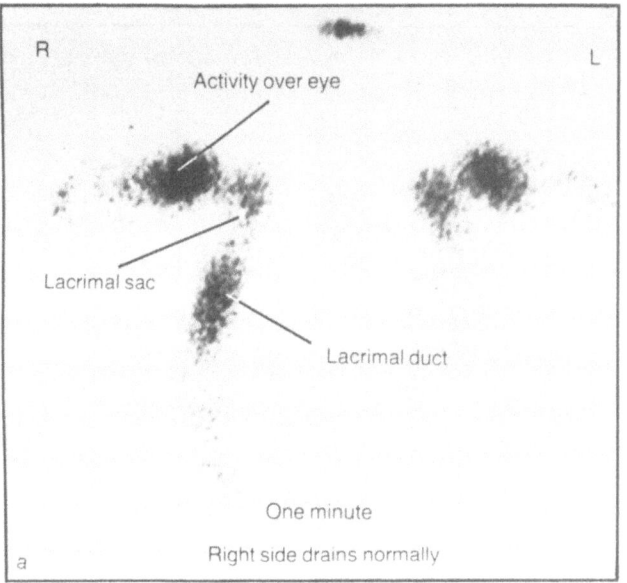

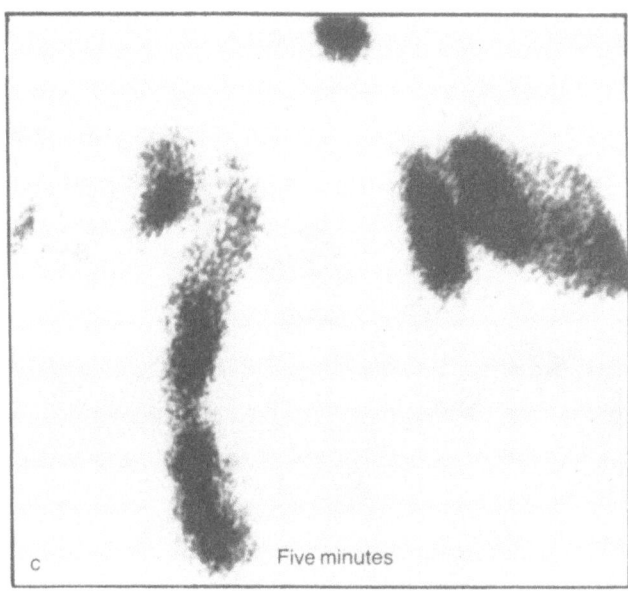

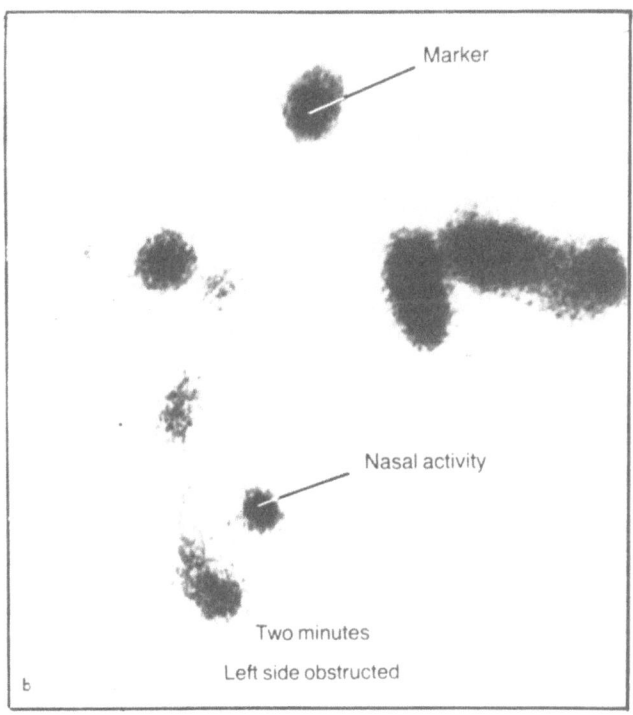

Figure 10.16 *A patient with unilateral epiphora. There is rapid transit of tracer through the right lacrimal system, but delay on the left side due to hold up at the lower end of the lacrimal sac.* **(a)** *One minute view,* **(b)** *two minute view and* **(c)** *five minute view.*

provided exactly this much needed technique. As with so many other examples, the standard radiographic method—the Dacrocystogram (DCG), which is excellent at demonstrating fine anatomy but poor at assessing physiological function—is now entirely complementary to the functional test. Lacrimal scintillography (LS) assesses the function of the entire lacrimal drainage system by monitoring the flow of tears across the eyes, through the lacrimal duct and into the nose.

Method

The patient is seated comfortably with the head held still in a cradle (Figure 10.15) facing the gamma camera which is fitted with a pinhole collimator for maximal magnification. A small drop (0.013 ml) of $^{99}Tc^m$-sulphur colloid, having the pH and viscosity of tears, is delivered simultaneously to the lower lid margins of each eye by automatic pipettes. A ^{57}Co solid marker is placed in the midline between the eyebrows for localization before the study starts and for subsequent monitoring of movement. The tracer then passes through the conjunctival sac into the punctum, via the upper and lower canaliculi to the common canaliculus, to the lacrimal sac and duct, and from there into the nose. The patient is allowed to blink normally during the procedure which takes about 10 minutes.

The camera may be linked to a data processing system for further refinement by quantitation. In most cases, adequate assessment can be made by taking one minute images for a total of 15 minutes (Figure 10.16, right-hand-side) following injection. However, measurement of the rate of passage using a data processing system increases the sensitivity of the method for the detection of minor degrees of obstruction. When a quantitative study is viewed on computer, regions of interest corresponding to the inner canthus, lacrimal sac and the naso-lacrimal duct are delineated and the activity in these areas is measured, plotted against time and visualized in graph form.

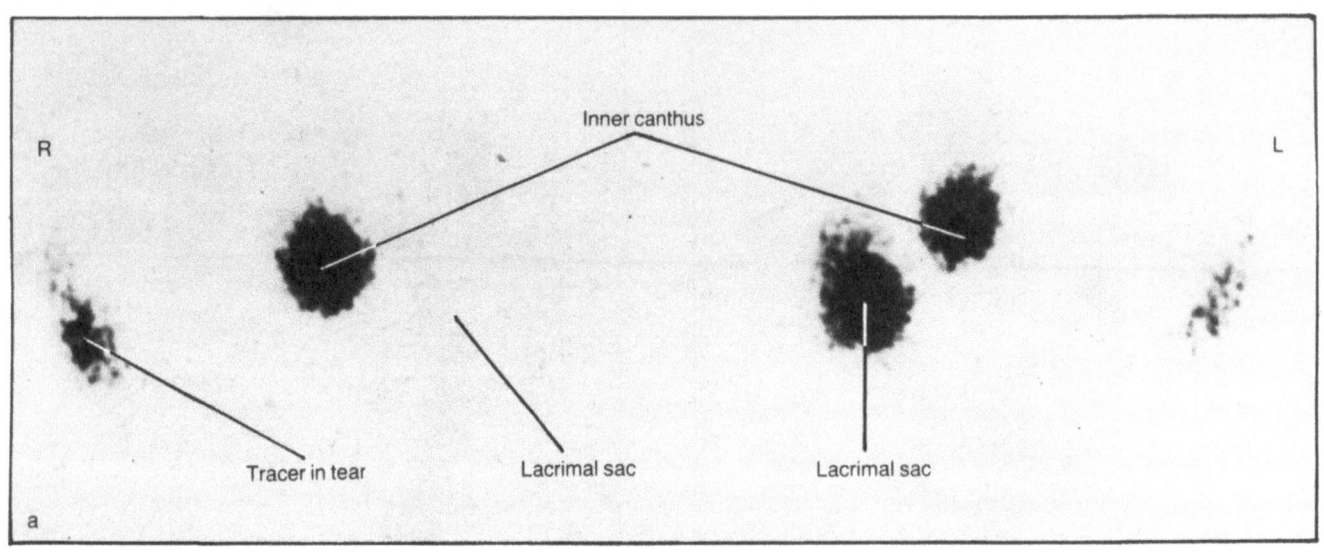

R — Inner canthus — L

Tracer in tear   Lacrimal sac   Lacrimal sac

a

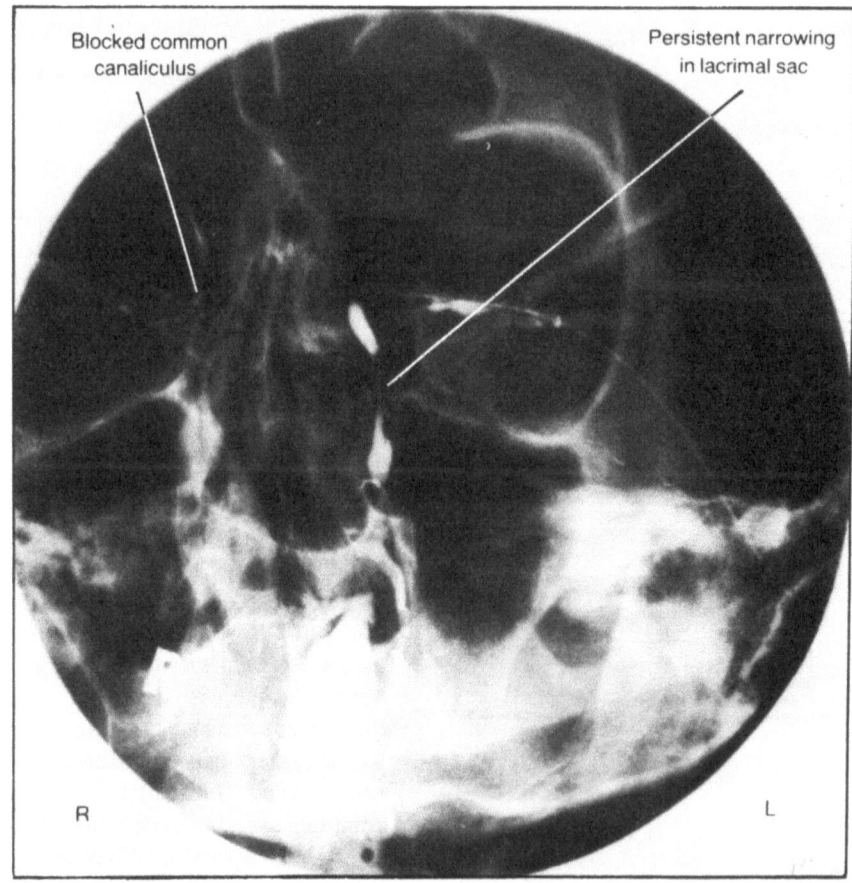

Blocked common canaliculus   Persistent narrowing in lacrimal sac

R   L

Figure 10.17a *A patient with bilateral epiphora. The lacrimal scan shows absence of tracer entering the right lacrimal sac and hold up at the lower end of the left lacrimal sac. (b) Dacrocystogram confirms obstruction at the right common canaliculus, and narrowing of the lower lacrimal sac on the left side.*

Clinical Indications

The problem usually is to differentiate between the patient with epiphora due to organic or functional obstruction of the lacrimal drainage system, and the patient with epiphora due to excessive tear production or an excess response to normal tear formation.

The correct way to use the method is as a screening

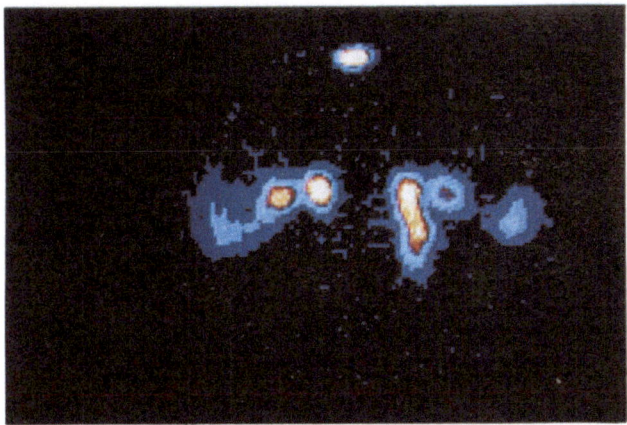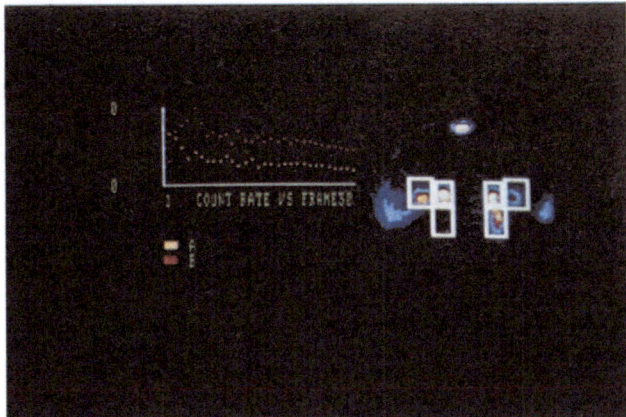

Figure 10.18a and b *A patient with unilateral epiphora due to a partially blocked right lacrimal system at the canaliculus.* **(a)** *Shows one frame from the computer processed image showing the difference between the two sides.* **(b)** *Shows the time activity curve generated by the computer at the lacrimal duct. There is rapid entry on the left and good clearance, but there is delayed entry and slow clearance on the right, partially obstructed side.*

test, because it is physiological, non-traumatic, simple and tests the whole system, whereas the DCG may overcome functionally significant blocks, but is relatively expensive, time-consuming and invasive, and in addition, as it requires cannulation of the puncta, it cannot test the drainage from the inner canthus to the canaliculae. When the lacrimal scintillogram is abnormal then one can proceed to the DCG with the specified question about the exact site and cause of the demonstrated obstruction.

Figures 10.17a and 10.17b show the scan and DCG of a patient with epiphora. The scan shows that no tracer passes from the inner canthus to the lacrimal sac on the right and on the left there is hold-up at the lower end of the lacrimal sac before it enters the lacrimal duct. The DCG shows complete occlusion of the common canaliculus on the right and a long thin obstruction between the lacrimal sac and duct on the left side. A perfect example of the complementary nature of the two techniques.

Figure 10.18a shows the scan of a patient with unilateral epiphora due to canalicular obstruction on the right. Quantitative scintigraphy in this case (Figure 10.18b) clearly shows the delay in drainage on the right.

This technique may also be used for the assessment of patients with persistent symptoms following surgical treatment for epiphora and as an objective assessment of patients with epiphora due to eyelid abnormalities and facial palsy. However, apart from the clear-cut clinical applications outlined here there is undoubtedly a tremendous scope for detailed assessment of the physiological mechanisms responsible for normal lacrimal drainage, which are ill understood.

CSF Cisternography

Introducing radioisotopes into the cerebrospinal fluid (CSF) to study flow was introduced by DiChiro in 1966. Although it remains a very elegant method of studying CSF dynamics under normal and pathological conditions, the clinical uses of this technique remain somewhat limited. There are two main clinical situations in which cisternography is of great importance, these are: CSF rhinorrhoea and for the diagnosis and assessment of communicating or abnormal pressure hydrocephalus.

Methods

The labelled chelate, ^{111}In-DTPA is now the radiopharmaceutical of choice for most purposes, and is used in preference to the previously popular radioiodinated human serum albumen which occasionally caused meningeal irritation and arachnoiditis. ^{111}In-DTPA diffuses quickly through the cisternal system, has a physical half-life of 2.8 days (so enabling delayed views to be taken at 48 and 72 hours), favourable physical properties and is non-irritating to the meninges and rapidly excreted by the kidneys by glomerular filtration.

One mCi of ^{111}In is injected into the cerebrospinal space via a normal lumbar puncture technique after which the patient must lie flat until the first views are taken one to two hours after injection. Ideally, the study should not be undertaken within two weeks of previous lumbar punctures as this seems to increase the likelihood of a poor technical result. The views, which are usually taken are: the anterior, lateral and posterior views. The normal study, which is seen in Figure 10.19,

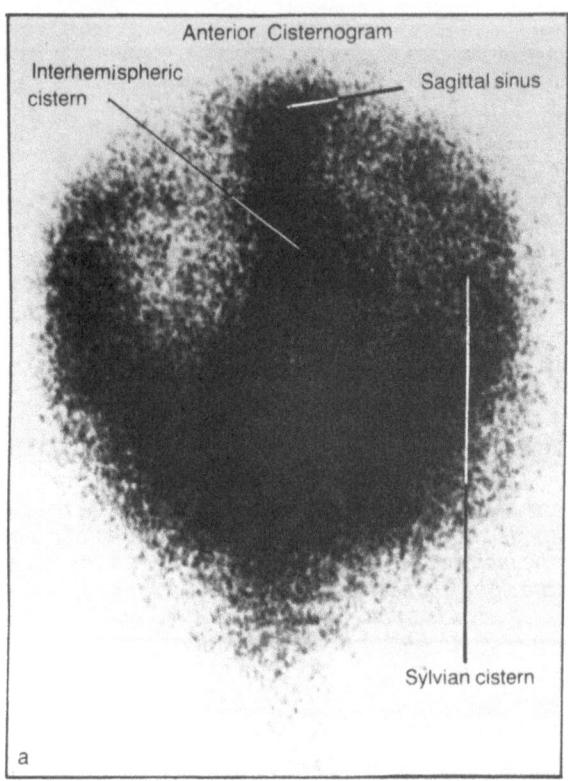

Anterior Cisternogram

Interhemispheric cistern

Sagittal sinus

Sylvian cistern

a

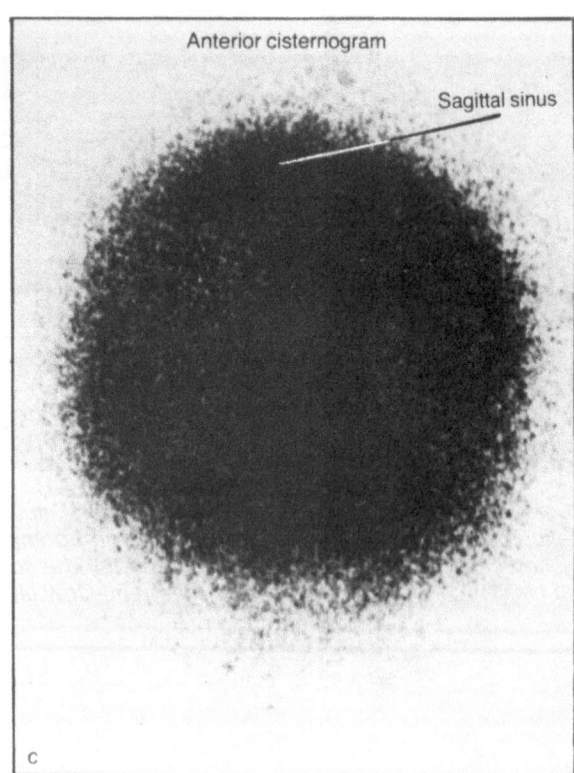

Anterior cisternogram

Sagittal sinus

c

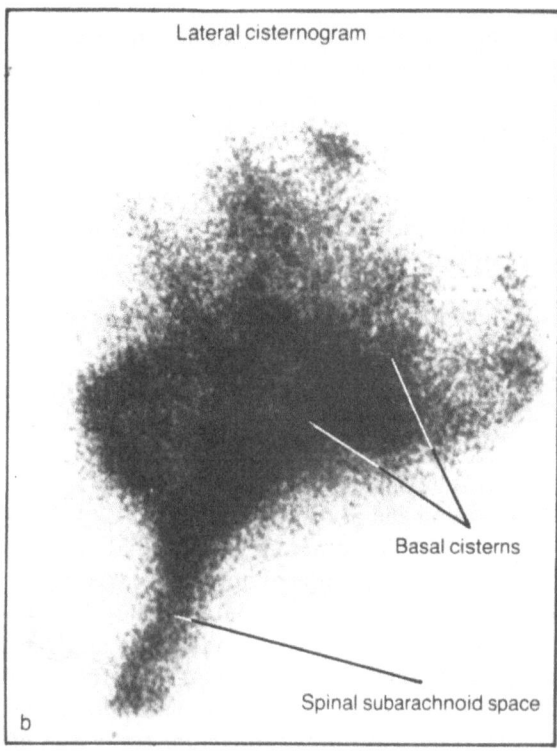

Lateral cisternogram

Basal cisterns

Spinal subarachnoid space

b

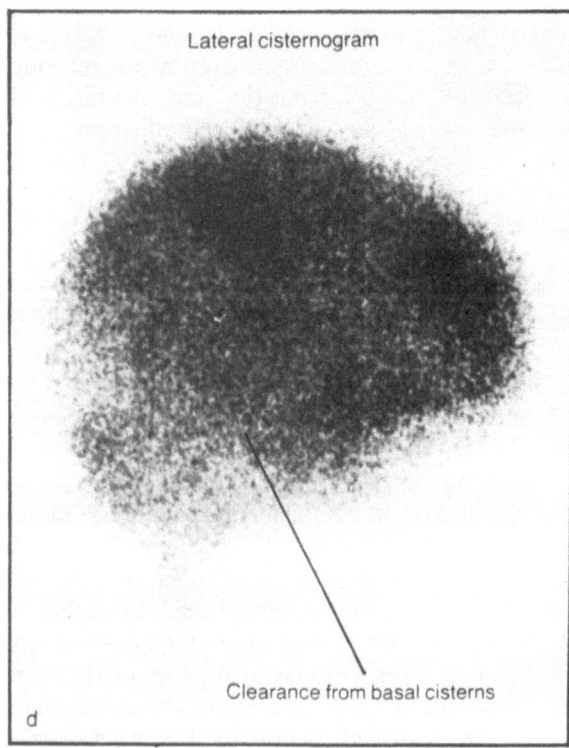

Lateral cisternogram

Clearance from basal cisterns

d

Figure 10.19 *A normal radionuclide cisternogram using a lumbar injection of indium-III DTPA. There is entry of tracer into the basal cisterns six hours after injection (a and b), with accumulation over the cerebral cortex at 24 hours (c and d). There is no entry into the ventricular system at any stage.*

shows only the anterior and lateral projections, but the main cisternae are clearly seen.

The normal cisternogram should show the basal cisterns after two hours, the interhemispheric and

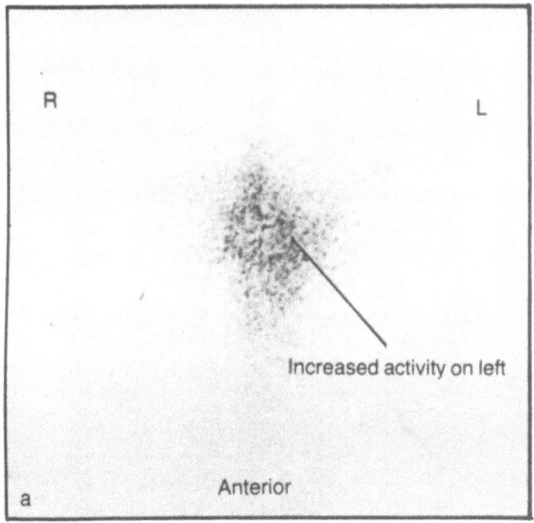

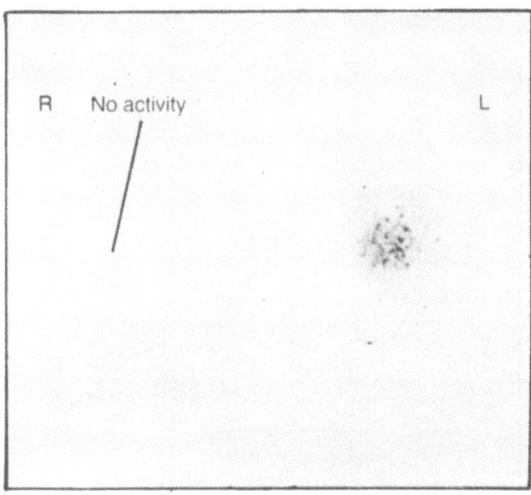

Figure 10.21 *The scan of each nasal pack (which were removed from the same patient—Figure 10.20—three hours afterwards), shows some activity from the left side but none from the right, confirming the clinical suspicion of a CSF leak.*

sylvian cisterns at six hours with all the activity over the cortex by 24 hours. At no point should the lateral ventricles be visualized as the CSF flow from normal sized ventricles is away from the ventricles and hence the tracer does not penetrate. It is only when the flow is very sluggish or the ventricles abnormally dilated that the tracer can diffuse into them. Abnormal findings,

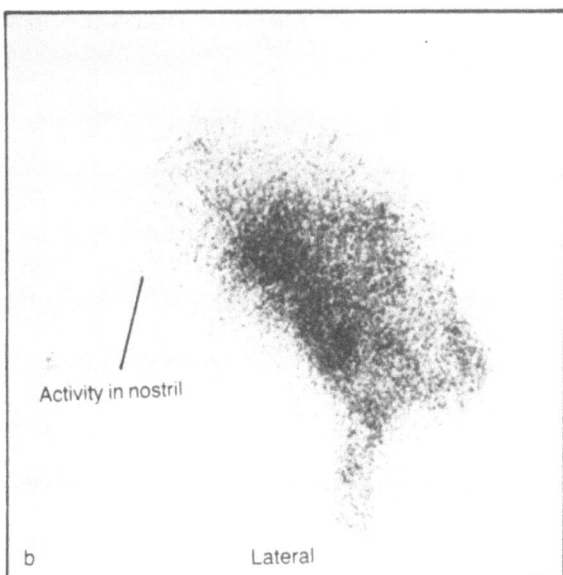

Figure 10.20 *Shows the anterior* **(a)** *and lateral* **(b)** *scans of a man with a CSF leak from the left side of the nose following trauma.*

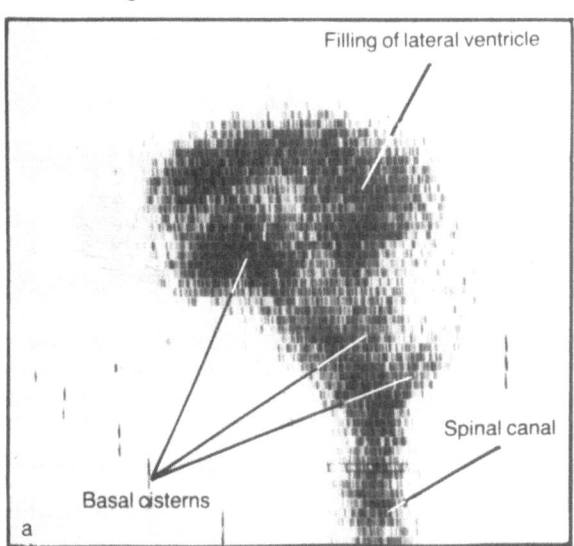

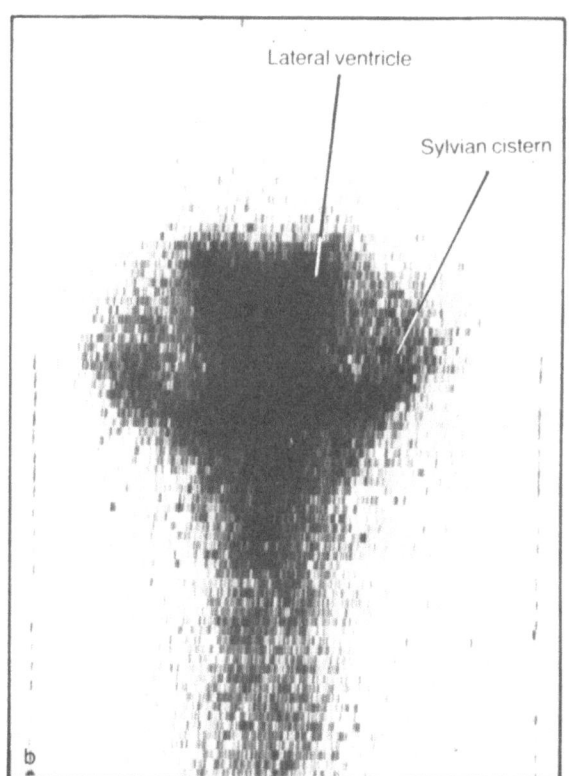

Figure 10.22 *Scan of a patient with communicating hydrocephalus, showing filling of the ventricular system.* **(a)** *Lateral view and* **(b)** *anterior view.*

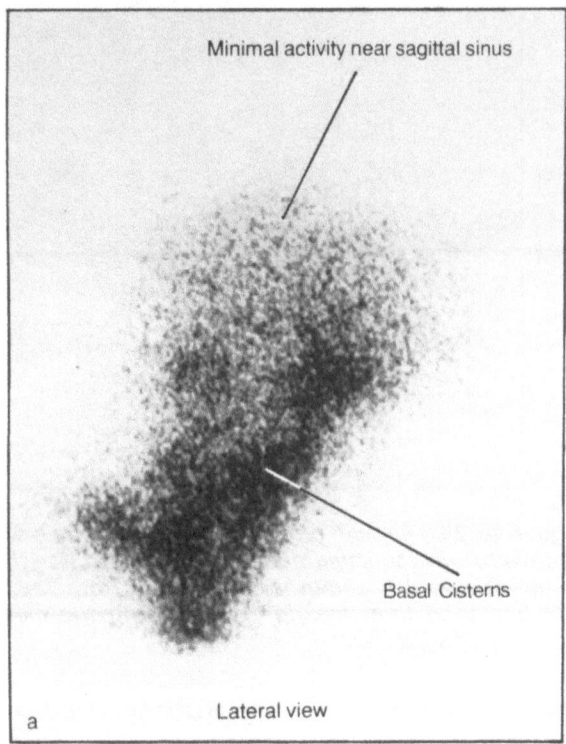

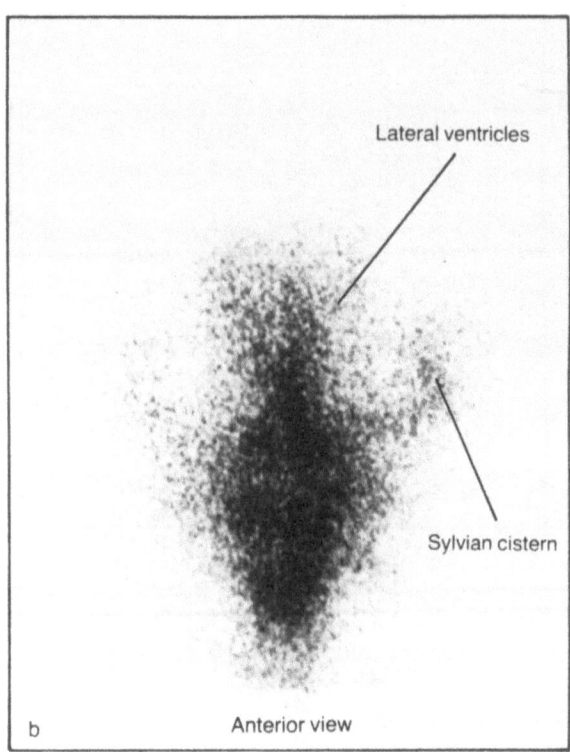

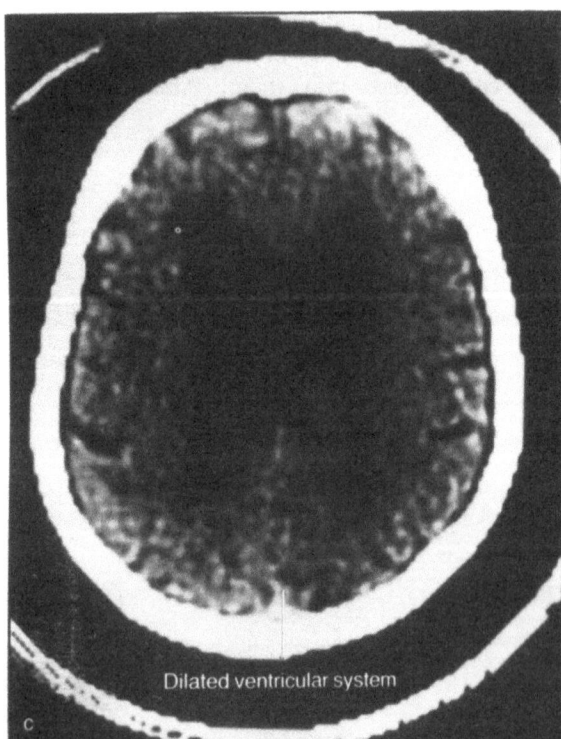

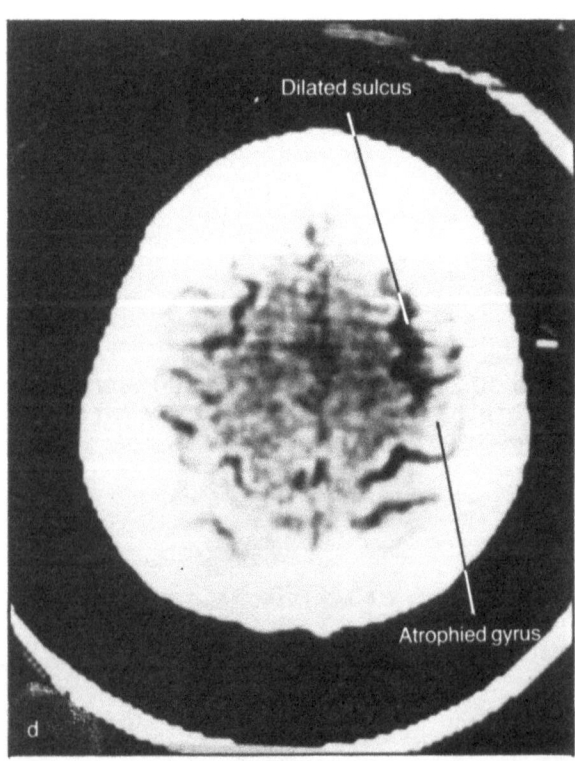

Figure 10.23 *Radionuclide cisternogram in a patient with dementia. There is abnormal entry of tracer into the enlarged ventricles at six hours (**a** and **b**). The ventricular dilatation and cerebral atrophy are confirmed by CT scan (**c** and **d**).*

therefore, included: delayed rate of flow into the basal cisterns and over the cortex, filling of the ventricular system, CSF leakage and rarely localized abnormalities, such as porencephalic cysts.

Clinical Applications

CSF Rhinorrhoea

If a CSF leak is suspected the patient should lie in the position in which the leak is thought to be maximal. Nasal pledgets or posterior nasal packs may be inserted to ascertain from which side the leak is coming and these may be scanned or counted after removal.

In this situation, the first pictures should be taken at one hour, the anterior and lateral views being all important. Nasal packs, if thought necessary, should be inserted at this stage and the patient re-scanned at three hours. The packs are then removed and the radioactivity measured and related to blood levels. Occasionally, the leak will be large enough for the fluid to be collected and counted separately. Figure 10.20 shows the anterior and lateral scans of a man with a CSF leak from the left side of the nose following trauma. The scans were taken one hour after injection. Activity can be seen in the left nostril, especially on the lateral view. Three hours later, the nasal packs were removed and the subsequent scan of each pack (Figure 10.21) shows some activity from the left side but none in the right, confirming the clinical suspicion of a CSF leak.

Presenile Dementia

This condition has a number of potentially reversible causes and cerebrospinal scintillography can help to delineate one of these causes, communicating hydrocephalus, and also one of the irreversible causes, namely cerebral atrophy.

Communicating hydrocephalus. Scanning may not only help in the diagnosis of this condition, but also may determine the site of the block to CSF flow and the likelihood of the patient benefitting from a shunting procedure. Delayed views are taken at 48 and 72 hours for a full study.

1. Diagnostic appearance. Penetration of the tracer into the ventricles is not seen in the normal scan but is seen in this condition (Figure 10.22) and there is delay of disappearance of the tracer from the ventricular system. The delayed views are, therefore, essential in assessing this slowing of tracer loss.

2. Location of the block. Sometimes the site of the block can be clearly delineated, the common sites of block being in the posterior fossa, the tentorial notch, the sylvian fissures and between the sylvian fissure and the sagittal sinus. In this situation, the tracer fails to penetrate beyond the point of obstruction.

Cerebral atrophy. Although this shows delay in the normal circulation of tracer, with tracer remaining in the basal cisterns and filling the ventricles (Figure 10.23a and b), the investigation of choice should really be a CT scan which shows up the dilated ventricles and atrophic gyri more clearly (Figure 10.23c and d).

Both communicating hydrocephalus and CSF rhinorrhoea are uncommon conditions, but both have a high morbidity untreated and are very amenable to treatment so that cisternography remains a useful investigation in carefully selected clinical situations. It is highly complementary to the air encephalogram or the CT brain scan, both of which elegantly demonstrate the abnormal anatomy associated with ventricular dilatation but only allow one to infer the likely abnormal flow mechanisms. The combination of the CT scan and the radioisotope cisternogram allows correlation of abnormal structure and function.

References

Blair, R. J., Beierwalters, W. H., Lieberman, L. M., Boyd, C. M., Cormsell, R. E., Weinhold, P. A. and Varma, V. M., *J. Nucl. Med.,* **12**, 176, 1971.

DiChiro, G., *Acta Radiol. Scanned,* 1966, **5**, 989.

Index